D1120539

OXFORD MEDICAL PUBLICATIONS

Oxford American
Handbook of
Surgery

Published and forthcoming Oxford American Handbooks

Oxford American Handbook of **Surgery**

Edited by

David L. Berger, MD

Associate Visiting Surgeon,
Massachusetts General Hospital
Assistant Professor of Surgery,
Harvard Medical School

with

Greg McLatchie

Neil Borley

Joanna Chikwe

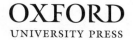

OXFORD
UNIVERSITY PRESS

OXFORD
UNIVERSITY PRESS

Oxford University Press, Inc., publishes works that further
Oxford University's objective of excellence
in research, scholarship, and education.

Oxford New York
Auckland Cape Town Dar es Salaam Hong Kong Karachi
Kuala Lumpur Madrid Melbourne Mexico City Nairobi
New Delhi Shanghai Taipei Toronto

With offices in
Argentina Austria Brazil Chile Czech Republic France Greece
Guatemala Hungary Italy Japan Poland Portugal Singapore
South Korea Switzerland Thailand Turkey Ukraine Vietnam

Copyright © 2009 by Oxford University Press, Inc.

Published by Oxford University Press, Inc.
198 Madison Avenue, New York, New York 10016

www.oup.com

Oxford is a registered trademark of Oxford University Press

Library of Congress Cataloging-in-Publication Data
Oxford American handbook of surgery / edited by David L. Berger ;
with Greg McLatchie, Neil Borley, Joanna Chikwe.
p. ; cm.
Adapted from: Oxford handbook of clinical surgery / edited by Greg McLatchie,
Neil Borley, Joanna Chikwe. 3rd ed. 2007.
Includes bibliographical references and index.
ISBN 978-0-19-530462-6 (flexicover : alk. paper)
1. Surgery—Handbooks, manuals, etc. 2. Surgery, Operative—Handbooks,
manuals, etc.
I. Berger, David L. (David Lawrence), 1964- II. McLatchie, Greg R. III. Borley,
Neil R. IV. Chikwe, Joanna. V. Oxford handbook of clinical surgery.
VI. Title: Handbook of surgery.
[DNLM: 1. Surgical Procedures, Operative—Handbooks. WO 39 O975 2009]
RD37.O84 2009
617—dc22   2008024755

9 8 7 6 5 4 3 2 1

Printed in China
on acid-free paper

Preface

Surgery and surgical knowledge continue to improve and evolve almost daily. The information required to stay abreast of the advances has increased exponentially. Surgeons themselves have tended to specialize or even subspecialize to advance their field. The medical student on surgical rotations or the surgical resident in their early years tends to rotate through different specialties on a monthly basis, requiring the student or resident to rapidly become proficient in another surgical subspecialty. This book is written as a resource for the surgical student and resident to ease these transitions. In a concise way it presents the integral information necessary to achieve as a student and function as a resident.

Thirty-five years ago it was written that "the acquisition of practical surgical knowledge is by nature fragmented and the student attains a unified understanding of the material only gradually."[1] This is even more applicable today. The body of medical knowledge continues to advance at a rapid rate and is so vast that it cannot all be committed to memory. Information, while easier to obtain, is even more fragmented than before, and the demands on the surgical student or resident continue to grow. Exposure to disease processes and the experience garnered take place in short snippets of time divided among many different patients and tasks. To maximize these short interactions, the basic principles must be readily available to provide the necessary building blocks for learning. This book is not meant to be an in-depth study of surgical disease but rather to provide these foundations to the surgical student or resident. The book is formatted to make the acquiring of this information easy and efficient. The book uses highlighted definitions, outlines of key points, and common pitfalls, presented concisely in a bulleted format. It would be very difficult to memorize all the information in this book, but it is possible with the aid of this information to maximize learning from the many interactions in the day of a student or resident.

1 Ottinger LW (1974). *Fundamentals of Colon Surgery*. Boston: Little, Brown and Company.

Contents

Detailed contents

19 Urology   **647**

Contributors

Joshua Alpert, MD
Sports Medicine Fellow

Peter Asnis, MD
Assistant in Orthopedic Surgery,
Massachusetts General Hospital
Instructor in Orthopedic Surgery,
Harvard Medical School

David L. Berger, MD
Associate Visiting Surgeon,
Massachusetts General Hospital
Assistant Professor of Surgery,
Harvard Medical School

Liliana Bordeianou, MD
Assistant in Surgery,
Massachusetts General Hospital
Instructor in Surgery, Harvard
Medical School

Mark Conrad, MD
Assistant in Surgery,
Massachusetts General Hospital
Instructor in Surgery, Harvard
Medical School

Marc DeMoya, MD
Assistant in Surgery,
Massachusetts General Hospital
Instructor in Surgery, Harvard
Medical School

Daniel P. Doody, MD
Visiting Surgeon,
Massachusetts General Hospital
Associate Professor of Surgery,
Harvard Medical School

Cristina Ferrone, MD
Assistant in Surgery,
Massachusetts General Hospital
Instructor in Surgery,
Harvard Medical School

Denise Gee, MD
Assistant in Surgery,
Massachusetts General Hospital
Instructor in Surgery,
Harvard Medical School
Massachusetts General Hospital

Martin Hertl, MD
Associate Visiting Surgeon,
Massachusetts General Hospital
Assistant Professor in Surgery,
Harvard Medical School

Matthew Hutter, MD
Assistant Surgeon,
Massachusetts General Hospital
Instructor in Surgery, Harvard
Medical School

Karen Kim, MD
Resident, Department of Surgery
Massachusetts General Hospital

Thomas E. MacGillivray, MD
Associate Visiting Surgeon,
Massachusetts General Hospital
Instructor in Surgery, Harvard
Medical School

Francis J. McGovern, MD
Assistant Clinical Professor
of Urology, Massachusetts
General Hospital
Assistant Clinical Professor
of Urology, Harvard Medical School

Michal Mekel, MD

Endocrine Surgery Fellow
Research, Department of Surgery
Massachusetts General Hospital

Sareh Parangi, MD

Associate Visiting Surgeon,
Massachusetts General Hospital
Assistant Professor in Surgery,
Harvard Medical School

Rubin Rodriguez, MD

Resident in Surgery
Massachusetts General Hospital

Warren S. Sandberg, MD, PhD

Assistant Anesthetist,
Massachusetts General Hospital
Associate Professor of Anesthesia,
Harvard Medical School

Michelle Specht, MD

Assistant in Surgery,
Massachusetts General Hospital
Instructor in Surgery, Harvard
Medical School

Patricia Sylla, MD

Instructor in Surgery, Harvard
Medical School
Massachusetts General Hospital

Jingping Wang, MD, PhD

Assistant in Anesthesia,
Massachusetts General Hospital
Instructor in Anesthesia, Harvard
Medical School

Jonathan M. Winograd, MD

Assistant Surgeon, Massachusetts
General Hospital
Assistant Professor of Surgery,
Harvard Medical School

Symbols and abbreviations

δ	decreased
↑	increased
↔	normal
→	leading to
⚠	warning
►	important
►►	don't dawdle
📖	cross-reference
♀	female
♂	male
AAA	abdominal aortic aneurysm
ABC	airway, breathing, circulation
ABG	arterial blood gas
ABPI	ankle–brachial pressure index
ACAS	Asymptomatic Carotid Artery Stenosis Study
ACE	angiotensin-converting enzyme
ACh	acetylcholine
AChE	acetylcholinesterase
ACL	anterior cruciate ligament
ACST	Asymptomatic Carotid Surgery Trial
ACTH	adenocorticotropic hormone
ACV	assist control ventilation
ADH	antidiuretic hormone
ADP	adenosine diphosphate
AF	atrial fibrillation
AFP	α-fetoprotein
AG	anion gap
AIDS	acquired immunodeficiency syndrome
AJCC	American Joint Committee on Cancer
AKA	above-knee amputation
ALI	acute lung injury
ALS	advanced life support
AMPLE	allergy, medication, past medical history, last meal, events of the incident
ANDI	abnormalities of normal development and involution (of breast)
ANF	antinuclear factor
AP	anteroposterior

APC	antigen-presenting cell; argon plasma coagulation
APR	abdominoperineal resection
APTR	activated partial thromboplastin time ratio
APTT	activated partial thromboplastin time
AR	aortic regurgitation
ARB	angiotensin receptor blocker
ARDS	acute respiratory distress syndrome
ARR	absolute risk reduction
ASA	American Society of Anesthesiologists
5-ASA	5-aminosalicylic acid
ASB	assisted spontaneous breathing
ATLS	Advanced Trauma Life Support (system)
ATN	acute tubular necrosis
ATP	adenosine triphosphate
AUR	acute urinary retention
AV	arteriovenous
AVM	arteriovenous malformation
AVR	aortic valve replacement
AZA	azathioprine
BCC	basal cell carcinoma
BCG	bacille Calmette–Guérin
BCR	B-cell receptor
bid	twice daily
BiPAP	biphasic positive airway pressure
BKA	below-knee amputation
BMI	body mass index
BP	blood pressure
BPH	benign prostatic hyperplasia
BS	blood sugar
BSA	body surface area
BXO	balanitis xerotica obliterans
CABG	coronary artery bypass graft
CAD	coronary artery disease
CAPD	continuous ambulatory peritoneal dialysis
CAVH	continuous arteriovenous hemofiltration
CBC	complete blood count
CBD	common bile duct
CCAM	congenital cystic adenomatoid malformation
CDH	congenital diaphragmatic hernia
CEA	carotid endarterectomy, carcinoembryonic antigen
CF	cystic fibrosis
CHF	congestive heart failure

CI	cardiac index
CIE	chemotherapy-induced emesis
CLI	critical limb ischemia
CMI	cell-mediated immune (reaction)
CMV	cytomegalovirus; controlled mechanical ventilation
CNS	central nervous system
CO	cardiac output
COAD	chronic obstructive airway disease
COPD	chronic obstructive pulmonary disease
CPAP	continuous positive airway pressure
CPB	cardiopulmonary bypass
CPK	creatine phosphokinase
C, P, & O	cysts, parasites, and ova
CPR	cardiopulmonary resuscitation
CRC	colorectal cancer
CRI	chronic renal insufficiency
CRP	C-reactive protein
CSF	cerebrospinal fluid
C-spine	cervical spine
C-T	chest tube
CT	computerized tomography
CTA	computerized tomography angiogram
CTPA	computerized tomography pulmonary angiography
CVA	cardiovascular accident; cerebrovascular accident
CVL	central venous line
CVP	central venous pressure
CVVH	continuous venovenous hemofiltration
CXR	chest X-ray
DA	dopamine
DALM	dysplasia-associated lesion or mass
DBP	diastolic blood pressure
DCD	donation after cardiac death
DCIS	ductal carcinoma in situ
DHS	dynamic hip screw
DHT	dihydrotestosterone
DIC	disseminated intravascular coagulation
DIEP	deep inferior epigastric perforator
DIPJ	distal interphalangeal joint
DM	diabetes mellitus
DMSA	dimercaptosuccinate
DNR	do not resuscitate
DP	distal phalanx; diastolic pressure

DPA	diagnostic peritoneal aspiration
DPL	diagnostic peritoneal lavage
DRUJ	distal radioulnar joint
DSA	digital subtraction angiography
DVT	deep venous thrombosis
EBV	Epstein–Barr virus
ECG	electrocardiogram
ECMO	extracorporeal membrane oxygenation
ED	erectile dysfunction; emergency department
EEG	electroencephalogram
EGD	esophago-gastro-duodenoscopy
EGDT	early goal-directed therapy
ELISA	enzyme-linked immunosorbent assay
EMD	electromechanical delay
EMG	electromyography
EPL	extensor pollicis longus
EPO	erythropoietin
ER	estrogen receptor; emergency room
ERCP	endoscopic retrograde cholangiopancreatography
ES	endoscopic sphincterotomy
ESR	erythrocyte sedimentation rate
ESWL	extracorporeal shock-wave lithotripsy
ETT	endotracheal tube
EUA	examination under anesthetic
EUS	endoscopic ultrasound
EVAR	endovascular aneurysm repair
EVLT	endovascular laser therapy
FAP	familial adenomatous polyposis
FAST	focused abdominal sonography for trauma
FBC	full blood count
FDP	flexor digitorum profundus; fibrin degradation product
FDS	flexor digitorum superficialis
FEV_1	forced expiratory volume in 1 second
FFP	fresh frozen plasma
FHH	familial hypocalciuric hypercalcemia
FLC	fibrolamellar carcinoma
FiO_2	fraction of oxygen in inspired air
FNA	fine needle aspiration
FRC	functional residual capacity
FSH	follicle-stimulating hormone
5-FU	5-fluorouracil
GA	general anesthetic

GANT	gastrointestinal autonomic nerve tumor
GCS	Glasgow Coma Score
GERD	gastroesophageal reflux disease
GFR	glomerular filtration rate
GI	gastrointestinal
GIP	gastric inhibitory polypeptide
GIST	gastrointestinal stromal tumor
γGT	gamma glutamyl transferase
GTN	glyceryl trinitrate
GVHD	graft vs. host disease
HAR	hyperacute rejection
Hb	hemoglobin
HCC	hepatocellular carcinoma
HCG	human chorionic gonadotropin
Hct	hematocrit
HCV	hepatitis C virus
HDU	high-dependency unit
HHD	hand-held Doppler
HIDA	carbamoylimino diacetic acid
HIT	heparin-induced thrombocytopenia
HITT	heparin-induced thrombocytopenia and thrombosis
HIV	human immunodeficiency virus
HLA	human leukocyte antigen
HMMA	4-hydroxy-3-methoxymandelic acid
HNPCC	hereditary non-polyposis colorectal cancer
HPV	human papillomavirus
HR	heart rate
HSV	herpes simplex virus
5-HT	5-hydroxytryptamine (serotonin)
HTLV	human T-cell lymphotropic virus
HVA	homovanillic acid
IABP	intra-aortic balloon pump
IBD	inflammatory bowel disease
IC	intermittent claudication
ICD	intracardiac defibrillator
ICP	intracranial pressure
ICU	intensive care unit
IF	intrinsic factor
IFN	interferon
IHD	ischemic heart disease
IL	interleukin
IM	intramuscular

IMA	inferior mesenteric artery; internal mammary artery
IMHS	intramedullary hip screw
IMV	intermittent mandatory ventilation
INPV	intermittent negative pressure ventilation
INR	international normalized ratio
IPJ	interphalangeal joint
IPPV	intermittent positive pressure ventilation
IPSS	International Prostate Symptom Score
IRV	inverse-ratio ventilation
ITA	internal thoracic artery
ITU	intensive treatment unit
IV	intravenous
IVC	inferior vena cava
IVIG	intravenous immunoglobulin
IVU	intravenous urogram
JVD	jugular vein distension
JVP	jugular venous pressure
KUB	kidney, ureter, bladder
LA	local anesthetic
LAD	left anterior descending (artery)
LAP	left atrial pressure
LatexAT	latex agglutination test
LDH	lactate dehydrogenase
LDL	low-density lipid
LES	lower esophageal sphincter
LFT	liver function test
LH	luteinizing hormone
LHRH	luteinizing hormone release hormone
LIF	left iliac fossa
LITA	left internal thoracic artery
LMA	laryngeal mask airway
LMS	left main stem
LMWH	low molecular-weight heparin
LSV	long saphenous vein
LUTS	lower urinary tract symptoms
LV	left ventricle
LVEDP	left ventricular end-diastolic pressure
LVEDV	left ventricular end-diastolic volume
LVEF	left ventricular ejection fraction
LVF	left ventricular failure
MAC	monitored anesthesia care
MAG3	99Tcm-mercaptoacetyltriglycine

MALT	mucosa-associated lymphoid tissue
MAO	monoamine oxidase
MAP	mean arterial pressure
MCPJ	metacarpophalangeal joint
M, C, & S	microscopy, culture, and sensitivity
MCV	mean cell volume
MELD	Model for End-stage Liver Disease
MEN	multiple endocrine neoplasia
MHC	major histocompatibility complex
MI	myocardial infarction
MMF	mycophenolate mofetil
MMR	mismatch repair (genes)
MMV	mandatory minute ventilation
MODS	multiple organ dysfunction syndrome
MR	mitral regurgitation
MRA	magnetic resonance angiography
MRCP	magnetic resonance cholangiopancreatography
MRI	magnetic resonance imaging
MRSA	methicillin (or multiply) resistant *Staphylococcus aureus*
MSU	midstream urine
MTA	motor traffic accident
MTC	medullary thyroid carcinoma
MTP	mid-thigh perforator
MTPJ	metatarsophalangeal joint
MV	mitral valve
MVC	motor vehicle collision
NA	noradrenaline (norepinephrine)
NASCET	North American Symptomatic Carotid Endarterectomy Trial
NEC	necrotizing enterocolitis
NG	nasogastric
NGT	nasogastric tube
NIH	National Institutes of Health
NIPPV	noninvasive intermittent positive pressure ventilation
NK	natural killer (cell)
NNT	number needed to treat
NO	nitric oxide
npo	nothing by mouth (nil per os)
NRFM	non-rebreathing face mask
NSAID	nonsteroidal anti-inflammatory drug
NSGCT	nonseminomatous germ cell tumor
NTG	nitroglycerin
NVB	neurovascular bundle

NYHA	New York Heart Association
OCP	oral contraceptive pill
od	once a day
OG	osmal gap
O & P	ova and parasite
OPCAB	off-pump coronary artery bypass
ORIF	open reduction and internal fixation
PA	pulmonary artery
$PaCO_2$	arterial carbon dioxide tension
PACU	post-anesthesia care unit
PADSS	Post-Anesthetic Discharge Scoring System
PAF	platelet-activating factor
PAK	pancreas after kidney transplant
PaO_2	arterial oxygen tension
PAP	pulmonary artery pressure; placental alkaline phosphatase
PAWP	pulmonary artery wedge pressure
PCA	patient-controlled analgesia
PCI	percutaneous coronary intervention
PCL	posterior cruciate ligament
PCNL	percutaneous nephrolithotomy
PCO_2	carbon dioxide tension
PCP	primary care physician
PCV	packed cell volume; pressure-controlled ventilation
PCWP	pulmonary capillary wedge pressure
PDGF	platelet-derived growth factor
PE	pulmonary embolism
PEA	pulmonary endarterectomy
PEEP	positive end-expiratory pressure
PEFR	peak expiratory flow rate
PEG	percutaneous endoscopic gastrostomy
PEJ	percutaneous endoscopic jejunostomy
PEP	post-exposure prophylaxis
PET	positron emission tomography
PFO	patent foramen ovale
PH	portal hypertension
pHPT	primary hyperparathyroidism
PICC	peripherally inserted central venous catheter
PID	pelvic inflammatory disease
PIP	peak inspiratory pressure
PIPJ	proximal interphalangeal joint
PMN	polymorphic neutrophils
po	orally (per os)

PO$_2$	oxygen tension
PONV	postoperative nausea and vomiting
PPH	procedure for prolapse and hemorrhoids
PPHN	persistent pulmonary hypertension of newborn
PPI	proton pump inhibitor
PPN	peripheral parenteral nutrition
PPOI	prolonged postoperative ileus
PR	per rectum
PRBC	packed red blood cells
prn	as required
PS	pressure support
PSA	prostate-specific antigen
PSARP	posterior sagittal anorectoplasty
PSV	pressure support ventilation
PT	prothrombin time; physical therapy
PTC	percutaneous transhepatic cholangiogram
PTE	pulmonary thromboembolism
PTH	parathyroid hormone
PTT	partial prothrombin time
PTU	propylthiouracil
PUJ	pelviureteric junction
PV	per vagina
PVD	peripheral vascular disease
PVR	pulmonary vascular resistance
PVRI	pulmonary vascular resistance index
qac	before each meal
q8hr	every 8 hours
qhs	at bedtime
qid	four times a day
RA	right atrial; rheumatoid arthritis
RAP	right arterial pressure
RAIR	rectoanal inhibitory reflex
RAP	right arterial pressure
RCT	randomized controlled trial
RIF	right iliac fossa
ROM	range of motion
RR	relative risk (or risk ratio); respiratory rate
RRR	relative risk reduction
RSTL	relaxed skin tension line
RTA	road traffic accident
RV	right ventricle
RVP	right ventricular pressure

SAH	subarrachnoid hemorrhage
SaO_2	arterial oxygen saturation
SBE	subacute bacterial endocarditis
SBO	small-bowel obstruction
SBP	systolic blood pressure
SCAT	sheep cell agglutination test
SCC	squamous cell carcinoma
SCM	sternocleidomastoid
SD	standard deviation
SDU	step-down unit
SEMS	self-expanding metal stenting
SEPL	subfascial endoscopic perforator ligation
SFJ	saphenofemoral joint
sHPJ	secondary hyperparathyroidism
SIMV	synchronized intermittent mandatory ventilation
SIRS	systemic inflammatory response syndrome
SL	sublingual
SLE	systemic lupus erythematosus
SMA	superior mesenteric artery
SNP	sodium nitroprusside
SOB	shortness of breath
SPJ	saphenopopliteal junction
STD	sodium tetradecyl sulphate; sexually transmitted disease
STI	sexually transmitted infection
SV	stroke volume
SVC	superior vena cava
SVI	stroke volume index
SvO_2	percentage oxygen saturation of mixed venous hemoglobin
SVR	systemic vascular resistance
SVRI	systemic vascular resistance index
SVT	supraventricular tachycardia
T_3	triiodothryonine
T_4	thryoxine
TB	tuberculosis
TBSA	total body surface area
TCC	transitional cell carcinoma
TCD	transcranial Doppler (ultrasound)
TCR	T-cell receptor
TCT	transitional cell tumors
tid	three times a day
TEDS	thromboembolic deterrent stockings
TEMS	transanal endoscopic microsurgery

TFCC	triangular fibrocartilage complex
TGF	transforming growth factor
TIA	transient ischemic attack
TIBC	total iron binding capacity
TIPS	transjugular intraparenchymal portosystemic shunt/stent
TKA	through-knee amputation
TNF	tumor necrosis factor
TNM	tumor nodes metastasis (cancer staging)
tPA	tissue plasminogen activator
TPN	total parenteral nutrition
TRALI	transfusion-related acute lung injury
TRAM	transverse rectus abdominis myocutaneous (flap)
TRUS	transrectal ultrasound
TSH	thyroid-stimulating hormone
TTE	transthoracic echocardiogram
TUIP	transurethral incision in the prostate
TURP	transurethral resection of the prostate
U	international units
U & E	urea and electrolytes
UC	ulcerative colitis
UES	upper esophageal sphincter
UFH	unfractionated heparin
URI	upper respiratory infection
US	ultrasound
UTI	urinary tract infection
UW	University of Wisconsin (solution)
VAC	vacuum-assisted closure
VACTERL	vertebral defects, anorectal atresia, cardiac defects, tracheoesophageal fistula ± esophageal atresia, renal anomalies, limb defects (syndrome)
VAD	ventricular assist devices
VATS	video-assisted thoracoscopic surgery
VF	ventricular fibrillation
VHL	von Hippel–Lindau (disease)
VIP	vasoactive inhibitory polypeptide
VMA	vanillylmandelic acid
VQ	ventilation/perfusion (scan)
VRE	vancomycin-resistant *Enterococcus*
VT	ventricular tachycardia
vWF	von Willebrand factor
WBC	white blood cell count

Principles of surgery

Patricia Sylla, MD

Terminology in surgery

How to describe an operation

The terminology used to describe all operations is a composite of basic Latin or Greek terms.

First, describe the organ to be operated on

Examples:
- lapar-, abdomen (laparus = flank)
- nephro-, kidney
- pyelo-, renal pelvis
- cysto-, bladder
- chole-, bile/the biliary system
- col(on)-, large bowel
- hystero-, uterus
- thoraco-, chest
- rhino-, nose
- masto/mammo-, breast

Second, describe any other organs or things involved in the procedure

Examples:
- docho-, duct
- angio-, vessel (blood- or bile-carrying)
- litho-, stone

Third, describe what is to be done

Examples:
- -otomy, to cut (open)
- -ectomy, to remove
- -plasty, to change shape or size
- -pexy, to change position
- -raphy, to sew together
- -oscopy, to look into
- -ostomy, to create an opening in (*stoma* = mouth)
- -paxy, to crush
- -graphy/gram, image (of)

Lastly, add any terms to qualify how the procedure is done

Examples:
- percutaneous, via the skin
- trans-, across
- antegrade (forward), retrograde (backwards)
- laparoscopic, endoscopic

Examples

- choledochoduodenostomy—an opening between the bile duct and the duodenum
- rhinoplasty—nose reshaping
- pyelolithopaxy—destruction of pelvic calyceal stones
- bilateral mastopexy—breast lifts

- percutaneous arteriogram—arterial-tree imaging by direct puncture injection
- loop ileostomy—external opening in a loop of ileum with two sides (afferent and efferent limbs)
- flexible cystourethroscopy—internal bladder and urethral inspection

Taking a history and writing notes

Medical note writing

All medical professionals have a duty to record their input and care of patients in the case notes. These form a permanent legal and medical document. There are some basic rules.

- Write legibly in blue or black ink; other colors do not photocopy well.
- Date, time, and sign all entries, identify your title (medical student, postgraduate year [PGY]).
- Write legibly, especially your name and contact number.
- Keep entries brief, concise and accurate.
- Avoid abbreviations (medications, units) and medical jargon (AVSS Afebrile and Vital Signs Stable).
- Clearly document information given to patients and relatives.
- Avoid nonmedical judgments of patients or relatives, and avoid documenting conflicts in opinions among various medical services.

Basics

- Always record name, medical record number, and date of birth on all documents.
- Review the medical history:
  - Chief complaint and history of present illness
  - Past medical history, review of systems
  - Previous surgeries, obstetric history, allergies, medications
  - Family history, social history (smoking, drinking, drugs, sexual history, living situation)

Chief complaint

This is a one- or two-word summary of the patient's main symptoms (abdominal pain, nausea, vomiting, rectal bleeding). In elective admissions it is reasonable to write, "elective admission for varicose vein surgery."

History of present illness

- This is a detailed description of the main symptom and should include relevant details (location, duration, timing, character and intensity of pain, alleviating or exacerbating factors, associated symptoms).
- Include pertinent positives and negatives.
- Document the time sequence of symptoms and events.
- In a complicated history with multiple prior episodes, summarize previous events and how they relate to the present episode, e.g., "episode of small bowel obstruction 6 months ago requiring lysis of adhesions…fine until today when developed crampy abdominal pain and nausea similar to last episode."
- Summarize the results of all investigations: blood tests, X-rays, ultrasound, computerized tomography (CT) scan, ultrasound, magnetic resonance imaging (MRI), angiogram, intraoperative findings, pathology.

Past medical history
- Include all medical problems (diabetes, hypertension, coronary artery disease, chronic obstructive pulmonary disease [COPD], arrhythmias, clotting disorders, blood clots, inflammatory bowel disease) and correlate with medications.
- List and date all previous operations, correlate with surgical scars.
- Ask about previous problems with any anesthetics.
- Asking the question "Have you ever had any medical problem, or been to the hospital for anything?" may elicit additional information.

Review of systems
This is extremely important and often neglected. It can help identify significant medical comorbidities and diagnose occult pathologies. A pulmonary and cardiovascular review may help identify patients at high surgical risk and who might benefit from a cardiac workup and potential therapeutic intervention. A review of the gastrointestinal (GI) system may identify acute exacerbations of an otherwise chronic condition (inflammatory bowel disease flare).
- Cardiovascular: Chest pain, palpitations, claudication, ulcers
- Respiratory: Dyspnea on exertion or at rest, cough, sputum, wheeze, hemoptysis
- Gastrointestinal: Anorexia, change in appetite, weight loss, diarrhea, constipation, bright red blood per rectum, black tarry stool
- Genitourinary: Sexual activity, dyspareunia, burning on urination, nocturia, abnormal discharge, last menstrual period
- Neurological: Transient ischemic attacks, weakness

Tips for case presentation
- Practice and get feedback from residents (maintain eye contact, avoid reading excessively from your notes and flipping pages, don't make up data, if you don't know or didn't ask, just say so).
- Start with name, age, and any key medical facts together with the main presenting complaint(s).
- Follow the time course of the presentation. Start at the beginning of any relevant prodrome or associated symptoms and bring the audience up to the current status.
- Be concise, especially with the past medical history. Only expand on things that you really feel may be relevant to either the diagnosis or management.
- For the physical exam, always summarize the general appearance and vital signs first.
- Describe the most significant exam findings first but be systematic— "inspection, palpation, percussion, and auscultation."
- Briefly summarize other physical findings. Only expand on them if they may be directly relevant to the diagnosis or management.
- Briefly summarize relevant laboratory and radiology findings (do not list every test result).
- Finally, summarize and synthesize, don't repeat. Try to group symptoms and signs together into clinical patterns and recognized scenarios.
- End with your assessment and plan: propose a diagnosis or differential and treatment alternatives, and be prepared to discuss what diagnostic or further evaluation tests might be necessary.

Common surgical symptoms

Pain

Every complaint of pain needs systematic assessment. The acronym SOCRATES can be used to elicit all important features.
- **S**ite. Where is the pain—is it localized, in a region or generalized?
- **O**nset. Is it gradual, rapid, or sudden? Intermittent or constant?
- **C**haracter. Is it sharp, stabbing, cramping, dull, aching, tight, or sore?
- **R**adiation. Does it spread to other areas (e.g., to shoulder tip in diaphragmatic irritation, to back in retroperitoneal pain, to jaw and neck in myocardial pain)?
- **A**ssociated symptoms. Is there nausea, vomiting, dysuria, or jaundice?
- **T**iming. Does it occur at any particular time (after meals, after exercise)?
- **E**xacerbating or relieving factors. Becoming worse with deep breathing, moving, or coughing suggests irritation of somatic nerves in either the pleura or peritoneum.
- **S**urgical history. Does the pain relate to surgical interventions?

Dyspepsia (epigastric discomfort or pain, usually after eating) What is the frequency? Is it always precipitated by food or is it spontaneous in onset? Is there relief from anything, especially milky drinks or food? Is it positional?

Dysphagia (pain or difficulty during swallowing) Is the symptom new or long-standing? Is it rapidly worsening or relatively constant? Is it worse with solid food or fluids? (Worse with fluids suggests a motility problem rather than a mechanical cause.) Can it be relieved by anything? Does it feel like food is "getting stuck" in the throat or chest? Is it relieved by vomiting? Is it associated with changes in eating habits? Weight loss?

Acid reflux (bitter- or acidic-tasting fluid in the pharynx or mouth) How frequently does this occur? What color is it? (Green suggests bile, whereas white suggests only stomach contents.) When does it occur (lying only, on bending, spontaneously when standing)? Is it associated with coughing? Is it worse with certain foods? Does the patient wake up with an acidic taste in their mouth?

Hematemesis (presence of blood in vomit) What color is the blood? (Dark red-brown "coffee grounds" is old or small-volume stomach bleeding; dark red may be venous from the esophagus; bright red is arterial and often from major gastric or duodenal arterial bleeding.) What volume has occurred over what period? Did the blood appear with the initial vomiting or only after a period of prolonged vomiting (suggests a traumatic esophageal cause).

Abdominal distension Symmetrical distension suggests one of the "five Fs" (fluid ascites, flatus due to ileus or obstruction, fetus of pregnancy, fat, or a "flipping big mass"). Asymmetrical distension suggests a localized mass. What is the time course? Does it vary? It is associated with vomiting? Relieved with stool or flatus?

Change in bowel habit There may be change in frequency, or looser or more constipated stools. Increased frequency and looser stools suggest a pathological cause. Is it persistent or transient? Are there associated symptoms? Is it variable?

Frequency and urgency of defecation New urgency of defecation is almost always pathological. What is the degree of urgency—how long can the patient delay? Is there associated discomfort? What is passed—is the stool normal?

Bleeding per rectum What color is the blood? Is it pink-red and only on the paper when wiping? Does it splash in the pan? (Both suggest the source is in the anal canal, i.e., hemorrhoids.) Is it bright red and coat the surface of the stool? (This suggests a lower rectal cause.) Is the blood darker, with clots or marbled into the stools? (This suggests a colonic cause.) Is the blood fully mixed with the stool or altered? (This suggests a proximal colonic cause.)

Tenesmus (desire to pass stools with either no result or incomplete satisfaction of defecation) Suggests rectal pathology.

Jaundice (yellow discoloration due to hyperbilirubinemia) How quickly did the jaundice develop? Is there associated pruritus? Are there any symptoms of pain, fever, or malaise? (These suggest infection.) What color is the stool? (Acholic stools suggest biliary obstruction.)

Hemoptysis (presence of blood in expectorate) What color is the blood? (Light pink froth suggests pulmonary edema.) Are there clots or dark blood (infection or endobronchial lesion), and how much blood? Moderate bleeds quickly threaten airways: get help quickly!

Dyspnea (difficulty in or increased awareness of breathing) When does it occur—quantify the amount of effort. Is it positional?
- **Orthopnea** is difficulty in breathing that occurs on lying flat. Quantify it by asking how many pillows the patient needs at night to remain symptom-free.
- **Paroxysmal nocturnal dyspnea** is intermittent breathlessness at night. Both orthopnea and paroxysmal nocturnal dyspnea suggest cardiac heart failure.

Claudication (presence of pain in the muscles of the calf, thigh, or buttock precipitated by exercise and relieved by rest) After what degree of exercise does the pain occur (both distance on the flat and gradients)? How quickly is the pain relieved with rest?

Rest pain (pain in a limb at rest without significant exercise) How long has the pain been present? Is it intermittent? Does it occur mainly at night? Is it relieved by dependency of the limb involved? Is it associated with discoloration or ulcerations?

Evaluation of breast disease

History

A thorough assessment of individual risk factors for breast cancer should be obtained, including any prior history of breast cancer, surgery for other breast lesions, nulliparity, age at birth of first child, and menopausal status. A family history of breast cancer including age at diagnosis should be elicited. Other questions should cover the following:

• Use of hormonal supplements, contraceptives
• Prior mammogram findings
• If the patient presents with a breast mass, how long has the mass been present? Is there any change in size or shape? With menstrual cycles?

Physical examination

All breast examinations should be performed with a chaperone present.

Positioning and inspection

Breasts are best examined with the patient in a supine position and then sitting upright. Initially the arms are by the side. After initial inspection the patient should be positioned with hands on hips, sitting upright (initially relaxed and then moving shoulders forward to tense the pectoral muscles) and finally abducted slowly above the head. For palpation, the hands should lie on the hips and the patient may lie back in the supine position again.

Inspection is critical and should concentrate on the following:

• Overall symmetry and position. Are the breasts the same size? Is there deformity due to underlying disease?
• Skin appearance. Is the skin erythematous or edematous? Is there fixed lymphedema of the skin ("peau d'orange")? Are there scars from previous surgery?
• Skin tethering. Does the skin move freely as the arms are raised? (Tethering suggests underlying intraparenchymal scarring or tumor.)
• Nipples. Are the nipples retracted, inverted, or ulcerated (suggestive of subareolar tumor or infection)? Is there any evidence of discharge?

Palpation

Use the flat of the fingers and all four fingers at once. Palpate the "normal" breast first. Be methodical and don't "knead" the breast. A common routine is upper outer quadrant; lower outer; lower inner; upper inner; central (subareolar), supraclavicular fossa, axilla. Features to look for include the following:

• Palpable mass. Is it hard, irregular, and tethered? (cancer), or smooth, rounded, and mobile (cysts or fibroadenoma)?
• Diffuse nodularity, diffuse tenderness. Typical of benign disease
• Nipple discharge on palpation of the central area. Bilateral in young women, serous or milky suggests benign cause; blood and spontaneous from single duct suggest malignancy, pus suggests infection
• Axillary and supraclavicular lymphadenopathy. Is it multiple and tethered (cancer)?

Investigations

Ultrasound
- Easy to perform and minimal pain, done in breast outpatient clinic
- Avoids radiation in young women
- Highly sensitive for differentiating between solid tumors and cysts (hypoechoic lesions with posterior shadowing are suspicious for malignancies)
- Ultrasound-guided aspiration and biopsy permit pathologic examination.

Mammography
- Used both for population screening and diagnostic testing
- Low radiation, uncomfortable for most women
- Able to identify nonpalpable lesions
- Able to identify premalignant lesions (ductal carcinoma in situ)
- Mammographic features of malignancy include spiculated microcalcification, irregularity, stellate outline

Fine needle aspiration biopsy
- Almost painless and easy to do (local anesthetic, 22-gauge needle and syringe, glass slide, fixative), can be performed in breast clinic
- Good sensitivity and specificity
- Provides cytology: cellular atypia suggests malignancy
- Does not provide histology, cannot differentiate between invasive and in situ carcinoma
- Primarily used to distinguish cystic from solid lesions and to drain cysts

Core needle biopsy
- Performed under ultrasound or mammographic guidance using a Trucut® device or 14-gauge needle
- Can be done with local anesthesia
- Provides histology
- Able to differentiate between invasive and in situ carcinoma
- Highly sensitive and specific, good alternative to surgical excisional biopsy

Stereotactic breast biopsy
- Used to localize and biopsy nonpalpable lesions using mammography
- Can be used to target a suspicious area just before surgical excisional biopsy

CT scanning and MRI
- Relatively nonspecific for local breast pathology
- Useful for assessment of extensive local invasion, regional and systemic staging, evaluation of recurrence

Clinical pearls—anatomy of the breast

- The breast comprises epithelial ductal tissue, epithelial secretory lobules, fat, and connective tissue.
- The areola is the pigmented area around each nipple.
- The arterial supply is from segmental perforators from the internal thoracic artery (ITA).
- Lymphatic drainage—important in breast cancer management
  - Nonpathological lymph drainage is almost entirely to the axillary nodes.
  - The medial half can occasionally drain to internal mammary nodes.
  - Lymph nodes are divided into three levels: 1, lateral; 2, posterior; 3, medial to the edge of the pectoralis minor.

Evaluation of the neck

History

- If the patient presents complaining of a neck mass, elicit all associated symptoms (pain, dysphagia, hoarseness, hemoptysis, otalgia, tremors, palpitations). Investigate time of onset, change and rate of change in size and symptoms, and systemic complaints (fever, night sweats, weight loss, anorexia).
- The medical history should elicit prior history of malignancy, radiation exposure, smoking and alcohol history, travel and family history, and risk factors for HIV.

Physical examination

Positioning and inspection

- Sit the patient upright at rest with the head looking straight ahead. Inspect the neck from the front and side.
- Observe the neck at rest, during swallowing, and when the patient protrudes the tongue.

Inspection includes looking for the following:
- Overall symmetry and lumps
- Are there obvious lumps?
- Are they single or multiple?
- Is the lump lying in or close to the midline?
- Does it move with swallowing or tongue protrusion?

Palpation

Systematically palpate the regions of the neck in order. Use both hands with the flats of the fingers to compare each side. A typical sequence of palpation is anterior triangle (bottom to top), submental area, submandibular area, posterior triangle (top to bottom), supraclavicular fossae. Repalpate the neck with the patient swallowing—particularly the anterior triangle (Fig. 1.1). Lastly, palpate carotid arteries.

- Lumps. Single or multiple (multiple suggests lymphadenopathy)? Is it tender? Is it strictly in the midline (likely to be related to the thyroid)? Does it move with swallowing? What are the general features?
- Thyroid lumps. Is it unilateral or bilateral? Does it move with tongue protrusion?
- Carotid arteries. Are they normal, ecstatic, or aneurysmal?
- Supraclavicular fossae. Is there associated lymphadenopathy (suggests malignancy)?

Auscultation

Listen to the carotid arteries and any large masses for bruits suggesting a hypervascular local circulation or stenosis.

Investigations

Ultrasound

- Easy to perform and painless
- Avoids radiation
- Highly sensitive for differentiating between solid tumors and cysts

Fine needle aspiration biopsy (FNA)
- Minimal pain, easy to perform and provides quick results, done as an outpatient (22-gauge needle and syringe, glass slide, fixative)
- First diagnostic test for solitary neck mass
- Performed under ultrasound guidance if mass is nonpalpable
- Provides only cellular information and relies on cellular atypia for a diagnosis of malignancy
- Does not provide histological information
- Occasionally therapeutic for cysts
- Good sensitivity and specificity
- Contraindicated where there is suspicion that the lesion may be vascular

CT scanning and MRI
- Useful for assessment of extensive local invasion and regional and systemic staging of tumors
- Allows evaluation of the thorax in some thyroid tumors

Additional investigations
- In the setting of a solitary neck mass, a complete head and neck examination should be performed, including indirect and direct visualization of the upper aerodigestive tract with a fiber-optic endoscope.

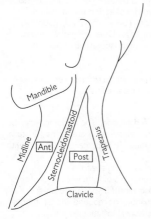

Fig. 1.1 Key points—triangle of the neck.

Evaluation of the abdomen

Positioning and inspection

The patient should be placed supine with arms at the sides and with headrest to ensure that abdominal muscles are relaxed. The patient may be rolled to the left or right lateral positions during palpation and percussion. Asking the patient to cough or lift the head off the table or bear down may accentuate abdominal wall hernias. When evaluating the groin, ask the patient to stand up and bear down (valsava maneuver) to help identify inguinal hernias.

Inspection should be done during both normal and deep respiration and include the following:

- General features. Is there evidence of jaundice? Does the patient look underweight, malnourished?
- Note the location and healing of all scars (keloid, hypertrophic), and whether hernias are visible with valsalva near the scars.
- Skin. Is there evidence of a fistula? Where is it, and what is the size of opening, quality and quantity of drainage?
- Is there a stoma? What type? Does it look healthy? Does it protrude or retract excessively? How does parastomal skin look? What is the content in the stoma appliance?
- Overall appearance. Is the abdomen symmetrical? Is there evidence of global distension (e.g., ascites, distended bowel)? Localized protrusion (mass or organomegaly)? Is there any discoloration (periumbilical bruising (Cullen's sign) or flank bruising (Grey Turner's sign), both of which suggest retroperitoneal hemorrhage? Does the patient appear uncomfortable with any type of movement (suggestive of peritoneal irritation)?
- Umbilicus. Is there a hernia?
- Pulsation. Is there visible pulsation? (Further assessment requires palpation to evaluate for aortic abdominal aneurysm.)

Palpation

Be methodical. Stand on the patient's right side. The abdomen can be divided into five "quadrants" (Fig. 1.2). Palpate each area gently in turn. Identify any masses or areas of tenderness. Repeat the examination with deeper palpation.

Palpation should be directed toward assessing the following:

- Signs of peritoneal irritation. Are there signs of local visceral peritoneal irritation (tenderness and pain on palpation)? If so, are there signs of mild parietal peritoneal irritation (guarding or rebound and tap tenderness) or signs of marked parietal peritoneal irritation (rigidity)?
- Masses. Assess their size, surface (smooth, lobulated), edge, mobility, pulsatile quality, tenderness, anatomic relation to adjacent organs.
- Organs
  - Liver. Palpate from right lower quadrant into right upper quadrant, feeling for the liver edge during inspiration every few centimeters upward until it is found. Assess the edges (smooth, nodular).

- Spleen. Palpate from right lower quadrant into left upper quadrant, feeling for the spleen edge during inspiration as for the liver. Assess the edge and any palpable surface.
- Kidneys. Palpate bimanually.

Percussion

- Percussion is used to identify the presence of excessive amounts of gas or fluid. It is also useful for confirming the presence of mild to moderate parietal peritoneal irritation ("percussion or tap tenderness").
- Gas (hyperresonance). Is it generalized or localized? Is there evidence of loss of dullness over the liver (suggestive of copious free intraperitoneal gas)?
- Fluid (ascites). Usually identified as "shifting dullness," dullness in the flanks in the supine position moves to the lower portion of the abdomen upon turning to the lateral position.

Auscultation

To fully assess bowel sounds, it is necessary to listen for at least 1 min. Bowel sounds can be described as

- Absent
- Normal
- Active
- Obstructive—characterized by high-pitched, frequent sounds often with crescendos of activity ("tinkling")

Abdominal assessment should always include a rectal examination in adults, but in children this is rarely useful and should usually be avoided.

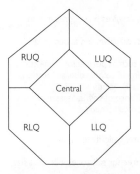

Fig. 1.2 The five quadrants: RUQ, right upper quadrant; LUQ, left upper quadrant; LLQ, left lower quadrant; RLQ, right lower quadrant; central quadrant.

Abdominal tests

Fecal occult blood testing
- May be chemical or immunological
- Of little value in hospital setting
- Most commonly used for colorectal cancer screening

Endoscopic gastroduodenoscopy
- Typically used for evaluation of esophageal, gastric, and duodenal pathology (bleeding, tumors, ulcers, strictures)
- Most commonly used for diagnosis and treatment of upper gastro-intestinal bleeding, evaluation of peptic ulcer disease
- Allows minor therapeutic procedures (biopsy, injection/cauterization of bleeding points)
- Allows major therapeutic procedures (percutaneous endoscopic gastrostomy feeding tube placement, dilatation of strictures, mucosal resections, endoscopic retrograde cholangiopancreatography)

Flexible sigmoidoscopy
- Outpatient procedure without sedation
- Very low risk of perforation (1/5000)
- Should visualize up to the descending colon
- Allows minor therapeutic procedures (decompression of sigmoid volvulus, polypectomy, injection/cauterization of bleeding points, marking of colonic disease location, biopsy, assessment of colonic mucosa and lesions)

Colonoscopy
- Outpatient procedure under sedation, requires bowel preparation
- Low risk of perforation (1/1000)
- Should visualize the entire colon, ileocecal valve, and appendiceal orifice (95% of the time)
- Allows minor therapeutic procedures such as polypectomy, injection/cauterization of bleeding points, marking of colonic disease location, biopsy, assessment of colonic mucosa and lesions
- Typically used for diagnosis and surveillance of colitis, assessment of colonic neoplasia, investigation of colorectal bleeding

Transabdominal ultrasound
- Easy, safe, and avoids radiation exposure, typically used for
  - Identification of ovarian disease
  - Primary investigation of the biliary tree for gallstones, bile duct size, and liver parenchymal texture
  - Investigation of suspected subphrenic or pelvic collections
  - Assessment of the splenic parenchyma
  - Identifying free fluid in abdominal trauma

CT scanning
- Easy and safe; requires significant radiation exposure and IV contrast
- Typical uses include the following:
  - Primary assessment of all intra-abdominal masses

- Staging of intra-abdominal and pelvic malignancy and evaluation of recurrence
- Investigation of choice in evaluating abdominal pain of unclear etiology
- Often the investigation of choice in suspected intestinal obstruction
- May be specifically tailored for pancreatic, biliary, visceral vessel evaluation (thin cuts, arterial and venous injection phases)
- Investigation of choice for suspected postoperative complications

MRI scanning

- Conventional body scanner with external coils
- Avoids radiation
- Test of choice in pregnant patients with suspected intra-abdominal pathology who refuse CT scan
- Typically used for the following:
  - Investigation of suspected bile duct disease
  - Assessment of pancreas
  - Assessment of pelvic and retroperitoneal soft tissue disease

Plain abdominal radiograph

- Limited use
- May identify intestinal obstruction, urinary tract stones, calcified gallstones, free intra-abdominal air, intra-abdominal fluid

Barium enema (single and double contrast)

- May be single contrast (contrast material filling the colon) or double contrast (dilute contrast and air to coat the mucosal surface of the colon)
- Requires bowel preparation and relatively mobile patient
- Single contrast used to identify strictures and obstructions (used to assess colorectal anastomoses in dilute or water-soluble form)
- Double contrast typically used to identify colonic neoplasia, assess colonic anatomy

Gastrointestinal transit studies

- Serial abdominal X-rays to identify the progress of ingested radio-opaque markers
- Used to assess intestinal motility and transit time

Positron emission tomography (PET) scanning

- Injection of radioactive metabolic substrate to identify metabolically active tissue. Typically used to
  - Identify tumor deposits
  - Assess central nervous system (CNS) disease

Gastrointestinal motility testing

- Manometry testing of the esophagus including lower esophageal sphincter (LES) and of the anal canal
- Pressure sensitivities of the esophagus and anal canal
- Ph testing of the contents of the esophagus (continuously for 24 hr)
- Used to assess anorectal function, esophageal motility and function, and gastroesophageal reflux

Evaluation of pelvic disease

Positioning and inspection

Examination is performed in up to three positions: supine (for trans-abdominal palpation), supine with hips flexed and abducted (for vaginal and bimanual palpation), and left lateral position with hips flexed (for rectal examination, rigid proctoscopy, or flexible sigmoidoscopy). *Any* pelvic examination should be performed with a chaperone present.

- Anus. Is the anus gaping (loss of internal sphincter muscle tone)? Is there mucosal or rectal prolapse? Is there vaginal prolapse or evidence of a cystocele? Are there scars from previous surgery, fistulous openings, or abscesses?

Palpation

- Palpate the lower abdominal quadrants.
- Rectal examination. Is the anal tone normal and squeeze normal and symmetrical? Is the prostate of normal size with a normal central sulcus? Does the rectal mucosa feel normal? Is there tenderness, lesions, a mass, or induration?
- Vaginal examination as needed (abdominal pain in sexually active female patients). Speculum exam: Is the cervix inflamed? Note the presence of purulent or foul-smelling discharge; send for Gram stain and cultures.
- Bimanual examination. Note tenderness along the perineal body, evaluate the presence of ovarian tenderness (suggestive of pelvic inflammatory disease or tubo-ovarian abscess).

Investigations

Anoscopy or rigid proctoscopy

- Performed in outpatients without sedation.
- Only visualizes the anal canal (anoscope) and rectum (proctoscope), which may be difficult to visualize without an enema
- Useful to identify the source of rectal bleeding or pain (fissure, hemor-rhoids, radiation proctitis) and anorectal pathology (anal and rectal cancers, infectious lesions, etc.) where biopsies can be performed

Flexible sigmoidoscopy

- Low-risk, outpatient procedure usually performed without sedation.
- Should visualize up to the descending colon
- Allows biopsy of lesions and minor therapeutic procedures

Transabdominal or transvaginal ultrasound

- Easy, safe, and avoids radiation
- Good for identification of ovarian disease (ovarian torsion, cyst, tubo-ovarian abscess, mass)

Endoanal or endorectal ultrasound

- 360° scanning endoanal/endorectal probe without sedation
- Endoanal ultrasound—for assessment of anal sphincter integrity, anal fistulas, and abscesses

- Endorectal ultrasound—for visualization and staging of rectal cancer (depth of invasion and lymph node status), prostate disease (including biopsy), and presacral lesions

CT scanning
- Easy, safe, but significant radiation exposure and intravenous (IV) contrast
- Investigation of choice for pelvic symptoms of unclear etiology and to evaluate postoperative complications

MRI scanning
- Usually via conventional body scanner with external coils (occasionally performed with endorectal coils)
- Investigation of choice for assessment of advanced rectal, gynecological, and urological cancer or complex pelvic sepsis
- Investigation of choice for complex pelvic and anal sepsis

Clinical pearls—pelvic anatomy

- The true pelvis lies between the pelvic inlet (sacral promontory, illiopectineal lines, symphisis pubis) and outlet (coccyx, ischial tuberosities, pubic arch).
- Pelvic floor muscles (levator ani) support and are integral to the function of the anorectum, vagina, and bladder. They are innervated by anterior primary rami of S2, S3, and S4.
- Anterior relations of the rectum (palpable during rectal exam) are as follows:
  - Women: vagina, cervix, pouch of Douglas
  - Men: prostate, seminal vesicles, rectovesical pouch

Evaluation of peripheral vascular disease

Positioning and inspection

Ideally the patient should be examined in a warm environment at rest. Inspect the limb at rest in the supine position first, then elevated (passively), and, finally, dependent. Be sure to expose the entire limb, including the foot or hand, to allow thorough inspection. It is important to remove all dressings for proper inspection. For venous disease, the patient should also be examined standing.

During supine inspection look for the following:

- Appearance. Does the skin look chronically ischemic (lack of hair, brittle nails, pale)? Are there areas of established skin necrosis (dry gangrene at apex of digits, between digits, heel of the foot)? Are there changes of chronic venous stasis (prominent veins, lipodermatosclerosis)?
- Color. Waxy white suggests acute severe ischemia; blue and mottled suggests acute irreversible ischemia; dark purple and shiny suggests chronic ischemia.
- Color changes during position. Note the presence and delay in change in color when the limb is dependent. Ischemic limbs slowly turn deep purple.
- Ulcers. What is the location (medial suggests venous disease, lateral or plantar suggests arterial disease)?
- Venous inspection. Have the patient stand up. Inspect for varicose veins. Are they in the long (greater) saphenous or short (lesser) saphenous distribution?

Palpation

- Temperature. Does the skin feel cold or warm? Is there a transition level?
- Skin capillary compression and refill. A delay of greater than 5 sec suggests significant ischemia.
- Peripheral pulses. Start with the most proximal (major) vessels (femoral) and work distally. Record if the pulse is hyperdynamic (+++), normal (++), reduced (+), or absent (−). Record if there are any thrills palpable.
- In venous disease, tests of venous competence may be performed.
- Surgical grafts. Palpate the course of any surgical grafts and record the presence of pulses if present

Percussion

Look for transmitted thrill. The course of varicose veins may be tracked by presence of a percussion thrill.

Auscultation

Listen for bruits. Are there bruits in the proximal vessels (suggestive of stenosis or previous surgery)?

Tests

Doppler ultrasound

- Easy to use. Can be carried and performed anywhere from the emergency room (ER) to the intensive care unit (ICU)
- May be simply diagnostic (confirm the patency of a graft or vessel)
- May be used to evaluate the relative flow in vessels by measuring the pressure at which detectable flow ceases, using a compression cuff. The most common example is the ankle–brachial pressure index (ABI).

Color flow Doppler

- Combined two-dimensional (2D) ultrasound image with Doppler-derived flow represented with color, superimposed in real time
- May be used to assess stenoses or flow characteristics in vessels or grafts
- May be used for assessment of reflux between deep and superficial veins

Direct angiography

- Either simple or, more commonly, digital subtraction angiography (DSA; used to reduce background image "noise" and convert the arterial images for easier viewing)
- Invasive, requires direct arterial puncture with associated risks (hematoma, pseudoaneurysm, dissection, abscess)
- Requires IV contrast with a small risk of allergic reaction (relatively contraindicated in renal dysfunction, may premedicate with gentle hydration and N-acetylcysteine)
- Gives direct views of arterial tree, may perform angioplasty

Magnetic resonance angiography (MRA)

- Provides images of an arterial tree, based on the presence of arterial flow during scanning
- Safe and noninvasive, requires no contrast but would required angiography for therapeutic intervention (angioplasty)
- Tends to overestimate degree of stenosis because very low flow is underrepresented

CT angiography

- Requires multi-slice rapid acquisition ("helical"/"spiral") scanner
- Images acquired in arterial phase after IV injection of contrast
- Three-dimensional (3D) reconstruction allows "virtual angiogram" images to be produced
- Easier to perform and safer than direct angiogram (visceral vessels)
- Requires dose of IV contrast

Evaluation of the skin and subcutaneous tissue disease

Assessment and description of a lump

Key features in the history include the following:
- Rate of growth. Rapid increase in size is suspicious of malignancy (primary or secondary).
- Recent change in size suggests malignant change or infection in a previously benign lesion.
- Associated symptoms. Paresthesia or weakness suggests involvement of nerves; reduced movement suggests involvement of muscle.
- History of local trauma may suggest cause, although a previously undiagnosed and asymptomatic underlying lump should always be ruled out.

The following features should be considered when examining the lump.

Basic facts
- Location
- Size
- Shape

Features of infection or inflammation
- Temperature
- Tenderness
- Color

Features of malignancy
- Surface (rugged)
- Edge (irregular)
- Consistency (hard)

Features of fluid or vascular lesions
- Fluctuant (fluid-filled)
- Transilluminates (fluid-filled)
- Pulsatile (arterial lesion)
- Presence of a bruit (arterial lesion)
- Expansibility (indicative of an arterial aneurysm)
- Presence of compressibility (venous lesion or arteriovenous malformation [AVM])

Features of locoregional invasion
- Tethering to surrounding structures
- Involvement of surrounding structures (e.g., nerves)
- Regional lymphadenopathy

Assessment and description of an ulcer

Key features in the history include the following:
- Is it painful? (Venous, diabetic, and neuropathic ulcers are painless.)
- Did it start as an ulcer or did a lump become ulcerated (suggests a malignancy in/of the skin)?
- Is there a history of underlying infection, e.g., of bone?

Describe the basic morphology of the ulcer.
- **Location**
  - Pressure points and bony prominences suggest pressure sores (decubitus ulcer).
  - Medial shin suggests venous ulcer.
  - Lateral shin, dorsum of foot, and toes suggest arterial ulcer.
- **Edge**
  - Sloping edge suggests conventional ulcer (can be many etiologies).
  - Rolled edge is typical of basal cell or squamous carcinomas.
  - Everted edge suggests squamous or metastatic carcinomas.
  - Vertical edge (punched out) suggests syphilis or chronic infection.
- **Base**
  - Friable, red, and bleeding suggests venous or traumatic
  - Green slough suggests infected
  - Black, hard eschar suggests chronic ischemia.
- **Discharge**. May suggest an underlying cause (intestinal fistula with enteric content, golden pus in chronic actinomycosis)
- **Surrounding tissue**. Erythema and swelling suggest secondary infection.

Surgery at the extremes of age

Surgery is being performed more frequently in older patients, and the range of procedures available to surgeons for both the very elderly and the very young and neonates is increasing. Minimally invasive surgery is increasingly being offered to older patients at risk from open surgery. Both of these groups need particular attention and have specific potential problems.

Surgery and the elderly

Common misconceptions

- Elderly patients benefit just as much from potentially curative cancer surgery as younger patients. Cancers demonstrate the same range of behaviors at all ages and are neither more "benign" nor less responsive to treatment in the elderly.
- Minimally invasive procedures in the elderly can offer all the benefits available to younger patients.
- "Palliative" procedures for benign disease (e.g., cholecystectomy, joint surgery, eye surgery) are just as important in the elderly as in younger patients, as they may allow preservation of independence and offer as much improvement in quality of life as in the young.

Common problems in the elderly

- Multiple comorbidities and polypharmacy increase the scope for potential complications and drug interactions.
- Comorbidities are often "silent," either due to atypical presentation or underreporting of symptoms (e.g., angina may not be manifest because of reduced mobility).
- Social, family, nursing, and medical support structures are often complex and easily lost during a hospital admission.
- Reduced or acutely impaired mental faculties may make history taking, consent, and identification of a health-care proxy and living will difficult.
- Reduced or acutely impaired mental faculties may reduce or blunt the manifestation and vocalization of severe illness.
- The elderly are particularly prone to mild or moderate chronic malnutrition, increasing general complication rates and the risk of pressure ulcers.

Strategies for management of the elderly

- Involve all the necessary specialties as soon as possible (social workers, physical and occupational therapists, hospitalists).
- Start to plan early for discharge and establish early the patients' needs and wishes and coordinate discharge plans with the family.
- Evaluate nutritional needs as soon as possible after surgery. Does the patient need a feeding tube or hyperalimentation?

Surgery and the young

Although most surgical procedures performed on neonates and very young children are done by specialized pediatric surgical and nursing teams, most surgeons will care for young children at some time, and the principles of care used in pediatric surgery can be usefully applied to older children.

Common problems in children

- Young children may not be able to accurately report symptoms and illness behavior is often nonspecific.
- Cardiovascular responses in the young are excellent. Tachycardia and particularly hypotension are (very) late signs of hypovolemia.

Tips for managing children

- Take the history from the parents or caretakers and the child.
- Infections are common and often present with nonspecific signs.
- Consider nonsurgical diagnoses at all times, e.g., meningitis, urinary sepsis, systemic viral infections.
- Examine the child as much as possible while they are sitting on a parent's lap. Use the same position for phlebotomy.
- Put local anesthetic cream on phlebotomy sites 30 min in advance.
- Some children are too young to cooperate with procedures under local anesthesia and will require general anesthesia for relatively minor procedures.
- Make sure all prescriptions for drugs and fluids are written according to weight to avoid inadvertent adult dosing—if in doubt, ask.
- Fluid balance may be critical, since small volume changes are highly significant in small children. Pay close attention to fluid resuscitation.

Ambulatory and minimally invasive surgery

Ambulatory surgery procedures

An increasing number of procedures in all aspects of surgery are being performed in the ambulatory setting. The key features that make a procedure suitable include the following:

• Low risk of major complications
• Predictable recovery period not requiring specialized postoperative therapy or treatment
• Postoperative analgesia that does not require prolonged therapy or opiates routinely
• Anesthetic technique not requiring invasive monitoring, prolonged muscle relaxation, or epidural or spinal anesthesia
• Low risk of difficult or unpredictable anesthetic technique

Many types of surgical procedures are now performed routinely as day-care surgery, including hernias, anorectal procedures, arthroscopy, and minor laparoscopic and endoscopic surgeries.

Selection of patients for day case surgery

Most hospitals have well-defined protocols to select patients for suitability for ambulatory surgery and most day-surgery units conduct their own preadmission assessment by either telephone or questionnaire. Typical criteria might include the following:

• Maximum age of 75 years
• Appropriate social support for the patient at home, including transport and a responsible adult to monitor progress
• No history of more than mild to moderate cardiac or respiratory disease (e.g., uncomplicated asthma or controlled angina)
• Non-insulin-dependent diabetes only (unless for procedures performed under local anesthesia)
• Body mass index (BMI) below 35 (typically)—higher than this is associated with increased risk of anesthetic and surgical complications

Minimally invasive surgical procedures

Minimally invasive surgery is becoming more common in many areas of surgery. It is a broad term that includes a wide range of procedures with varying degrees of overlap with conventional "open" surgery and should also include interventional radiological procedures. A useful definition of minimally invasive surgery is a procedure that can be performed by a technique involving fewer and/or smaller incisions than alternative "conventional" open surgery, or under less invasive anesthetic techniques. This includes most laparoscopic and thoracoscopic surgery (cholecystectomy, gastric fundoplication, gastric bypass, small-bowel resection, colectomy, lobectomy, nephrectomy, adrenalectomy, hernia repair). It also includes flexible and rigid endoscopic procedures (diagnostic and therapeutic colonoscopy, cystoscopy, transurethral prostate surgery, hysteroscopic surgery) and several procedures using specific techniques or equipment (e.g., transanal endoscopic microsurgery, subfascial endoscopic venous surgery).

Advantages of minimally invasive surgery

Many minimally invasive surgical techniques require specific training to perform and expensive equipment. There are, however, a number of benefits associated with minimally invasive surgery.

Patient benefits
- Smaller, fewer, or no scars
- Reduced postoperative pain
- Reduced length of hospital stay
- Fewer postoperative complications (particularly wound and respiratory)
- Faster return to normal daily activities

Surgeon benefits
- Reduced length of hospital stay
- Avoid the need for specialized analgesia such as patient-controlled analgesia (PCA), epidurals

Hospital benefits
- Improved turnover
- Reduced postoperative complications

To whom should minimally invasive surgery be offered?

The advantages of minimally invasive surgery give it a wide application:
- Young patients—small scars and short hospital stays
- Elderly—reduced postoperative complications and shortened hospital stay are critical in patients who often have multiple comorbidities
- Unfit patient—easier anesthetic techniques and reduced surgical stress may reduce the perioperative risk

Surgery during pregnancy

Pregnancy testing

- Urinary dipstick. human chorionic gonadotrophin (HCG) is 91% sensitive (even lower for women self-testing). Specificity ranges from 61% to 100% if tested from the first day of the first missed period (2 weeks after ovulation).
- Blood. HCG is almost 100% sensitive and specific, and able to detect pregnancy 6–8 days after ovulation.
- False negatives and positives are most commonly due to user error.

Changes in anatomy and physiology

First trimester

- Drugs may have a teratogenic effect.
- Reduced lower esophageal sphincter tone, increasing the risk of gastroesophageal reflux and aspiration when supine

Second trimester

- Drugs may have an adverse effect on fetal development or metabolism without causing gross malformation.
- Increased susceptibility to urinary tract infections, particularly ascending renal infections and pyelonephritis
- Increased risk of venous thromboembolism rises in the second trimester and remains constantly raised in the third
- Increased susceptibility to superficial infections

Third trimester

- Drugs may cause labor.
- Displacement of mobile abdominal viscera superiorly and behind the enlarging uterus (appendix comes to lie in the right upper quadrant)
- Risk of hypotension in supine position (inferior vena cava [IVC] compression by gravid uterus): positioning the patient in slight left lateral decubitus

Common surgical diseases in pregnancy

These include appendicitis, biliary disease (biliary colic, cholecystitis, choledocholithiasis, gallstone pancreatitis), ovarian disorders (torsion, neoplasm), trauma, breast or cervical disease, and bowel obstruction.

Appendicitis

- The pain is within a few centimeters of McBurney's point in the vast majority of pregnant women, regardless of the stage of pregnancy.
- Leukocytosis may not be a sign of appendicitis (common in pregnancy).
- Graded compression ultrasound > MRI (when available) > CT scan
- Differential diagnosis: ectopic pregnancy, pyelonephritis, threatened miscarriage/placental abruption, round ligament syndrome

Biliary disease
- Hormonal changes in pregnancy predispose to develop cholelithiasis.
- In most cases, episodes resolve with supportive care.
- Surgery is indicated for intractable pain, clinical deterioration.

Trauma
- Resuscitate and stabilize maternal vital signs (air, breathing, circulation [ABC]).
- Indications for surgical exploration: penetrating abdominal injury, intraperitoneal hemorrhage, bowel perforation, injury to the uterus or fetus
- C-section is indicated only if there is evidence of fetal distress that fails to respond to maternal resuscitation.

Bowel obstruction
- More likely to occur as uterus enlarges into the upper abdomen
- Common causes include adhesions, volvulus, and intussusception.
- Diagnosis and treatment are similar to that for nonpregnant patients, but aggressive intervention is recommended (delay in treatment increases maternal and fetal morbidity and mortality).

Risks of miscarriage and imaging

The risk of miscarriage related to surgical pathology and surgery varies according to trimester. It is highest in the first trimester, and the risk of a viable premature labor rises in the third trimester. The risk of miscarriage induced by general anesthesia and surgery should be balanced against increased maternal and fetal morbidity and mortality from untreated surgical pathology. This is a common dilemma in surgical practice. CT scanning is contraindicated due to radiation dose. Ultrasound imaging may be less useful because it provides poor views, but MRI is a safe imaging modality. The only way to a diagnosis may be surgery, once nonsurgical diagnoses have been excluded.

Steps to minimize fetal risks of surgery

Although surgery and anesthesia are not associated with adverse effects in early pregnancy, the rates of low–birth weight infants and early neonatal death are increased among women who have had surgery. Steps to minimize fetal risks include the following:
- Delay elective surgery (until second trimester).
- Avoid use of potentially harmful agents during organogenesis (first trimester).
- Use regional anesthesia, if possible.
- Position mother in slight left lateral decubitus (gestation >20 weeks).
- Use continuous fetus monitoring (gestation >23–24 weeks).
- Laparoscopic surgery: keep intra-abdominal pressure as low as possible (<15 mmHg), avoid Veress needle

Prescribing drugs in pregnancy

It is clearly unethical to screen drugs for harmful effects on the human fetus; many new and commonly used drugs have therefore never been used in pregnancy. Some older drugs have been used in pregnancy and are regarded as safe in the absence of any reports of fetal harm. Generally:
- Avoid prescribing drugs if at all possible.
- Know the stage of the pregnancy; many drugs are only approved in particular trimesters.

Check every drug that you prescribe. If in doubt, seek specialist advice.
- Important teratogens include thalidomide, carbamazepine, and sodium. Valproate, isotretinoin, tetracycline, warfarin, ACE-inhibitors, lithium, methotrexate, cyclophosphamide

Surgery in endocrine disease

Diabetes

Specific perioperative risks

- Hypoglycemia, hyperglycemia, or ketoacidosis
- Underlying diabetes-related comorbidities (nephropathy, small-vessel coronary and cerebrovascular disease, autonomic neuropathy with reduced cardiovascular homeostasis responses) are often overlooked.
- Poor wound healing and increased risk of infections (necrotizing fasciitis)
- Increased susceptibility to skin pressure necrosis

Management of the diabetic patient

- Involve endocrinology and nephrology staff as needed to assist in the patient's care.
- Clarify whether the patient is on oral glycemic agents or is insulin-dependent (determine amount and type of insulin preparation), since the risk of perioperative complications correlates with the degree of blood glucose control.
- Surgery should not be delayed for prolonged periods of time to avoid fluctuations in blood glucose.
- Ketoacidosis in the perioperative period is associated with a very high morbidity and mortality rate and should be avoided at all costs.

Minor surgery

- Oral glycemic agent–controlled: Continue normal regimen.
- Insulin-controlled: Omit preoperative insulin on day of surgery, monitor blood sugar qac and qhs (before each meal and at bed time), restart normal insulin regimen once oral diet is established.

Major surgery

- Oral glycemic agent–controlled: Omit long-acting glycemic agents preoperatively. Monitor blood sugar qac and qhs; if blood glucose >200, cover with regular insulin (sliding scale) either subcutaneous (SC) or IV drip, restart oral agents when oral diet is resumed.
- Insulin-controlled: Monitor blood sugar qac +qhs, start insulin on sliding scale preoperatively once patient is npo and continue until normal diet is reestablished. Restart normal insulin regimen (start at half dose) once oral diet is resumed.

Glycemic control in critically ill patients

- Tight glycemic control with IV insulin (blood glucose 80–110) confers survival benefit in critically ill surgical patients.
- Normoglycemia has significant survival benefits in acute myocardial infarction (MI).

Emergency surgery

- Rule out ketoacidosis. If present, use medical treatment algorithm to control blood glucose and postpone surgery until blood glucose is <200 mg/dL unless the condition is life threatening.

Insulin coverage
- IV insulin drip is preferable to SC injections because of erratic absorption and unreliable therapeutic levels.
  - Run IV insulin along with dextrose-containing IV fluids, follow institutional protocol for titration.

Steroids
Specific perioperative risks
Chronic steroids are used to treat a number of chronic illnesses (rheumatoid arthritis, severe asthma and COPD, temporal arteritis, polymyalgia rheumatica, inflammatory bowel disease [IBD]). Steroids reduce neutrophil and fibroblast function and lead to irreversible changes in connective tissue. Long-term use of systemic steroids results in adrenal suppression. Long-term steroid use is associated with the following:
- Addisonian (hypoadrenal) crisis (see Box 1.1)
- Susceptibility to infection
- Poor wound healing (increased risk of anastomotic failure)
- Increased friability of skin and other tissues (hernia repair failure)
- Osteoporosis, fractures
- Increased risk of gastrointestinal hemorrhage or ulcer

Box 1.1 Addisonian (hypoadrenal) crisis

Stresses (surgery, sepsis) require increased adrenal secretion of corticosteroids; failure to mount this response (due to suppression of the hypothalamic–pituitary–adrenal axis by chronic steroids) can result in an Addisonian crisis. The following groups of patients are at high risk:
- Any patient currently taking >5 mg prednisone for >2 weeks
- Any patient who reduced their long-term steroids within 2–4 weeks
- Patients who have undergone adrenalectomy

Clinical features
- Lethargy and malaise
- Abdominal pain often poorly localized (may present as acute abdomen)
- Nausea and vomiting
- Hypotension
- Hypoglycemia, hyponatremia
- Coma, death

Management
- Treat with IV hydrocortisone 100 mg q8hr
- Fluid resuscitation with normal saline
- 50% dextrose IV to treat hypoglycemia (titrate against blood sugar)

Management of the patient on chronic steroids
- Glucocorticoid equivalences: 20 mg prednisone = 20 mg prednisolone = 16 mg methylprenisolone = 3 mg dexamethasone = 80 mg hydrocortisone
- Wean steroids preoperatively if possible.
- For minor procedures or procedures under local anesthesia, take usual oral daily dose.
- For moderate surgery, take usual daily dose, give hydrocortisone 50 mg IV before induction, 25 mg q8hr × 24 hr, resume baseline dose thereafter
- For major surgery, take usual daily dose, give hydrocortisone 100 mg IV before induction, 50 mg q8hr × 24 hr, taper dose by half per day to baseline dose
- Provide GI ulcer prophylaxis while the patient is on high-dose steroids
- Follow glucose levels, cover with insulin as needed

Surgery and heart disease

Ischemic heart disease

Risk factors for perioperative cardiac events include clinical markers and surgery-specific risks. According to the Revised Cardiac Risk Index for General Surgery, risks for adverse cardiac events include high-risk surgery, known ischemic heart disease, history of heart failure, history of cerebrovascular disease, diabetes, and renal dysfunction.

- Assess risk factors and quantify exercise tolerance; enquire about palpitations, orthopnea, use of anti-anginals, and previous MI, percutaneous coronary intervention (PCI), or coronary artery bypass surgery (CABG).
- Asymptomatic patients undergoing major surgery should be evaluated by a cardiologist to optimize anti-anginal medications and determine whether further evaluation such as stress testing and angiography are warranted.

Myocardial infarction

The risk of a perioperative MI relates to past history and risk factors.
- Overall population incidence after abdominal surgery, 0.5%
- Incidence with preexisting cardiovascular symptoms, 2%
- Incidence with previous MI (old), 5%–10%
- Incidence after recent MI, 25% (70% will die with reinfarction)

Strategies to reduce risk

- Non-urgent surgery should be delayed for at least 4–6 weeks following acute MI and, if possible, for 6 months. Cancer surgery may be undertaken if the risk of disease progression is felt to outweigh the increased perioperative mortality rate.
- Ensure that all normal cardiovascular medications are continued up to and through surgery. Control any new symptoms of angina if surgery is urgent.
- Perioperative beta-blockers should be used only in high risk patients.
- Resume antiplatelet medication as soon as deemed safe from a surgical bleeding perspective.
- Consult cardiology during the perioperative period.

Valvular heart disease

Cardiac murmurs are common. Request a transthoracic echo to evaluate the lesion and consult cardiology.
- Severe aortic stenosis carries a serious risk of mortality.
  - Elective surgery should be postponed; severe aortic stenosis carries an associated mortality of 10% with noncardiac surgery.
- Severe mitral stenosis can lead to pulmonary edema and heart failure.
  - Major elective surgery should be postponed until the lesion is corrected.
- Aortic regurgitation requires attention to fluid and rate control.
- Mitral regurgitation (MR) should be managed with diuretics and vasodilators.
  - Beware: left ventricular (LV) function is frequently overestimated in MR.

- Prosthetic valves have several associated issues:
  - Mechanical valves require anticoagulation. Stop warfarin 5 days preoperatively, and admit patient early for IV heparinization.
  - Do not heparinize if the INR will be subtherapeutic only briefly.
  - Stop IV heparin 6 hr before surgery and resume as soon as surgical bleeding is no longer a problem until INR is therapeutic on warfarin.
  - Thrombosis is most likely in mechanical mitral valves, atrial fibrillation (AF), poor LV function, previous embolus, ball-and-cage valves.
  - if surgery performed for life-threatening bleeding, e.g., bleeding peptic ulcer, intracranial hemorrhage, it may be necessary to reverse anticoagulation for several days. Involve cardiology early for risk assessment.
  - All prosthetic valves require antibiotic prophylaxis for procedures that can cause bacteremia: bladder catheterization; dental work; colorectal or abdominal surgery. If in doubt, discuss with cardiology.

Arterial hypertension

Control of blood pressure (BP) preoperatively may reduce the risk of perioperative ischemia. Always note BP and, if severe (>180 mmHg), surgery should be delayed until control is obtained.
- Review existing antihypertensive management, or start treatment.
  - Beta-blockers (e.g., metoprolol 25 mg po q6hr, titrate dose to heart rate [HR] of 60) reduce BP and perioperative ischemia and mortality.
- Look for evidence of end-organ damage and associated heart disease.
- Rule out rare but important causes: pheochromocytoma, hyperaldosteronism, coarctation of the aorta, renal artery stenosis.

Congestive cardiac failure

Heart failure is associated with a poor prognosis in noncardiac surgery. Risk factors include ischemic and valvular heart disease.
- Listen for S_3, as well as pedal edema, raised jugular venous pressure (JVP), and bibasilar crackles.
- Chest X-ray may show cardiomegaly or pulmonary edema.

Cardiac arrhythmias

Arrhythmias and conduction defects are common. Asymptomatic arrhythmias are not associated with an increase in cardiac complications, but look for underlying problems, e.g., ischemic heart disease, drug toxicity, metabolic derangements.
- High-grade conduction abnormalities, e.g., complete heart block, should be assessed by a cardiologist. Pacing may be indicated.
- Patients with known AF and either a history of embolic stroke or associated structural cardiac defect should take warfarin.
- Request a cardiology consult preoperatively if rate control is poor.
- Beware of the patient with the permanent pacemaker or intracardiac defibrillator (ICD). Diathermy may cause the pacemaker to reset, or completely inhibit pacing, and trigger ICD discharge.
  - Pacemakers and ICDs should be evaluated by a cardiac technician preoperatively and postoperatively.

- Pacemakers should be changed to fixed-rate pacing for surgery, and then reprogrammed after surgery.
- ICDs should be switched off to prevent discharge, and external fibrillator pads positioned on the patient.
- if defibrillation or synchronized cardioversion is required, place the paddles as far from the pacemaker or ICD as possible.

Surgery and respiratory disease

Surgery and smoking

Smoking tobacco is associated with significant anesthetic and surgical risks. There is a six-fold increase in postoperative respiratory complications among patients smoking in excess of 10 cigarettes per day.

Effects of smoking

- Reduction in general and specific immune function via reduced neutrophil chemotaxis and reduced natural killer (NK) cell efficacy
- Increased platelet aggregation (probably explaining the increased risk of perioperative acute MI and cerebrovascular accident in smokers)
- Reduced oxygen-carrying capacity of blood per unit volume due to the presence of carboxyhemoglobin increasing the risk of tissue hypoxia in susceptible organs
- Increased upper-airway mucosal secretions. This worsens initially after stopping smoking, until the chronic effects on the mucosa wear off.
- Reduced mucociliary clearance
- Reduced lung compliance and increased "closing volume" of the small airways, increasing the risk of air trapping, especially while the patient is supine in the postoperative period.

Stopping smoking

- Within 48 hr: Carboxyhemoglobin is cleared from the blood, platelet aggregation begins to return to normal.
- Within 7 days: Neutrophil, macrophage, and NK cell function improve.
- Mucus production temporarily increases but mucociliary clearance takes up to 6 weeks to recover, leading to a "rebound" effect.
- Within 6 weeks: Upper airway function returns to underlying level; lung dynamics improve to "normal" levels (depending on the extent of fixed parenchymal disease).

The optimal time for stopping smoking is at least 6 weeks prior to surgery, but a minimum of 7 days is required to reduce the "rebound" effects of stopping on upper-airway function.

Mitigating the effects of smoking in the postoperative period

Active smokers and those who have recently stopped should receive extra attention to prevent the risks associated with smoking and surgery:

- Use preoperative chest physiotherapy, incentive spirometry, and education on breathing and coughing techniques.
- Mobilize as soon as possible postoperatively.
- Consider the use of epidural anesthesia to improve compliance with postoperative physiotherapy.
- Use pre- and postoperative saline nebulizers or bronchodilators if wheezing occurs.
- Ensure that postoperative analgesia is effective.

Respiratory conditions

Respiratory tract infection

An active upper respiratory tract infection is sufficient reason to cancel elective surgery, so ask patients about cough, colds, and sputum.

- If you suspect the patient has an upper respiratory tract infection, check their temperature and white blood cell count (WBC) early.
- Elective surgery should be cancelled, and patients asked to return in 2 weeks if their symptoms are better.
- Reserve antibiotics for patients with suspected bacterial infections; most acute upper respiratory tract infections are viral.

Asthma

- Assess severity of asthma by asking about hospital admissions, intubations, inhalers, nebulizers, peak expiratory flow rates (PEFR), and use of home oxygen.
- Elective surgery should ideally coincide with remission of symptoms.
- Identify patients on long-term steroid therapy.
  - Attempt to time surgery to coincide with a reduction in steroids.
  - Any patient taking more than 5 mg daily prednisone and undergoing inpatient surgery, or presenting with sepsis should be started on an equivalent dose of IV hydrocortisone; adrenal suppression may otherwise result in an Addisonian crisis.
- Patients receiving a general anesthetic generally experience deterioration in lung function. Prophylactically increase their normal therapy by converting inhalers to frequent nebulizer treatments.

Chronic obstructive pulmonary disease (COPD)

- If dyspnea is a prominent symptom in the setting of COPD, obtain preoperative pulmonary lung function tests and an arterial blood gas on room air.
- Optimize patients with preoperative physiotherapy and nebulizers.
- Prophylactically increase patients' normal therapy by converting inhalers to nebulizers and increasing the frequency.
- Provide humidified oxygen (to prevent mucus plugging).
- Ensure that the patient gets twice-daily chest physiotherapy and use incentive spirometry.
- Ensure that the patient is on their usual inhalers and consider converting these to nebulizers for major surgery.

Surgery in renal and hepatic disease

Renal insufficiency

Renal insufficiency covers a spectrum ranging from subclinical dysfunction (normal serum creatinine and urea, but borderline creatinine clearance) to end-stage renal failure. It is helpful to consider these patients in two main groups: patients with chronic renal impairment and dialysis-dependent patients.

Chronic renal impairment

Surgery may precipitate acute renal failure in patients with chronic renal impairment.

- Avoid hypovolemia and hypotension. Ensure that these patients receive adequate IV hydration if they are to be npo for any length of time.
- Avoid nephrotoxic drugs wherever possible, including nonsteroidal anti-inflammatory drugs (NSAIDs), aminoglycosides, angiotensin-converting enzyme (ACE)-inhibitors, diuretics, and radiological contrast.
- Reduce doses of drugs with renal elimination, e.g., morphine, digoxin, most antibiotics, and request trough levels frequently.

Patients with end-stage renal failure

- Discuss perioperative management following major surgery with anesthesiologists and nephrologists early.
- If major surgery and large fluid shifts are anticipated, plan central venous monitoring.
- Dialysis should be performed the day before surgery.
- Minimize perioperative fluids, monitor electrolytes closely.
- Reduce doses of drugs with renal elimination and request appropriate levels frequently.
- Use DDAVP perioperatively if there is uremic platelet dysfunction.
- Note the sites of arteriovenous (AV) fistulas. *Never* use them for blood draws or cannulation and avoid using BP cuffs on that side.
- Avoid complications such as hyperkalemia and other electrolyte disturbances, metabolic acidosis, pulmonary edema, anemia, hypertension, coagulopathy, and infections.

Hepatic impairment

- Patients undergoing surgery should be screened for liver disease by careful history (blood transfusions, IV drug use, alcohol use) and physical exam (ascites, jaundice, spider telangectasia, hepatosplenomegaly, asterixis).
- Surgery is associated with significant morbidity in patients with chronic liver failure. Perioperative mortality and morbidity in patients with cirrhosis can be evaluated using the Child-Turcotte grading (see Box 1.2).
- Liver failure can be associated with the following complications:
  - Hypoglycemia
  - Hepatic encephalopathy
  - Coagulopathy

- Electrolyte and acid–base disturbances
- Infections
- Respiratory failure
- Renal failure (hepatorenal syndrome)
- Several factors may cause acute decompensation of mild hepatic disease and should be avoided or treated aggressively in this group:
  - Infection, especially bacterial peritonitis
  - Diuretics and other hepatotoxic medications
  - Electrolyte imbalance
  - Dehydration and hypotension
- Optimize medical therapy preoperatively:
  - Request liver ultrasound in newly diagnosed hepatic impairment (rule out portal vein or hepatic artery thrombosis).
  - Avoid or reduce doses of hepatotoxic drugs and drugs with hepatic clearance.
  - Correct elevated PT with vitamin K and fresh frozen plasma preoperatively.
  - Control ascites preoperatively with aggressive diuresis.
  - Correct electrolyte abnormalities, follow renal function.

Box 1.2 Child-Turcotte classification of surgical risk in hepatic dysfunction

A (minimal risk)	B (moderate risk)	C (advanced risk)
• Serum bilirubin <2 mg/dL	• Serum bilirubin 2–3 mg/dL	• Serum bilirubin >3 mg/dL
• Serum albumin >3.5 g/dL	• Serum albumin 3.0–3.5 g/dL	• Serum albumin <3.0 g/dL
• No ascites	• Easily controlled ascites	• Poorly controlled ascites
• No encephalopathy	• Mild encephalopathy	• Advanced encephalopathy
• Excellent nutrition	• Good nutrition	• Poor nutrition

In one study, perioperative mortality rates were 10%, 31%, and 76% in patients with predominantly alcoholic cirrhosis undergoing abdominal surgery who were Child-Turcotte class A, B, and C, respectively.

Surgery in neurological disease

Cerebrovascular accidents

The presence of cerebrovascular disease is often a marker for coexisting cardiovascular disease. A thorough cardiac workup is indicated.

Workup for ischemic stroke includes the following:

- Non-contrast head CT or MRI, electrocardiogram (ECG), hypercoagulable workup
- Carotid Doppler ultrasound, carotid endarterectomy (CEA) indicated for symptomatic stenosis ≥70%
- Transcranial Doppler (TCD) ultrasound for vertebrobasilar disease
- Holter monitoring or telemetry to assess paroxysmal AF
- Echocardiography with bubble study to rule patent foramen ovale (PFO) or atrial septal aneurysm, cardiac thrombus, valvular vegetations
- Ischemic events are associated with a risk of reinfarction or extension of the infarct area due to interference with cerebrovascular autoregulation by anesthetic agents. Autoregulation is reestablished in ~6 weeks.

Workup for hemorrhagic stroke includes the following:

- Laboratory (coagulation function, platelet count), blood pressure
- Non-contrast head CT or MRI
- Angiography or MRA (aneurysm, AVM)
- Hemorrhagic infarcts are associated with a small, increased risk of further bleeding, especially if the patient is given thromboprophylaxis.

Strategies to reduce risk

- Delay non-urgent surgery for 6 weeks following infarcts, especially ischemic ones.
- Consider omitting thromboprophylaxis in patients with a recent hemorrhagic event.
- Ensure that blood pressure is well controlled (prevention of both hypotension and hypertension) in the perioperative period to reduce fluctuations in cerebral blood flow.
- Avoid positioning the patient head down on the operating table, as this increases cerebral venous pressure.

Seizures

Paroxysmal neuronal discharge from various areas of the brain causes a range of disturbances that may affect consciousness (grand mal seizures, and petit mal or absences), movement, or sensory perception. In addition to epilepsy, cerebral space-occupying lesions, metabolic disturbances (uremia, hypercalcemia, hyponatremia, hypoglycemia), cerebral edema, drug and alcohol withdrawal, and drug toxicity (including anesthetic agents) may induce seizures perioperatively. In patients with known epilepsy,

- Establish the frequency, severity, and typical features of seizures (prodrome).
- Ensure that the correct equivalent dose of anticonvulsant medication is continued during hospitalization. If this is not possible or the patient is npo, phenytoin and sodium valproate can be given IV.
- Phenytoin interacts with a number of drugs—check for specific drugs.

Status epilepticus

Call neurology. Complications include neuronal death, rhabdomyolysis, and lactic acidosis. Management includes the following:

- Airway. Place patient in semi-prone position to decrease risk of aspiration, remove dentures, insert oral or nasopharyngeal
- Breathing. Give high-flow oxygen, suction airway. If prolonged, intubate
- Secure IV access, start fluids, check fingerstick blood glucose, send stat labs (electrolytes, urine toxicology screen, anticonvulsant levels)
- Give dextrose (50 g IV push) if low blood glucose
- Give lorazepam 2–4 mg IV pushes *or* diazepam 5–10 mg IV pushes over 2 min, repeat once if seizures do not stop
- If seizure persists, give phenytoin 1–1.5 g IV over 20 min. Consider electroencephalographic (EEG) monitoring and ICU admission.

Parkinson's disease

This disease is marked by a slowly progressive degenerative process involving depletion of dopamine in dopaminergic neurons. Clinical features include tremor, rigidity, bradykinesia, impaired postural reflexes, and autonomic dysfunction (orthostatic hypotension, inability to control temperature, abnormal sweating). Perioperative issues in management include assessment of swallowing to avoid aspiration and of respiratory function. Specifically,

- Patients with swallowing difficulties preoperatively should undergo barium-swallow evaluation.
- Pulmonary function tests and arterial blood gas should be performed preoperatively. Postoperative management includes aggressive incentive spirometry, chest physiotherapy, and nebulizer treatments.
- Anti-parkinsonian medications need to be resumed as soon as possible.

Malignant hyperthermia

This is a rare autosomal dominant, genetic disorder characterized by a hypermetabolic response to inhaled anesthetics or depolarizing muscle relaxants (most commonly halothane and succinylcholine). Before surgery, all patients should be asked about the following:

- A family history of unusual reactions or death from anesthesia
- A history of unexplained muscle cramps or weakness with febrile responses

Intraoperative clinical signs include

- Skeletal muscle rigidity, persistent sinus tachycardia, blood pressure instability, rise in PCO_2, fever, hypotension, and, finally, cardiovascular collapse

Management includes

- Dantrolene sodium IV, supportive therapy, cooling measures

Myasthenia gravis

In this autoimmune disease, antibody is directed against muscle acetylcholine receptors, leading to muscle weakness. It usually occurs in young females, presents with extraocular (ptosis, diplopia), bulbar (dysphagia, dysarthria), and limb weakness (proximal is worse than distal). Perioperative management includes the following:

- Continued anticholinesterase medication
- Immunosuppression (prednisone, azathioprine, cyclophosphamide)
- Postoperative respiratory failure may be triggered by surgical stress, upper respiratory infections, over- or undertreatment, and medications.
- Myasthenic crisis: treat precipitant, aggressive immunosuppression, IV immunoglobulin (Ig), plasmapharesis, thymectomy

Fluid management

Fluid management is aimed at making sure the patient is neither fluid depleted nor fluid overloaded.

Maintenance fluids

The goal is to replace normal daily losses of water and electrolytes, including sensible losses (urine, stool) and insensible losses (sweat, breath). The average water loss is 2500 cc/day. Additional losses that might need to be taken into account include those from vomiting, diarrhea, high-output fistulas, stomas, and "third-spacing" such as edema and ascites.

The 24-hr volume of maintenance fluids is calculated on the basis of weight (1) or the 4–2–1 rule for hourly rate of maintenance fluids (2):
- (1) 100 mL/kg/day for the first 10 kg of weight, 50 mL/kg/day for the second 10 kg of weight, 20 mL/kg/day for each kg above 20 kg of weight (e.g., a 70-kg patient will require 2500 cc/day of maintenance fluids)
- (2) 4 mL/kg/hr for the first 10 kg, 2 mL/kg/hr for the next 10 kg, 1 mL/kg/hr for each additional kg above 20 kg (e.g., a 70-kg patient will require 110 mL/hr of maintenance fluids)

The electrolyte composition of maintenance fluids is based on the anticipated daily loss of electrolytes. Under normal conditions, the average daily electrolyte requirement includes 1–2 mEq/kg/day of Na^+ and 0.5–1 mEq/kg/day of K^+ and the minimal amount of glucose necessary in a 70-kg adult to avoid proteolysis is 150 g. Replacement of calcium, magnesium, and phosphorous is usually not needed in short-term maintenance requirements. An appropriate IV maintenance solution includes
- $D_5 0.45\%$ NaCl (5% dextrose solution and half isotonic normal saline) with 20 mEq/L Kcl in an adult
- $D_5 0.2\%$ NaCl with 20 mEq/L KCl in a child

Identifying patients with volume deficit

In addition to preoperative and postoperative patients in need of aggressive fluid resuscitation, other conditions are associated with significant fluid losses that need to be recognized and treated early. These include the following:
- Conditions associated with significant fluid losses (diarrhea, vomiting, nasogastric, ostomy and enterocutaneous fistula, diabetes insipidus)
- Large third-space fluid loss (inflammatory conditions, e.g., pancreatitis, infections with fevers, bowel obstruction, burns, ascites)
- Elderly patients in whom reduced creatinine clearance makes them more susceptible to dehydration and electrolyte imbalances
- Drugs that impair renal responses to fluid changes (diuretics)

Assessing fluid deficit

The severity of the fluid deficit can be grossly estimated on the basis of duration and severity of symptoms (npo, vomiting, diarrhea) or magnitude of gastrointestinal losses (ostomy, fistula output). However, the history provided by patients is typically misleading and often grossly underestimates the severity of hypovolemia. Useful indicators of fluid deficit include the following:

- **Symptoms**: dizziness, syncope, somnolence, stupor, and coma
- **Physical findings**: hypotension, tachycardia, narrowed pulse pressure, orthostatic changes in heart rate and blood pressure, oliguria, dry mucous membranes, sunken eyes, atonic muscles, poor skin turgor and weight loss, low central venous pressure (CVP)
- **Lab values**: elevated hematocrit, Na^+, K^+, BUN:creatinine ratio >20, and a fractional excretion of sodium (FeNa) <1 ($U_{Na}/P_{Na} \times P_{Cr}/U_{Cr} \times 100$) suggesting hypovolemia, electrolyte imbalances

Fluids used for resuscitation

In most situations, hypovolemia should be treated with isotonic crystalloids.

- Lactated Ringer's (Na^+ 130 mEq/L, K^+ 4 mEq/L, Ca^{2+} 2.7+, Cl^- 109 mEq/L, HCO_3. 28 mEq/L), whose composition most closely resembles that of extracellular fluid (Na^+ 142 mEq/L, K^+ 4 mEq/L, Ca^{2+} 5+, Cl^- 103 mEq/L, HCO_3. 27 mEq/L)
- Isotonic 0.9% NaCl ("normal saline") may be preferable in specific situations (hypovolemia with hypochloremic metabolic alkalosis; gastric losses)
- Colloids (blood products, albumin, hextastarch, dextran) can be helpful if lower volume is required to correct fluid deficits and produce a more lasting expansion of intravascular volume than with crystalloids, which rapidly enter the interstitial tissues. Use is limited by cost and side effects (coagulopathy, anaphylactic reaction, no increase in survival).
- Other fluids can be used in very specific circumstances, including hypertonic saline for hyponatremia, hypotonic saline, or D5W for hypernatremia, but must be used carefully because of the risk of significant fluid shifts in and out of cells, which can cause cellular injury particularly to neurons.
- K^+ should only be added if there is significant hypokalemia.

How to administer fluids

The rate and amount of fluid infusion depend on the severity of hypovolemia, hemodynamic status, age, and cardiac status of the patient.

- In young, fit patients with normal cardiac and renal function, an initial IV bolus of 10 mL/kg of either Lactated Ringer's or 0.9% NaCl is appropriate and should be repeated as necessary to correct hemodynamic instability.
- Boluses and/or infusions of fluids can be subsequently titrated to correct the volume deficit.
- Goal of fluid resuscitation: normalize vital signs and mental status, achieve urine output of 0.5 mL/kg/hr in adults and 1–2 mL/kg/hr in children
- Elderly patients and patients with renal or cardiac dysfunction should have fluid deficits repleted more slowly to prevent intravascular volume overload. When intravascular fluid status and response to repletion is difficult to assess, CVP and pulmonary-artery wedge pressure monitoring might be required (central line, Swan Ganz® catheter)

Identifying patients with volume overload

Fluid overload may result from excessive fluids or inadequate output (renal insufficiency, urinary retention), or is cardiac related (congestive heart failure).

- Physical exam: elevated JVP (or CVP), dependent edema, crackles on lung auscultation, shortness of breath (SOB) when lying flat (orthopnea)
- Other studies: may have low Na^+, peripheral vascular congestion, edema, or effusions on chest X-ray
- Order strict ins and outs (fluid balance chart): follow fluid balance hourly or per shift. Add up all fluid loss (urine output, wound, stoma, and fistula drainage) and subtract from all IV, nasogastric (NG), and oral fluids given.

Nutrition in surgical patients

Also see Enteral support. Nutrition is critical to the recovery of surgical patients. It has a direct impact on postoperative morbidity and mortality. Patients with underlying nutritional deficits are susceptible to develop complications, and prolonged food deprivation affects overall healing and recovery. Patients with nutritional deficits and those anticipated to have higher than normal nutritional requirements postoperatively should be identified early and provided with nutritional support to prevent acute catabolism (severe burns, sepsis, major trauma, large open wounds, intestinal fistulas, malignancy, immunosuppression).

Assessment of nutritional status

Patients' overall nutritional status should be assessed from the history, physical exam, and labs. Findings suggestive of significant malnutrition:
- Decrease in appetite, history of non-intentional weight loss, muscle wasting, ascites, peripheral edema, inability to perform daily activities
- 10%–15% weight loss within 4 to 6 months
- Baseline serum albumin level <3.0 g/dL

Effects of protein–calorie malnutrition

- Reduced neutrophil and lymphocyte function (anergy to skin antigens)
- Impaired albumin production
- Impaired wound healing and collagen deposition

Micronutrient deficiencies may cause specific clinical syndromes.

Indications for nutritional support

The goal is to prevent muscle breakdown and maintain lean body mass (avoid negative nitrogen balance). Patients who should receive nutritional support, either preoperatively and/or postoperatively, include
- Severely malnourished patients. If possible, surgery should be delayed for a minimum of 5 to 7 days to provide nutritional support.
- Patients with insufficient oral intake 7 to 10 days postoperatively
- Patients with significant metabolic needs postoperatively (severe trauma, large wounds, sepsis)

Nutritional requirements

The caloric requirement can be estimated using the following formula:

25 Kcal/Kg/day + stress factor.

The stress factor can vary from 15% to 20% following elective abdominal surgery to 100% in severe burn patients. A more accurate determination of basal caloric needs is obtained from the Harris-Benedict formula.
- Males: basal energy expenditure (kcal/day) = 66 + [13.7 (weight in kg)] + [5 (height in cm)] − [6.8 (age in years)]
- Females: basal energy expenditure (kcal/day) = 655 + [9.6 (weight in kg)] + [1.8 (height in cm)] − [4.7 (age in years)]
- An activity component of 15% should be added; sepsis and major trauma can double the basal rate and a major burn can triple the basal rate.

Other requirements include (for adults)
- Protein: 0.8–1.5 g/kg/day (increased with stress)
- Carbohydrates: 450 g of glucose/day

- Fat: 30% of total calories should be in the form of fat
- Electrolytes, vitamins, and trace elements (zinc, copper, chromium, manganese, selenium)

Types of nutritional support

The oral route is always the preferred route. Enteral feeding is more physiologic, it promotes the normal health of gut mucosa, maintains gut barrier function, stimulates biliary secretion, and has fewer metabolic and infectious complications than with parenteral nutrition.

- Oral supplementation: high-calorie, high-protein nutritional supplements
- NG or duodenal tube feeding is typically used for temporary oral nutrition (feeding tubes should be placed beyond the pylorus, although the risk of gastric feed aspiration is the same as that of duodenal feeds).
- Feeding gastrostomy/jejunostomy—endoscopically or surgically placed tube. This is reserved for long-term feeding of patients whose GI tract is functioning but who cannot tolerate oral intake (dysphagia, neurologic impairment) or whose intake is persistently inadequate (feeds can be cycled at night to improve daytime appetite).
- Parenteral nutrition. May be central or peripheral. See below.

Total parenteral nutrition (TPN)

TPN is a major advance in the treatment of surgical malnutrition but has serious potential complications.

Routes of administration for TPN

- Peripheral (PPN)—Maximum calorie input is limited by the maximum osmolarity of solution given into a peripheral vein. Avoids risks of central venous cannulation. Usually used for short-term supplementation
- Central (TPN)—through the superior vena cava (SVC) or brachiocephalic vein via a tunneled Hickman catheter, central line, or a peripherally inserted central venous catheter (PICC line). Maximum calorie input is limited only by the volume of fluid that can be infused.

General risks of TPN/PPN

- Hyperosmolarity, poor glycemic control, micronutrient deficiencies, electrolyte imbalances, liver dysfunction (fatty liver), cholestasis, and acalculous cholecystitis

Catheter-related risks of TPN

- Complications of central line insertion (air embolism, pneumothorax, vascular injury), catheter thrombosis and thromboembolism, line sepsis, bacterial endocarditis

Care of TPN patients

Patients on TPN require regular review and monitoring, including
- Glucose, electrolytes, liver function tests (LFTs), micronutrients
- Central venous catheters should not be used for non-TPN infusions and *never* used for phlebotomy, as this increases the risk of catheter sepsis dramatically. Dressings should be changed regularly and the catheter entry site kept clean.

Preparing the patient for the OR

Preparation of the patient for a surgical procedure should follow specific protocol. All efforts should be made to minimize oversights and errors to avoid potentially harmful consequences for the patient.

Booking

Make sure the patient is on the operating room schedule or waiting list. Check that patient's name, medical record number, location, listed procedure(s), and attending surgeon are correct

Preoperative checklist

- Confirm that the medical history, physical exam, blood work, chest X-ray, and ECG (when indicated) are available for review and up-to-date.
- Check that specific tests and reports, including coagulation tests in patients on chronic anticoagulation, K^+ in renal failure patients, Ca^{2+} in parathyroidectomy patients, glucose level in diabetics, stress tests, cardiac catherization reports and medical clearance notes, are available for review by anesthesiology.
- Review all relevant radiological studies and make sure they are available in the operating room (arteriograms, CT scans, barium enema, GI series).
- Confirm that the surgical consent form has been signed.
- Communicate to the preoperative team and anesthesiologists specific medications to be administered (deep venous thrombosis [DVT] and antibiotic prophylaxis).
- Contact the surgical ICU team to book a bed if it is anticipated that the patient will be in critical condition postoperatively.

Patient preparation

- Check that the correct side(s) of the planned surgery, when relevant, is specified on the OR list and surgical consent. This should be confirmed by the preoperative nursing staff and the correct side should be marked in ink with the patient still awake in the preoperative area.
- Prepare the patient for stoma creation by consulting the enterostomal service for marking of a stoma site, and for amputation by consulting prosthetics.
- As part of the preoperative check list, ensure that the patient has been consented for a possible blood transfusion, and blood typed (for all procedures), and crossed for 2 units of blood (for major procedures).

Bowel preparation

The large majority of patients undergoing elective colorectal resections receive mechanical bowel preparation preoperatively. Because they are associated with varying degrees of dehydration, inform the anesthesiologists of their preoperative use. The most common types of bowel preparation include the following:

- Isoosmotic solution containing polyethylene glycol (Golytely®) is osmotically balanced, nonabsorbable, and cleans the bowel by washout of ingested fluid without significant fluid and electrolyte shifts.

- Hyperosmotic solution, e.g., sodium phosphate (Fleets phosphosoda®), osmotically draws plasma water into the lumen to promote evacuation and can be associated with significant fluid and electrolyte shifts. It is commonly used for preoperative preparation for colon surgery, colonoscopy, and CT colonography. It is contraindicated in chronic renal insufficiency.
- Hyperosmotic saline laxative (magnesium citrate). Magnesium citrate increases intraluminal volume, resulting in increased intestinal motility, and stimulates the release of cholecystokinin, which causes intraluminal accumulation of fluid and electrolytes and promotes small-bowel and, possibly, colonic transit. It should be used with caution in patients with renal insufficiency.
- Stimulant colon preparation, e.g., sodium phosphate enema (Fleets® enema) is used in preparation for anorectal examination or procedures and flexible sigmoidoscopy.
- Recent evidence suggests that mechanical bowel preparation might be associated with more infectious complications than unprepped bowel. In addition, bowel preparation is associated with significant side effects:
  - Electrolyte imbalances
  - Renal failure in patients with renal insufficiency (magnesium citrate)
  - Hypovolemia especially in the elderly
  - Nausea and vomiting (particularly with the large-volume osmotic preparations)

Anesthetic premedication
Principles
Anesthetic premedication is used for the following reasons:
- Relaxing patient to reduce anxiety during preparation for anesthesia
- Relaxation decreases the amount of anesthetic agent required for induction of general anesthesia.

Typical agents used for premedication
- Benzodiazepines (midazolam)

Antibiotic prophylaxis and thromboprophylaxis

Antibiotic prophylaxis

- Basic principles and practices are known to reduce the risk of surgical site infections and include basic antiseptic precautions, normoglycemia, perioperative normothermia, and prophylactic antibiotics.
- Prophylactic antibiotics administered preoperatively have been shown to reduce surgical site infections. The goal of antibiotic prophylaxis is to eradicate the growth of endogenous microorganisms and counter the effect of potential spillage of organisms from colonized organs such as the bowel.

Basic principles for antibiotic prophylaxis include the following:

- It is most important to achieve high drug tissue levels at the time of incision, therefore antibiotics should be given within 60 min of surgical incision.
- Repeat intraoperative dosing is recommended for procedures lasting more than 4 hr.
- Prophylaxis rarely needs to extend postoperatively unless risk factors are identified, such as gross contamination. In this case, one to three additional prophylactic doses might be administered, with discontinuation within 24 hr postoperatively.
- Patients with clean wounds, e.g., excision of skin lesions or breast surgery, do not require routine prophylaxis because of the low risk of skin infection.
- High-risk patients may require an extended prophylactic course (3 or more days): neutropenic or immunosuppressed patients, severely malnourished patients, patients with prosthetic implants, e.g., heart valves.

Prophylactic regimens

Most hospitals have established guidelines for prophylaxis. See Table 1.1 for an example of standard recommendations.

Thromboprophylaxis

Types of thromboprophylaxis

Mechanical devices

- Graduated compression stockings or TEDS (thromboembolic deterrent stockings). Reduce venous stasis in infrapopliteal veins by continuous direct compression. Reduce incidence of postoperative venous thrombosis only in low-risk and selected moderate-risk general surgical patients
- Intermittent pneumatic compression. Reduces venous stasis in infrapopliteal veins by intermittent compression. Also reduces plasminogen activator inhibitor-1 levels, thereby increasing endogenous fibrinolytic activity

Table 1.1 Prophylactic preoperative antibiotic regimen

Indication	Typical prophylaxis (single dose)
"Clean" bowel surgery, e.g., acute non-perforated appendicitis, elective colonic resection	Cefazolin 1–2 g IV + metronidazole 500 mg IV or cefoxitin 1–2 g IV or cefoxitin 1–2 g IV
"Clean" hepatobiliary surgery, e.g., ERCP, open biliary surgery	Cefazolin 1–2 g IV
"Clean" gynecological and obstetric surgery	Cefotetan 1–2 g IV or cefoxitin 1–2 g IV or cefazolin 1–2 g IV or unasyn 3 g IV
Elective genitourinary surgery	Ciprofloxacin 400mg IV
"Clean" vascular surgery	Cefoxitin 1–2 g IV or cefuroxime 1–2 g IV

ERCP, endoscopic retrograde cholangiopancreatography

Drugs acting on the clotting cascade
- Unfractionated heparin. Activates antithrombin III
  - Prophylaxis: 5000 U SC q8hr
  - Therapeutic: IV 10,000 U loading dose, 1000 U/hr, check aPTT 6 hr after starting and q6hr thereafter. Titrate to aPTT 60–85
- Low molecular-weight heparin (LMWH). Activates antithrombin III. Given SC:
  - Prophylaxis: enoxaparin 20–60 mg SC qd, deltaparin 2500–5000 SC qd
  - Therapeutic: 1 mg/kg SC bid, deltaparin 200 IU/kg SQ

Anti-platelet drugs
- Aspirin, dipyridamole, clopidogrel

Direct thrombin inhibitors
- Argatroban, lepirudin (used in patients with heparin-induced thrombocytopenia [HIT])

Synthetic heparin pentasaccharide
- Prophylaxis: fondaparinux 5–10 mg SC qd

Risk assessment
Specific patient factors and surgical procedures increase the risk of postoperative DVT and warrant specific prophylaxis. Patients are stratified according to their estimated risk.

Low risk (venous thromboembolism <1%)
- Minor surgery in patients <40 years of age with no additional risks

Recommendations: TEDS, early ambulation

Moderate risk (DVT 2%–4%, pulmonary embolism [PE] 1%–2%)
- Major surgery in patients <40 years of age, no risk factors
- Minor surgery in patients 40–60 years of age *or* with risk factors (cancer, prior DVT, obesity, heart failure, paralysis, or hypercoagulable state)

Recommendations: TEDS, intermittent compression, prophylactic LMWH or unfractionated heparin

High risk (DVT 4%–8%, PE 2%–4%)
- Minor surgery in patients >60 years of age *or* with risk factors
- Major surgery in patients <40 years of age *or* with risk factors
- MI, CVA, bed rest, chronic illness

Recommendations: TEDS, intermittent compression, higher prophylactic dose LMWH or unfractionated heparin

Highest risk (DVT 10%–20%, PE 4%–10%)
- Orthopedic surgery, trauma
- Major surgery in patients >40 years of age with risk factors
- Acute spinal cord injury

Recommendations: TEDS, intermittent compression, highest prophylactic dose LMW or unfractionated heparin

Positioning the patient

Getting the patient on to the operating table

The surgical team is in part responsible for the safety of the patient all the way on to and off the operating table. Be sure the basic rules of safety are being observed. See Figure 1.3 for some typical patient positions in surgery.

- The anesthesiologist is responsible for the patient's airway and should make sure it is always maintained during positioning of the patient (never move the patient without the anesthesiologist's approval).
- Be sure not to dislodge IV lines, epidurals, or drains.
- Use a sliding device rather than lifting the patient, if possible.
- Be aware if extra care or padding is needed during positioning, e.g., prosthetic joints, artificial hips, unstable fractures, pressure ulcers.
- Document any preexisting burns, wounds, and bruises to ensure they did not occur intraoperatively.
- When placing legs in stirrups, position both legs simultaneously to avoid strain on hip joints. Make sure that the leg and heel rest right against the padding of the stirrup.

Once in position

- Ensure that no points on the patient are in contact with the metal of the operating table to prevent diathermy exit point burns.
- Make sure bony prominences and delicate areas are well padded, e.g., hands, elbows, the neck of the fibula in leg stirrups.
- Ensure that any diathermy pad is correctly applied and not liable to be affected by disinfectant.
- Ensure that tubes, drains, and operative equipment (retractors) do not rest directly onto the skin (place padding in between).
- Ensure that the patient is well secured to the table, particularly if the table is tilted and rotated during the procedure (arm, chest, and abdominal support for lateral positions; shoulder bolsters if the patient is in Trendelenburg position, leg support if the patient is in reverse Trendelenburg).
- For procedures requiring access to the perineum, be sure that the pelvis is properly supported but that the perineum extends beyond the edge of the operating table.
- Avoid leaning onto the patient during the procedure.
- Make sure energy sources (cautery, vessel sealing devices) and light sources (laparoscopic light source) do not rest directly onto the skin or onto the drape covering the patient (avoid inadvertent burns).

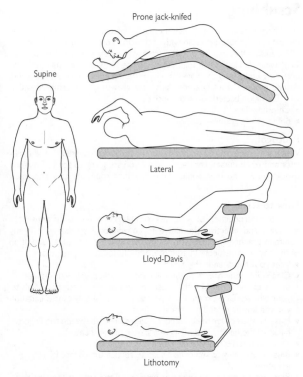

Fig. 1.3 Typical positions for surgery. Supine (most abdominal surgery); prone jack-knifed (some rectal or vaginal procedures); lateral (thoracotomy); Lloyd–Davis (pelvic surgery); lithotomy (most perineal procedures).

Scrubbing

Scrubbing is designed to reduce the risk of infection from the surgeon to the patient. A thorough clean with bactericidal soaps reduces the number of organisms that can be cultured from skin swabs but the skin (particularly sweat glands and hair follicles) cannot be sterilized. Moisture and heat occurring under surgical gloves quickly raise the bacterial count again and, despite modern cleaning agents, significant growth can be achieved within 2 hr. Common bactericidal soaps include
- Chlorhexidine®
- Betadine® (povidone–iodine)

Protocol

When you come to the operating room, introduce yourself to the circulator and scrub nurses. Let them know if you are going to scrub. Everyone should know who the people in the operating room are and what their role is.

How to scrub

Since the introduction of waterless, scrubless, alcohol-based antiseptics as a safe and effective alternative to conventional scrubbing, it is still common practice to scrub with antimicrobial soap for the first operation of the day and use alcohol-based preparations for subsequent cases.
- Wet your hands and arms first.
- Clean under the nails with the nail cleaner. Lather well with disinfectant soap and scrub with the brush and sponge from your fingernails to your elbows. Don't scrub too vigorously, as this simply causes irritation without any increased bactericidal effect.
- Make sure to cover the commonly missed areas (between the fingers, backs of the hands, under fingernails, base of the thumbs).
- Your total scrub time should be no less than 5 min.
- Rinse thoroughly to remove all soap to reduce the chance of skin irritation.
- Rinse off, trying to ensure the water runs off the arms at the elbows.
- Dry hands completely with a towel. Be sure your hands are completely dry before gowning and gloving.

For alcohol-based antiseptic solutions (liquid or foam):
- Apply a generous amount in the palm of your hand and clean from your fingertips and nails to your elbows.
- Hands and arms must be air dried before gowning and gloving.

How to gown and glove

- Be sure to open the gown without touching the outer "face."
- Don't push your hands through the cuffs.
- If gloving yourself, pick up the right glove with your left hand "through" the cuff of the gown, holding it by the bottom edge of the glove.
- Still holding firmly with your left hand, slide your right hand into the glove.
- Slide your right hand into the glove.

- Once on, pick up the left glove with your right hand holding it by the rolled up edge and pull it over your left hand.
- Slide your left hand into the glove and adjust glove position.

Universal precautions should always be taken. Eye protection is necessary, and it is good practice to wear two of gloves to reduce the risk of exposure to infectious agents.

Sterilization, disinfection, and antisepsis

Definitions

- *Sterilization* is removal of all viable microorganisms, vegetative and spores.
- *Disinfection* is the removal of actively dividing vegetative microorganisms.
- *Antisepsis* is the process whereby the risk of medical cross-infection by microorganisms is reduced.

Sterilization

Heat

- Dry heat (incineration, flaming to red hot) is effective but rarely useful. Dry heat requires temperatures of 160°C for at least 60 min.
- Moist heat (autoclave heating using pressurized steam 121°C at 15 lb/in^2 for 15 min) is effective and useful especially in operating rooms.

Irradiation Gamma radiation—effective for inorganic materials

Filtration Air or fluids can be sterilized by ultrafine membrane filters but are rarely useful in hospital practice.

Disinfection

Chemical

- Acids/alkalis (bleach). Effective for nonhuman contact use
- Alcohols/phenols
  - Ethyl alcohol—skin swabs
  - Alcohol solutions—hand disinfection
  - Carbolic
  - Chloroxylenols
  - Phenol
- Oxidizers
  - Povidone–iodine (Betadine®)—skin disinfection/surgical scrubbing
  - H_2O_2—superficial wound cleansing
  - Aldehydes (Cidex®)—surgical instruments such as endoscopes
- Cationic solutions, e.g., Chlorhexidine®—antiseptic washes
- Organic dyes

Antisepsis

Principles of antisepsis include the following:

- Always remove gross contamination with simple soap first.
- Use high-potency acid/alkali disinfection on inert surfaces.
- Use less corrosive oxidizers on delicate inert materials.
- Use weak alcohols, oxidizers for skin cleansing.

Surgical instruments

Blades
- Scalpels: There are two sizes of handle (4 and 6). Blade sizes include no. 11 (used for stab incisions), no. 10 (most skin incisions), no. 15 (fine incisions), and larger (no. 22, no. 23).
- Scissors: dissecting or for suture cutting. Dissecting scissors may be straight (Mayo), curved (curved Mayo, Metzenbaum), or angled (Potts).

Forceps
- Non-toothed. Fine non-toothed (DeBakey, Adson) forceps are used for handling delicate tissues such as vessels and bowel. Heavy non-toothed forceps are used for general handling, including specimens and sutures.
- Toothed. Fine toothed (Gillie's, McIndoe's) forceps are used for handling skin, and occasionally for precise hold of delicate tissues. Heavy toothed (Bonnie) forceps are used for holding heavy tissues such as fascia and scar tissue.
- Ring-tipped and microforceps are used in microvascular anastomoses.

Clamps
- Vascular clamps (Dunhill's, Mosquito) have serrated jaws.
- Tissue clamps
    - Lahey clamp—similar to a curved arterial clip
    - Doyen bowel clamp—non-crushing atraumatic
    - Kocher, Satinsky bowel clamps
    - Babcock, Pennington (Duval) clamp—non-toothed, semi-atraumatic tissue-holding clamp
    - Allis clamp—heavy, toothed, traumatic tissue-holding clamps
    - Right angle, Mixter, Kelly, Tonsil, Schnidt—hemostatic clamps

Retractors
- Self-retaining retractors:
    - Bookwalter, Goligher, Balfour, omni (Thompson)—large retractors for abdominal incisions
    - Finichetto—retractor for thoracic incisions
    - Norfolk-Norwich, Gelpi, Weitlaner (Travers), Beckmann—retractors for small skin and abdominal incisions
- Handheld retractors:
    - Large (Deaver, Kelly, Morris);
    - Small (Langenbeck, Senn, Hill-Ferguson (anorectal), Army-Navy (bladed retractor), Rake (forked retractor)

Incisions and closures

Incisions

- Laparotomy. Any incision to gain access to the peritoneal cavity or retroperitoneal space. Incisions are named according to their location on the abdomen, tissues crossed, or the individuals who described them (Fig. 1.4).
- Thoracotomy. Accessing the chest cavity, typically the pleural space or posterior mediastinum. Median sternotomy is a type of thoracotomy for access to the anterior and middle mediastinum.
- Craniotomy. Accessing compartments of the skull

Incision closures

Incisions are closed, following basic principles:

- Fascial layers are the strongest tissue for durable apposition and are used for primary closure when available. Fascial closure is usually achieved with heavy-weight, slowly absorbable sutures.
- In critical patients, when the fascia cannot be apposed and complex abdominal wound closure or use of a prostheses is not recommended, fascial closure can be achieved with retention sutures (avoid evisceration).
- Large cavities and potential spaces between tissues should be avoided to reduce the risk of fluid accumulation and risk of infection. Following extensive abdominal wall dissection, closure in multiple layers is recommended with or without external drain placement, and external compression (binder) to avoid rapid fluid accumulation.
- Bony defects, such as in a craniotomy, should be apposed to allow minimal movement.
- Defects in fascial or bony tissues should be replaced with either transposed tissues (skin, fascia, muscle flaps) or biological or synthetic prostheses (polypropylene mesh, Surgisis®, dual meshes, etc.).
- Following surgery in a grossly contaminated field, following fascial closure, wounds should be left open to heal by secondary intention.

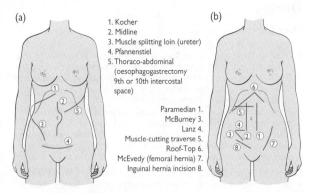

(a)

1. Kocher
2. Midline
3. Muscle splitting loin (ureter)
4. Pfannenstiel
5. Thoraco-abdominal
   (oesophagogastrectomy
   9th or 10th intercostal
   space)

(b)

Paramedian 1.
McBurney 3.
Lanz 4.
Muscle-cutting traverse 5.
Roof-Top 6.
McEvedy (femoral hernia) 7.
Inguinal hernia incision 8.

Fig. 1.4 Incisions. Taken from Longmore M, et al. (2007). *Oxford Handbook of Clinical Medicine*, 7th ed. Oxford: Oxford University Press.

Drains

Uses and complications

Drains can serve multiple purposes:
- Drain existing collections of fluid, blood, pus, or air (e.g., drainage of a subphrenic abscess, evacuation of pneumothorax, intracranial bleed)
- Prophylactically prevent the accumulation of physiologic fluid in a large, potential dead space (e.g., seroma after extensive subcutaneous tissue dissection, particularly in obese patients)
- Prophylactically prevent the accumulation of potentially symptomatic collections (pelvic hematoma following rectal surgery)
- Alert to and achieve control of leaking fluid (anastomotic leak following intestinal anastomoses, bile leak after cholecystectomy, pancreatic leak after distal pancreatectomy)

Drains can cause complications that should be balanced against their use
- Insertion percutaneously under ultrasound or CT-guidance or fluoroscopy can result in injury to adjacent organs (splenic injury during subphrenic abscess drainage, bowel perforation by abdominal drains).
- Drains provide a potential route for infection, especially external drains that remain for longer than a few days.
- Drains can erode through adjacent structures, especially if kept for more than a week, and if placed on wall or bulb suction and if large in caliber (enteric fistula).
- Drains do not always drain adequately and tend to clog easily, thus giving a false sense of security when drainage is minimal.

There is no place for "routine" use of drains after surgery unless there is a clear indication "Better no drainage than ignorant use of it" (Halstead).

Types of drain

Materials include latex rubber (T tubes), silastic rubber (long-term urinary catheters), polypropylene (abdominal drains), and polyurethane (NG tubes). Types of drains are listed in Box 1.3.

Box 1.3 Types of drains

Open passive drains
These provide a conduit around which secretions may flow.
- Penrose drain
- Draining setons for fistulas-in-ano and perianal abscesses

Closed passive drains
These drain fluid by gravity ("siphon effect") or by capillary flow.
- Percutaneous drains (placed by interventional radiology)
- Ventriculoperitoneal shunt

Closed active drains
These generate active suction (low or high negative pressure)
- Hemovac, Jackson Pratt, Blake drains

Other drains are connected to wall suction for more effective drainage:
- Nasogastric tube, thoracostomy tube, axiom sump drain

Stomas

The term *stoma* is applied to an external opening (temporary or permanent) created in a lumen of an organ. If creation of a diverting stoma is anticipated preoperatively as part of a surgical procedure, make sure that the patient is prepared. Consult an enterostomal nurse to prepare the patient emotionally and mark the stoma site for an ideal fit based on body habitus.

- Ileostomy. Formed from any part of the distal small bowel. The more proximal, the more copious and erosive the stoma output. It may be fashioned as
  - A loop ileostomy (with afferent and efferent limbs, not a complete diversion of enteric contents, does not typically require laparotomy for reversal, used when anticipating prompt reversal)
  - An end-ileostomy (complete diversion, requires laparotomy for reversal, used when not anticipating prompt reversal)
- Colostomy. Formed from any part of the large bowel. It may be fashioned as
  - A loop (with afferent and efferent limbs, not a complete diversion, typically used when expected to be temporary)
  - An end-colostomy (complete diversion, performed as part of a Hartmann's procedure)
- Urostomy. Formed from a short length of disconnected ileum into which one or both ureters are connected (following radical cystectomy)
- Gastrostomy. Either a surgically or endoscopically created connection between the anterior stomach and anterior abdominal wall. Used for gastric decompression (gastroparesis) or enteral feeding
- Jejunostomy. Either a surgically or endoscopically created connection between the proximal jejunum and anterior abdominal wall. Used as permanent access for enteral feeding

Features of stoma

- Ileostomies are usually "Brooked" so they protrude well above the skin, have prominent mucosal folds, are dark pink to red, and are most commonly located on the right side of the abdomen. A loop ileostomy has two lumens. Contents are typically bilious.
- Colostomies are usually flush against the skin, have flat mucosal folds, and are light pink and most commonly on the left side of the abdomen. Contents are feculent.
- Urostomies (end) are usually spouted, have prominent mucosal folds, are dark pink to red and most commonly in the right side of the abdomen. They are distinguishable from end ileostomies by the urinary output.
- Gastrostomies and jejunostomies are usually narrow caliber, flush with little visible mucosa, and most commonly in the left upper quadrant. They are usually fitted with indwelling tubes or access devices.

Examining stomas

Construction

- Ileostomies should be matured in a Brook fashion, e.g., protruding well above the skin to avoid retraction of the stoma back into the abdominal cavity and drainage of enteric content onto the skin when a stomal appliance is properly applied.
- Colostomies should be flush against the skin. Ileostomies and colostomies should not be prolapsing (protruding excessively) or retracted (with opening well below the skin).

Peristomal skin

- Assess irritation and ulcerations related to poor skin care and poor fit of the stomal appliance.

Stomal contents: Examine the type (flatus, bilious, feculent, bloody), consistency (liquid, semi-solid, hard) and volume.

Knots and sutures

Types of suture

See Table 1.2 for types of suture material and Fig. 1.5 for types of suturing used.

- Nonabsorbable sutures tend to be used where any loss of strength might compromise the future integrity of the tissues being joined, e.g., vascular anastomoses, hernia mesh fixation, tendon repairs, and sternal wiring.
- Absorbable sutures tend to be used where the persistence of foreign material would cause unnecessary tissue reaction or increased risk of infection, e.g., bowel anastomoses, skin, and subcutaneous tissues.
- Monofilaments have the advantage of smooth tissue passage and minimal tissue reaction but tend to have a crystalline structure that increases the "memory" effect of the suture, making knotting less secure and increasing the risk of suture "fracture."
- Braided polyfilaments exert more tissue friction during passage through but are intrinsically more flexible and knot securely more easily.

Size of suture

Size is denoted by imperial sizes ranging from 11–0 (smallest, invisible to naked eye, used in ophtalmology) through 6–0 (vascular anastomoses), 2–0 (bowel anastomoses), #1 (fascial closure), to #5 (largest, sternal wires).

Types of needle

Needles may be curved (ranging from half-curved to 5/8 circle) or straight.

- Blunt (Relatively safe, as it has low tissue penetrance)
- Taper (sharp pointed but smooth, round, cross-sectional profile). This type "pushes" tissue apart, so it is often used for delicate tissues such as bowel and blood vessels.
- Cutting (sharp point with triangular cross-section). This type slices through tissues, and is often used for dense structures such as fascia and tendons.
- Reverse cutting (cutting edge on the outside)

Table 1.2 Types of suture material

	Material	Absorption time
Nonabsorbable monofilament	Silver/steel wire	Permanent
	Nylon, Ethilon®	Permanent
	Prolene® (polypropylene)	Permanent
Braided monofilament	Surgidac®, Ethibond® (polyester)	Permanent
Nonabsorbable braided polyfilament	Silk	Permanent
Gut	Chromic gut	Within 90 days
	Plain gut	
Absorbable monofilament	Monocryl®, Caprosyn®	56 days
	Biosyn®, Monocryl®	90–110 days
	Maxon®, PDS II®	180 days
Absorbable braided polyfilament	Vicryl®, Polysorb®	56–70 days
	Dexon®	60–90 days

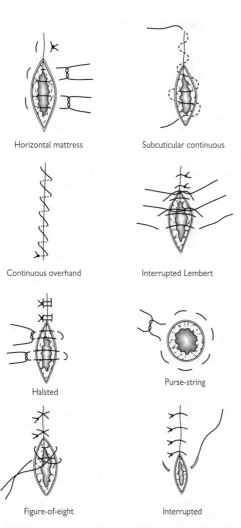

Horizontal mattress

Subcuticular continuous

Continuous overhand

Interrupted Lembert

Halsted

Purse-string

Figure-of-eight

Interrupted

Fig. 1.5 Types of suturing used (illustrated as skin sutures). Taken from McLatchie G, et al. (2008). *Oxford Handbook of Clinical Surgery*, 3rd ed. Oxford: Oxford University Press.

Postoperative management

Routine tests

Protocols vary widely according to the complexity of surgery and patients' comorbidities. This is a guideline to postoperative management following major surgery.

Blood tests

Complete blood count (CBC), coagulation, electrolytes (POD1 and subsequently based on course

- Anemia: Consider surgical bleeding, hemodilution, and gastrointestinal bleeding.
- Leukocytosis: Evaluate other signs of infection.
- Monitor coagulation daily if patient is on anticoagulation and before interventional procedures (insertion of drains, central lines) or reoperation.
- Check electrolytes if the patient is npo for a prolonged period of time, and adjust type of IV fluids.
- Monitor BUN and creatinine in patients with renal dysfunction, following cardiac and aortic surgery, and if the patient is receiving nephrotoxic drugs (NSAIDs, ACE-inhibitors, vancomycin/gentamicin).

ECG

An ECG is important in assessing cardiac surgical and vascular patients, and any patient with symptomatic ischemic or vascular heart disease. Look for rhythm disturbances such as atrial fibrillation and flutter and/or evidence of ischemia.

Chest X-ray

This should be done daily if there are chest or mediastinal tubes, after drain removal, and to check the position of newly placed central lines (including PICC lines). Look for the following:

- Position of indwelling lines and chest tubes
- "White out of lung" (hemothorax), pneumothorax, pleural effusions

Doing rounds

Check on patients a minimum of twice a day. On evening rounds, results from all completed tests should be reviewed.

- Divide tasks among the team, e.g., one person should write the note summarizing the team's evaluation and plans for the day while others review vital signs, labs and other tests, examine the patient, and write orders.
- Review the day's events (fever, nausea, vomiting) and progress (response to treatment, new issues) with the patient.
- Review oral intake, ambulation, pain control, and bowel habits.
- Check the chart for vital signs (maximum and current temperature, trends in blood pressure and heart rate, oxygen saturations), ins (oral intake, IV fluids and drips), and outs (urine, stool, drain outputs, vomiting).
- Check that all indwelling tubes and catheters are in position and patent.
- Check IV sites for erythema or purulent drainage.
- Check for edema (pitting edema of lower extremities).
- Check for pressure ulcers (buttock, back, heels) in bed-bound patients.
- Vascular patients: Assess pulses (Doppler grafts).

- Wounds: Change dressing and check for erythema and check drainage (purulent, bilious, serous, sanguinous, feculent).
- Thoracic patients: Check for air leaks from chest tubes.
- Auscultate all patients, check for crackles and wheezing, review most recent chest X-ray.
- Check finger-stick values and doses of insulin administered.
- Review all medications. Restart regular oral medication as soon as possible. Convert IV to oral where appropriate. Look actively for drugs that can be discontinued to minimize interactions and side effects. Adjust doses according to renal function and set hold parameters for blood pressure medications.
- Review all laboratory, radiological, and other diagnostic studies, pathology, microbiology, and consultant's reports.
- Review the nutritional status of the patient.
- Make a problem list and a clear plan.

Special cases

Surgery for cancer

Review pathology as soon as it is available. Arrange for follow-up with oncology or inpatient consultation if the patient is admitted for a prolonged period. It is always preferable to discuss final stage, prognosis, further treatment and adjuvant therapy during outpatient follow-up.

Plastic and reconstructive surgery

- Check perfusion of flaps daily.
- Check take of split-thickness skin grafts on POD5.

Orthopedic surgery

- Check X-rays of prosthesis to assess position and fraction reduction.

Vascular surgery

- Check distal pulses, capillary refill, and swelling and check for severe pain on passive extension (rule out compartment syndrome) in patients status post (s/p) reconstructive surgery.
- Perform neurological examination in patients s/p carotid endarterectomy.
- Arrange prosthesis fitting for amputees.

Cardiac surgery

- Check sternal stability daily (ask the patient to cough while you feel for abnormal sternal movement).
- Request transthoracic echo for POD4–5 s/p valve repair and auscultate daily.

Discharge

- Plan discharge from the day of admission. Touch base with social workers to identify patients who will require specialized care (home-care nurse services, wound care, physical therapy, rehabilitation).
- Make sure the patient understands what operation they have had.
- Instruct patient in how to look out for common problems such as wound infections and tell them who to contact if any issues arise.
- Go over follow-up instructions (appointments, diet, wound care, drain care, medications, etc.).
- Tell patients when they can expect to go back to work and resume activities.
- Write a concise discharge summary.

Drain management

Also see Drains.

Chest tubes

Chest tubes should always be connected to a pleurovac chamber (underwater sealed container).

Management of chest tubes inserted for pneumothorax

- Connect the pleurovac to low wall suction (−20mm Hg) initially.
- Request and review chest X-rays daily.
- Bubbling in the underwater seal, either continuously or only when the patient coughs, means that there is an air leak in the system and implies that there is either a leak in the tubing (check that all the connections are air-tight and no air is being sucked into the system) or the lung parenchyma has not healed. You can only remove the drain when there is no air leak; otherwise a pneumothorax will rapidly re-form.
- When no air leak is detectable, take the drain off suction for 4 hr and repeat the chest X-ray. If the lung is still expanded with no evidence of pneumothorax, the drain can be removed.
- Seal the chest opening quickly with an air-tight dressing after removing the chest tube (and make sure the patient doesn't suck air in during removal of the chest tube).
- Get a chest X-ray after drain removal to check for a pneumothorax.

Management of chest tubes inserted to drain collections

- There is no evidence that suction improves outcome.
- Make sure that the nursing staff measures chest-tube output: hourly in the postoperative or trauma patient, every shift if the drain has been in place longer.
- Trauma patients in whom the initial chest tube insertion drains ≥1.5 L blood, hemodynamically unstable postoperative or trauma patients, or patients draining more than 200 cc blood/hr should be evaluated promptly for the need to go or return to the OR for exploration.
- Postoperative thoracic drains showing no drainage for 2 consecutive hours should be suspected as clogged. In that case, they should be removed promptly.
- Drains for pleural effusions can be removed when they drain less than 250 cc in 24 hr.
- Drains for empyemas can be removed when they stop draining.
- Always request and review a chest X-ray after drain removal to check for pneumothorax.

Clamping chest drains

Clamping of drains when transferring patients stems from the days of TB treatment with caustic solutions, and was aimed at preventing drain effluent from draining back into the chest. In modern practice the *only* indications to clamp a drain are (1) in the trauma setting if the patient is exsanguinating through it, and (2) under specialist supervision in patients with chronic air leaks or pneumonectomy.

- Clamping a thoracic drain in a patient with an air leak may rapidly result in a **tension pneumothorax.**
- Clamping a mediastinal drain in a patient who is bleeding may rapidly result in **cardiac tamponade**.
- The safest mode is an **unclamped** drain connected to an underwater seal that is kept **below** the level of the patient at **all** times.
- Connecting the drain to wall suction without turning the wall suction on effectively clamps the drain. If you and the nurses do not know what you are doing, *ask for help*.

Acid–base balance

The pH of arterial blood is maintained at 7.36–7.44. Normal functioning of the body's complex enzyme systems depends on this stability. Derangements may be primarily due to *respiratory or metabolic* dysfunction (see Box 1.4). Compensatory mechanisms are also divided into metabolic and respiratory mechanisms.

Metabolic acidosis

- Check the anion gap (AG), the difference between unmeasured anions and unmeasured cations = $Na^+ - (Cl^- + HCO_3^-)$; it is dependent on serum albumin, expected value is albumin × 2.5.
- An *anion gap metabolic acidosis* may be caused by ketoacidosis (diabetes, alcohol, starvation), lactic acidosis (sepsis, ischemic bowel, short bowel syndrome, medications), renal failure, methanol, ethylene glycol, paraldehyde, salicylates, or acetaminophen.
- With an anion gap metabolic acidosis, check urine and plasma ketones, toxicology screen, lactate, and osmolal gap (OG; values >10 suggest a toxic ingestion).
- A *non-anion gap metabolic acidosis* may be caused by GI loss of bicarbonate (diarrhea, high-output ileostomy, pancreatic fistula), renal tubular acidosis, ingestion, post-hypocapnia, ureteral diversion, and dilution (excess administration of bicarbonate free IV fluid). The etiology can be suggested by evaluating the urinary anion gap.

Box 1.4 Workup for acid–base abnormalities (Table 1.3)

pH <7.36 is acidosis; pH >7.44 is alkalosis

- Determine primary disorder by checking pH, $PaCO_2$, and HCO_3.
- Determine whether compensation is appropriate.
- The *Flenley nomogram* (Fig. 1.6) is a useful diagnostic aid when mixed metabolic and respiratory derangements are present.

Table 1.3 Primary acid–base disorders with respiratory or metabolic compensation

Primary disorder	Problem	pH	HCO_3	P_aCO_2
Metabolic acidosis	Gain of H^+ or loss of HCO_3	Low	Low	*High*
Metabolic alkalosis	Gain of HCO_3 or loss of H^+	High	High	*Low*
Respiratory acidosis	Hypoventilation	Low	*Low*	High
Respiratory alkalosis	Hyperventilation	High	*High*	Low

Metabolic alkalosis

- May be saline responsive (U_{Cl} <20 mEq/L) or saline resistant (U_{Cl} >20 mEq/L)
- Saline-responsive causes include GI losses (vomiting, nasogastric tube drainage, villous adenoma), diuretic use
- Saline-resistant causes include mineralocorticoid excess, severe hypokalemia, exogenous alkali ($NaHCO_3$, citrate in blood transfusions), and Bartter's or Gitelman's syndrome.

Respiratory acidosis

- Etiologies include respiratory failure or hypoventilation, CNS depression, neuromuscular disorders, and airway obstruction (sleep apnea, obstructive lung disease, etc.).

Respiratory alkalosis

- Etiologies include hyperventilation due to hypoxia or due to CNS disorders, drugs, pregnancy, sepsis, or liver failure.

Consequences of acid–base disorders

Severe acidosis (pH <7.20)

- Decreased cardiac contractility, arteriolar vasodilatation, decreased cardiac output and mean arterial pressure (MAP), increased risk of arrhythmias
- Hyperventilation, change in mental status

Severe alkalosis (pH >7.60)

- Arteriolar vasoconstriction, increased risk of arrhythmias, decreased coronary blood flow
- Hypoventilation, change in mental status, seizures

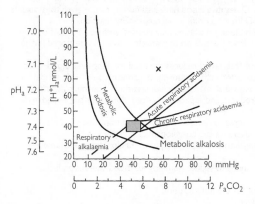

Fig. 1.6 Flenley nonogram. Taken from Longmore M, et al. (2007), *Oxford Handbook of Clinical Medicine*, 7th ed. Oxford: Oxford University Press.

Blood products

Box 1.5 Indications for transfusion of blood products

- Young, fit patients tolerate hemodilution much better than elderly patients with multiple comorbidities (particularly cardiovascular and respiratory disease).
- **Blood**. In general, transfuse for hemoglobin (Hb) <7.0 g/dL (goal is 7–9.0 g/dL); in patients >65 and/or those with cardiovascular or respiratory disease, transfuse when Hb <8.0 g/dL (goal is 10–12.0 g/dL); transfuse for acute blood loss ≥30% blood volume (>1500 cc); transfuse to increase O_2-carrying capacity if end-organ ischemia is present.
- **Fresh frozen plasma (FFP)**. Massive blood transfusion or bleeding from deficiency in multiple coagulation factors, active bleeding or pre-procedure with INR >2.0
- **Platelets**. Platelets <10,000/µl or <20,000 with increased bleeding risk or <50,000 with active bleeding or pre-procedure bleeding (lower threshold if the patient was on aspirin or clopidogrel within 5 days and is actively bleeding)
- **Cryoprecipitate**. Massive blood transfusion, deficiency in fibrinogen (<100 mg/dL), factors XIII, VIII, and von Willebrand factor (vWF)

Blood

- 1 unit of blood transfusion increases Hb by ~1 g/dL in a 70-kg adult.
- A large volume of blood transfusion can deplete Ca, lower K^+ levels, cause metabolic alkalosis, dilute clotting factors, and cause hypothermia.
- Blood is normally provided as packed red blood cells (1 unit = 250 cc).
- In trauma, O-negative blood (universal donor) can be given to recipients of any ABO Rh group without incompatibility reaction.
- Autologous blood transfusion may be used with up to 2 units of blood withdrawn from patients preoperatively, which may be stored for up to 5 weeks.
- Cell salvage (cell saver) reduces the need for allogeneic blood. Shed blood is collected intraoperatively, heparinized, spun with normal saline to remove all material including residual heparin, platelets, and clotting products, and repackaged as red blood cells suspended in saline for transfusion.
- Simple measures to reduce need for blood transfusion include
  - Treating anemia and coagulopathies preoperatively
  - Stopping warfarin, heparin, aspirin, and clopidogrel in a timely fashion
- Special methods to reduce homologous blood transfusion include the following:
  - Autologous blood transfusion
  - Cell saver
  - Procoagulants (see next page)
  - Erythropoietin (EPO) stimulates erythrocyte production.
  - Platelets

- 6 units increases platelet count by 30,000–60,000/μL in a 70-kg adult.
- Platelets are provided as units (1 unit = 50 mL).
- Platelets do not need to be cross-matched but they should be ABO compatible (and rhesus-matched in females of childbearing age).

Fresh frozen plasma

- 1 unit of FFP contains all the coagulation factors except platelets.
- 1 mL of FFP/kg will raise most clotting factors by 1% in a 70-kg adult.
- 1 unit of FFP = 250 mL
- FFP does not need to be cross-matched but should be ABO compatible (and rhesus matched in females of childbearing age).
- FFPs must be thawed, usually over 20 min before infusion, and discarded if not used within 2 hr.

Cryoprecipitate

- One bag of cryoprecipitate (cryo) contains 150–250 mg fibrinogen, and factors VIII, XIII, and vWF.
- If cryo is unavailable, 5 units of FFP contain the same amount of fibrinogen as 10 units of cryo.
- 10 bags of cryo raise the fibrinogen level to about 70 mg/dL in a 70-kg adult.
- One bag of cryo = 10–15 cc: 5–10 pooled bags are normally given.
- ABO and rhesus compatibility are not relevant.

Antifibrinolytics (e.g., aprotinin and tranexamic acid)

- **Action**. Inhibit plasminogen and plasmin; reduce active fibrinolysis
- **Indications**. Prophylaxis against bleeding in cardiovascular surgery, especially high risk. Some studies suggest they are useful in "high-risk" orthopedic surgery. They are used for treatment of excessive bleeding postoperatively (cardiac surgery).

Clinical pearls—physiology of blood groups

- **ABO antigens** preexist on red cells. **ABO antibodies** preexist in the circulation and will cause an immediate reaction if incompatible.
- **Anti-rhesus (D/E) antibodies** only develop following exposure to the RhD antigen, e.g., during blood transfusion or delivery.
- O Rh-negative donors are **universal donors** (red cells carry no ABO/Rh antigens).
- AB Rh-positive donors are **universal recipients** (serum contains no A, B, RhD antibodies).
- **Blood grouping** involves adding A, B, RhD agglutinins to donated blood to determine blood type—it takes less than 5 min.
- **Cross-matching** involves mixing donated blood with the intended recipient serum.

Transfusion reactions

Acute hemolytic reaction

ABO incompatibility as a result of clerical, bedside, sampling, or laboratory error is the most common cause. It may also be caused by incompatibility within other antigen systems (Duffy/Kidd). Donor erythrocytes carrying either A and/or B erythrocyte antigens bind to the recipient's anti-A or anti-B antibodies, resulting in complement formation, membrane attack complex, and immediate intravascular hemolysis. Cytokine and chemokine release mediates a systemic inflammatory response characterized by sudden onset of hypotension, tachycardia, fever, tachypnea, and back pain. Hemolysis may result in anemia, hemoglobinuria, disseminated intravascular coagulation (DIC), shock. and acute renal failure.

- Stop the transfusion immediately and provide supportive care.
- Keep the bag for analysis and inform hematology and the blood bank.
- Start crystalloid infusion with diuretic to promote diuresis.
- Dialysis may be required.

Anaphylaxis and allergic reactions

Allergic reactions are caused by IgE antibody–mediated histamine release in response to soluble allergenic substances in infused plasma, platelets, and red blood cells. These reactions are usually mild, characterized by erythematous papular rashes, wheals, pruritus, and fever. They are treated by stopping the transfusion and administering diphenhydramine (oral or IV).

Anaphylaxis often occurs in IgA-deficient recipients with preformed anti-IgA antibodies. Anaphylaxis is characterized by hypotension, bronchospasm, angioedema, and shock, which can occur within a few seconds to minutes of transfusion.

- Stop the transfusion immediately and disconnect connection tubing.
- Supportive care, crystalloid infusion
- Treat bronchospasm and angioedema with epinephrine (0.3 cc of a 1:1000 IV) ± hydrocortisone (100 mg IV).

Nonhemolytic febrile reaction

This is the most common transfusion reaction, caused by recipient antibodies directed against donor human leukocyte antigen (HLA) and leukocyte-specific antigen on leukocytes and platelets. Cytokine release causes fevers, typically occurring within 1–6 hr after transfusion of red cells or platelets is started. Severe reactions include rigors, nausea, and vomiting.

- Stop the transfusion and rule out a hemolytic reaction.
- Give antipyretics (acetaminophen) and meperidine for severe chills and rigors.

The severity of symptoms is proportional to the number of leukocytes in the transfused blood and the rate of transfusion. Leukocyte-depleted blood helps prevent these reactions.

Delayed extravascular hemolytic reaction

Although pre-transfusion antibody testing is negative (a satisfactory cross-match), patients with this reaction experience accelerated destruction of transfused red blood cells 5–10 days following transfusion. This is an antibody-mediated reaction, usually by a patient antibody (commonly rhesus E, Kell, Duffy, and Kidd) present in levels too low to be detected clinically until produced in larger amounts on exposure to circulating antigen. As hemolysis is extravascular, hemoglobinuria and myoglobinuria are uncommon: it is characterized by an unexpected fall in hematocrit a few days post-transfusion, hyperbilirubinemia, and a positive Coombs' test. No specific treatment is needed, but future transfusions containing the implicated red cell antigen need to be avoided.

Transfusion-related acute lung injury

Noncardiogenic pulmonary edema, typically within 6 hr of transfusion, is mediated by recipient antibodies against donor HLA. Activated recipient leukocytes migrate to the lung, releasing proteolytic enzymes that cause a localized capillary leak syndrome and pulmonary edema. Treatment is similar as for acute respiratory distress syndrome (ARDS).

Infection

Bacterial

Serious bacterial contamination of stored blood may occur, although platelets, which are usually stored at room temperature, are at greater risk of this. Common organisms include *Staphylococcus*, *Enterobacter*, *Yersinia*, and *Pseudomonas* spp. Contamination is difficult to detect. The recipient becomes febrile and hypotensive. This may occur during the transfusion or hours after completion and, unlike febrile transfusion reactions, is not self-limiting.

- Volume resuscitation
- Send blood cultures and send the bag to microbiology.
- Start empirical broad-spectrum antibiotics.

Nonbacterial

Pre-transfusion testing includes screening for hepatitis B (HbsAg, anti-HBc), hepatitis C (anti-HCV), HIV (anti-HIV-1/2, HIV-1 p24 antigen), human T-cell lymphocytotrophic virus (HTLV; anti-TLC-1/2), and syphilis. HIV can be transmitted by an infective but seronegative donor ~15 days after infection. The HCV window is 20 days. Cytomegalovirus (CMV) is common in the donor population (40%–60%); immunocompromised donors must receive leukocyte-depleted or CMV-negative blood.

- Infection risk (hepatitis B 1:220,000; hepatitis C 1:1,600,000; HIV 1:1,800,000)

Fluid overload

This is characterized by hypertension, high filling pressures, dyspnea, and pulmonary edema, particularly in elderly patients, small children, or patients with compromised cardiac function. Treatment consists of limiting the volume of blood transfusions and using diuretics between transfusions and supplemental O_2.

Massive transfusion

- Replacement of the patient's circulating volume in ≤24 hours
- Stored red cells are depleted of adenosine triphosphate (ATP), 2,3 DPG, are stored in a citrate solution, and leak potassium. Large-volume blood transfusion has poor O_2-carrying capacity, causes hypokalemic metabolic alkalosis (citrate is metabolized to bicarbonate),

hypothermia, and depletion of coagulation factors. To reduce the effect of massive transfusion:
• Use infusion warmers and a warming blanket
• Monitor central circulation and respiratory function closely
• Follow coagulation, fibrinogen, and K^+

Shock

Definition
Shock is inadequate tissue perfusion and oxygenation that, if untreated, can lead to cell death, end-organ damage, multi-organ failure, and death (see Box 1.6).

Box 1.6 Recognizing the stages of shock

- Pre-shock (warm or compensated shock): especially in young patients in whom the only signs may be decreased pulse pressure, mild tachycardia, modest hypotension, peripheral vasoconstriction
- Shock: hypotension, tachycardia, and *usually* the patient is cold, clammy, pale, oliguria, metabolic acidosis, confusion (agitation or obtundation)
- End-organ dysfunction: anuria, coma, acidosis, multiple-organ failure

---

Emergency management
- Assess the airway: if patent, give high-flow O_2 by face mask
- Check carotid or femoral pulses
- Secure IV access and bolus with crystalloid
- Monitor BP; if low and falling, prepare the crash cart
- Take a rapid history and examine patient to differentiate between the types of shock
- If intravascular volume is difficult to assess, or if the type of shock is difficult to assess, the patient may need pulmonary artery catheter placement for accurate hemodynamic measurements (Table 1.4)

Hypovolemic shock (decreased preload)
Causes
- Hemorrhagic (trauma, ruptured aortic abdominal aneurysm [AAA], ruptured ectopic, postoperative hemorrhage) or from severe fluid loss (profound dehydration, burns, pancreatitis)

Treatment
- Have the patient lie flat or in Trendelenburg position; high-flow O_2; IV access, aggressive fluid resuscitation, check for adequate hemodynamic response (rise in BP, urine output)
- Cross-match blood, send CBC, coags, electrolytes, blood gases
- Insert a Foley catheter, correct electrolyte imbalances
- If the patient does not respond promptly to fluid resuscitation with crystalloids or blood transfusions, look for other causes.

Distributive shock
- Includes anaphylactic, septic, Addisonian, and neurogenic shock
- Treatment begins with volume but can require adrenergic agents

Anaphylactic shock
Causes
- Drug allergy, blood-product reaction, latex allergy

Clinical features

- History of sudden onset after administration of drug or exposure to material (stridor or bronchospasm, angioedema, urticaria, pruritus, rash)
- Treatment
- Sit the patient up; give high-flow O_2; call anesthesia if stridor
- Secure IV access, epinephrine 0.3 cc of 1:1000 ± corticosteroids, antihistamines
- Nebulized beta-agonist treatment for wheezing

Septic shock

Causes

- Overwhelming sepsis

Clinical features

- May be the same as hypovolemic shock or, if established, with circulatory collapse. In the early course, the patient may look "septic," i.e., febrile, flushed, with bounding pulses and hyperemic skin.

Treatment

- As for hypovolemic shock
- Send blood cultures, give broad-spectrum antibiotics

Cardiogenic shock (pump failure)

Causes

- Rapidly reversible causes are cardiac tamponade (trauma, post-cardiac surgery), arrhythmias, and tension pneumothorax.
- Other causes are cardiomyopathy, MI, valvular heart defects, and pulmonary embolus.

Clinical features

- History of recent surgery or trauma, chest pain, dyspnea, palpitations

Treatment

- Give high-flow O_2
- Morphine IV (anxiolytic, venodilator, analgesic, anti-arrhythmic)
- 12-lead ECG, chest X-ray, blood gases, CBC, electrolytes, coagulation, cardiac enzymes
- Treat arrhythmias, MI, pneumothorax, or cardiac tamponade
- ICU admission, place arterial line and Foley catheter
- Aggressive diuresis if fluid overload
- Consider central venous and pulmonary artery catheter (to follow cardiac output, systemic vascular resistance)
- Transthoracic echo to exclude pericardial effusion and valvular lesions, and to assess LV function

Table 1.4 Hemodynamic profiles associated with different types of shock

Type of shock	CVP/PCWP	CO	SVR
Hypovolemic	Decreased	Decreased	Increased
Cardiogenic	Increased	Decreased	Increased
Septic/neurogenic	Decreased or unchanged	Increased	Decreased

CVP, central venous pressure; PCWP, pulmonary capillary wedge pressure; CO, cardiac output; SVR, systemic vascular resistance

Postoperative bleeding

Postoperative bleeding may be arterial or venous. Significant arterial bleeding is rare and can result from disrupted vascular anastomoses or unrecognized solid-organ injury. It is rapid, bright red in color, and often pulsatile. Venous bleeding is more common and usually originates from unsecured venous channels or unrecognized liver, splenic, or mesenteric laceration. Although it is nonpulsatile, low pressure, and dark in color, it can be profuse. Most postoperative bleeding is not overt and is contained within body cavities, causing delays in diagnosis. Even when correctly positioned, drains are unreliable markers of profuse bleeding and a high index of suspicion is required for prompt diagnosis and treatment.

Causes and features
- Primary hemorrhage: occurs immediately after surgery or represents ongoing bleeding noted during surgery. It is usually due to unsecured blood vessels (e.g., liver bleeding following trauma).
- Reactionary hemorrhage: occurs within first 24 hr postoperatively. Usually due to venous bleeding, it is commonly thought to result from increased venous pressure unmasking disrupted vessels previously in vasospasm (delayed splenic bleeding following minor trauma at laparotomy, delayed bleeding from abdominal port site in laparoscopy).
- Secondary hemorrhage: occurs up to 10 days postoperatively. It is usually due to infection of operative wounds or raw surfaces, causing clot disintegration and bleeding from exposed tissues.

Symptoms
- When rapid and massive, postoperative bleeding can lead to confusion, anxiety, and agitation (from cerebral hypoxia secondary to hypotension).

Signs
- Overt signs of bleeding are rare—soaked dressings, blood in drains
- Pallor, sweaty, tachypnea, tachycardia, hypotension (a late sign in children and young adults)

Emergency management
Resuscitation
- Place a large-gauge IV (16 gauge or larger). Start infusion with crystalloids and bolus with 1 L if the patient is hemodynamically unstable. Central lines should be placed only if rapid IV access is critical (arrest), pressors are needed, or peripheral access cannot be obtained.
- Control superficial bleeding with direct compression.
- Quickly cross-match blood if not already done and have at least 2 units of packed red blood cells available, send stat CBC and coagulation.
- If there is significant blood loss, alert the attending surgeons and possibly the OR and surgical ICU.
- Do not use O Rh-negative blood for resuscitation unless the patient is in extremis.
- Place the patient on a cardiac monitor, insert a Foley catheter, and follow ins and outs closely (to evaluate response to resuscitation).

Establish a diagnosis

The cause may be obvious from the bleeding or the operation.

- Review the operative report, and review CBC, coagulation function, and perioperative anticoagulation regimen.
- If the bleeding is severe, the only way to establish a diagnosis and control the bleeding is to re-explore the patient.

Definitive management

Most postoperative bleeding does not require reoperation. If bleeding is not associated with hemodynamic instability, or if fluid or blood resuscitation results in normalization of vitals signs, attempts at supportive care may be warranted and consist of

- Close observation (cardiac monitoring, hourly ins and outs, CBC q6 hr)

If coagulopathy is suspected as contributing to surgical bleeding, attempts at aggressive correction are indicated:

- Vitamin K, FFP, cryoprecipitate
- If a minimally invasive diagnostic or therapeutic alternative is available, it may be used as long as the patient is hemodynamically stable.
- Endoscopic management of bleeding staple line after colorectal resection
- Radiologically guided embolization

Wound hematoma

This is a localized collection of blood beneath the wound, usually characterized by swelling and discoloration of overlying skin.

- If this occurs after vascular surgery, flap surgery, or procedures on the limbs or neck, urgent surgical exploration and evacuation may be required to avoid ischemia, compartment syndrome, airway obstruction, flap failure, or ongoing hemorrhage.
- Apply firm pressure, followed by a pressure dressing.
- Check coagulation function and CBC.
- Hold anticoagulation.
- The patient may need to be evacuated electively to relieve pain and infection.

Cardiac complications

Chest pain

Taking a careful pain history should help differentiate between the causes of chest discomfort listed Box 1.7.

> **Box 1.7 Causes of postoperative chest pain**
>
> *Dull, central ache or pressure*
> - Myocardial ischemia (usually brought on by exertion)
> - Gastric distension
>
> *Central pain radiating through to back*
> - Thoracic aneurysm or dissection
> - Peptic ulcer disease, esophagitis, rarely pancreatitis
>
> *Pain on movement*
> - Musculoskeletal pain
> - Chest drains
>
> *Pleuritic pain*
> - Chest infection
> - Pneumothorax
> - Hemothorax, pleural effusion, empyema
> - Chest drain in situ
> - Pulmonary embolism

Diagnosis
- Take a careful history and examine the patient.
- A chest X-ray will demonstrate most lung pathology.
- A 12-lead ECG should help exclude myocardial ischemia.
- Recent WBC and C-reactive protein (CRP) values help identify sepsis.
- Review previous medical history for peptic ulcer disease and the drug chart for NSAID use.

Myocardial ischemia

Patients, particularly in vascular surgery, may have preexisting ischemic heart disease. Surgery can precipitate ischemia through the following:
- Stress response to major surgery (endogenous catecholamine release triggered by anxiety, pain)
- Fluid overload postoperatively
- Profound hypotension
- Failing to restart anti-anginal medication postoperatively

Diagnosis
Take a history, particularly of chest discomfort brought on by exertion and relieved by nitroglycerin (NTG). Check that the patient is back on any regular cardiac medication. The physiotherapists may report bradycardia upon exercising. A 12-lead ECG will confirm the presence of myocardial

ischemia. Cardiac enzymes (CKMB and troponin I and T) may be slightly raised postoperatively, but serial measurements showing a continued rise would suggest ongoing myocardial damage.

Management
- Sit the patient up; give high-flow O_2.
- Ensure that the patient is on aspirin 81 mg po qd.
- Give NTG sublingually.
- Restart preoperative anti-anginal medication.
- Discuss urgently with a cardiologist regarding the use of anti-thrombotic or anti-platelet medications.

Perioperative myocardial infarction

Perioperative MI may be difficult to diagnose (see Box 1.8) because the patient may be unable to give a good history or distinguish between chest and upper abdominal pain.
- The presentation is similar to that of myocardial ischemia, but the duration is longer (>20 min) and may be associated with hemodynamic instability, nausea, vomiting, confusion, and distress.
- The patient will be cold and clammy and may be hypoxic.

Box 1.8 Diagnostic criteria for myocardial infarction

In the setting of symptoms suggestive of acute coronary syndrome:
- ECG shows ST segment elevation: ST segment elevation MI (STEMI)
- No ST elevation, but elevated CKMB and positive troponin in non-Q wave or non-ST segment elevation MI (NSTEMI)

Management
- Attach an ECG monitor and pulse oxymeter, and get a 12-lead ECG.
- Make sure the defibrillator trolley is close at hand.
- Give high-flow O_2.
- Get IV access.
- Give morphine 5 mg IV.
- Give aspirin 325 mg po/pr and NTG 0.5 mg sublingually (SL).
- Give IV or po beta-blocker, titrated to heart rate of 60.
- Contact cardiologists urgently to discuss the use of anti-thrombotic or anti-platelet medications.

Clinical pearls—physiology of coronary blood flow

- Myocardial cells extract up to 70% of O_2 from blood.
- Coronary blood flow occurs during diastole.
- Tachycardia reduces the diastolic interval and increases O_2 demand, which may reveal occult ischemia.
- Coronary vasodilatation is mediated by adenosine, K^+, hypoxia, and β_2 stimulants and the N_2O pathway.

Respiratory complications

Postoperative pulmonary complications are an important cause of morbidity and mortality. Complications include the following:
- Respiratory failure requiring mechanical ventilation, upper-airway obstruction, infection, exacerbation of underlying COPD, atelectasis

Definite risk factors for postoperative pulmonary complications include
- Age >50, COPD, congestive heart failure (CHF), ASA class >2, serum albumin <3.5 g/dL, upper abdominal, thoracic, or aortic surgery, neurosurgery and AAA surgery, OR time >3 hr, emergency surgery, use of long-acting neuromuscular blockade

Other contributing factors include obstructive sleep apnea, general anesthesia (relative to epidural), $PaCO_2$ >45mm Hg, abnormal chest X-ray, smoking within previous 8 weeks, current upper respiratory infection.

Respiratory failure

Respiratory failure is a clinical diagnosis (failure to ventilate appropriately). Objective criteria can be used to guide the need for mechanical ventilation:
- Hypoxia: PaO_2 <60mm Hg, hypercarbia: PaC_2 >55mm Hg, respiratory rate (RR) >35/min

In general, mechanical ventilation is required for apnea, to improving gas exchange (increase oxygenation or alveolar ventilation), to relieve respiratory distress (decrease the work of breathing and relieve respiratory muscle fatigue), to protect the airway (change in mental status, etc.), and for aggressive pulmonary toilet (aspiration, pneumonia, etc.).

Basic assessment and management of respiratory failure
- Check mental status; if the patient is nonresponsive or quickly deteriorating, immediate intubation is warranted. Consider Narcan if opiate overdose is suspected.
- If the patient is alert and cooperating, sit patient up and administer high-flow O_2 through a non-rebreathing face mask.
- Check pulse oximetry readings on room air and on supplemental O_2.
- Auscultate the chest: Check for bilateral and equal breath sounds, poor air entry, wheezing, bronchial breathing, and crackles.
- Treat bronchospasm with nebulized beta agonists (albuterol).
- Get a chest X-ray, check blood gas. Look for consolidation, edema, effusions, and pneumothorax; calculate A-a gradient.

Postoperative pulmonary complications
Preoperative preventive strategies
- Smoking: cessation at least 8 weeks before surgery
- COPD: aggressive treatment with bronchodilators ± antibiotics, systemic steroids, smoking cessation, chest physical therapy (PT) for best possible status before surgery
- Asthma: minimize wheezing with inhaled beta-agonists or systemic corticosteroids (if peak flow rate or FEV1 <80% of predicted)
- Upper respiratory infection (URI): delay elective surgery until resolved

Intraoperative preventive strategies
- Recommend minimally invasive alternatives, if possible.
- Anesthesia: use spinal or epidural anesthesia for upper abdominal and thoracic procedures; use short- or intermediate-acting neuromuscular blockers instead of long-acting agents.

Postoperative preventive strategies
- Lung expansion maneuvers: chest PT, incentive spirometry, continuous positive airway pressure (CPAP)
- Humidified O_2 to prevent mucous plugging
- Adequate pain control to allow earlier ambulation and deep breaths
- Avoid use of nasogastric tube (NGT), if possible (increases risk of pneumonia and atelectasis)

Upper airway obstruction
- Occurs in the immediate postoperative period (laryngeal edema, cord paralysis, laryngospasm, soft-tissue obstruction, e.g., tongue)
- Manifests as stridor; reintubate if the patient fails to improve with bronchodilators

Postoperative pneumonia
- Presentation: cough with purulent sputum (or purulent aspirate if intubated), fevers, dyspnea, reduced air entry, leukocytosis, raised CRP, consolidation on chest X-ray, positive sputum cultures, dyspnea
- Most common etiology of nocosomial pneumonia is gram-negative bacteria and *Staphylococcus aureus*, often polymicrobial (*Enterobacter* + *Staphylococcus aureus* or streptococci) and highly resistant
- Most commonly occur within first 5 postoperative days
- Risk factors: NGT, head injury (*S. aureus*), prolonged antibiotics (methicillin-resistant *Staphylococcus aureus* [MRSA], *Pseudomonas*), prolonged intubation or COPD (*Pseudomonas, Acinetobacter*)
- Management: chest PT, empiric treatment of nocosomial pneumonia until organism sensitivities are known
- Aspiration pneumonia: abrupt onset of dyspnea, hypoxemia, tachycardia, fever, bronchospasm, infiltration in one or both lower lobes within 24 hr, may progress to ARDS
- Aspiration pneumonia most commonly occurs during tracheal extubation and may require intubation (if unable to protect the airway).

Exacerbation of COPD
- Ensure that all patients are on preoperative beta-agonist inhalers (albuterol) and that anti-cholinergics (ipratropium) are resumed; start chest PT.
- In hypoxic patients with COPD give maximal O_2 by CPAP and titrate against $PaCO_2$ and PO_2: do *not* restrict oxygen empirically, add systemic steroids, and consider antimicrobial therapy if you suspect superimposed infection.

Atelectasis

This is common, especially following abdominal and thoracoabdominal procedures.

- When clinically significant, it presents with increased work of breathing and hypoxemia (from decline in functional residual capacity [FRC]).
- Management: Prevention (see previous pages). Aggressive incentive spirometry, ambulation, CPAP (to prevent intubation in patients with severe atelectasis), mucolytic therapy (N-acetylcysteine), and bronchoscopy

Clinical pearls—monitoring and measuring lung function

- Pulse oximetry estimates % of saturated hemoglobin in capillary blood by the change in wavelength ratios of absorbed red light. It is inaccurate in CO poisoning, cold extremities, low-flow states, and tachydysrhythmias.
- PaO_2 can be approximately *estimated* from the SaO_2 (from the oxygen dissociation curve), 95%, >80 mmHg; 85%, 50 mmHg; 75%, <40 mmHg.

Renal failure and urinary complications

Oliguria

Urine ouput is an indicator of glomerular filtration rate (GFR), which is an indicator of renal plasma flow and renal perfusion. Hence, urine output is an indirect measure of renal (and thus systemic) blood flow as well as renal function. Patients with normal renal function usually maintain a urine output of at least 0.5 mL/kg/hr.

Management of oliguria

- Check that the Foley catheter is not the problem. The urine catheter may be obstructed, leaking, or malpositioned. Is the bed or floor wet? Flush the catheter with saline—can you draw this amount back without difficulty? If not, change the catheter.

Optimize cardiac function and intravascular volume

- Patients markedly hypertensive preoperatively may require high blood pressures to maintain satisfactory renal perfusion and urine output.
- Is the patient overfilled or underfilled?
- Make sure the patient is adequately filled by giving fluid challenges to achieve CVP of 14–16 mmHg, or raise the JVP moderately.
- Make sure the patient is not overfilled. If the CVP rises to >16 mmHg, or if the BP falls, the patient may be overfilled and need diuretics.
- Invasive monitoring. If the patient does not rapidly respond to fluid boluses and intravascular volume is difficult to assess, a central line for CVP measurements might be required.

Acute renal failure

- Cr increase by ≥0.5 mg/dL or by ≥20% if baseline Cr >2.5 mg/dL in ≤2 weeks
- Oliguria: urine output <0.5 cc/kg/hr
- Anuria: urine output <100 cc/24 hr

Etiology of renal failure

Prerenal process

- Decreased systemic perfusion (hypotension, hypovolemia, low-flow state, e.g., cardiogenic failure, vasodilatory shock, i.e., sepsis)
- Renal vasoconstriction (NSAIDS, ACE inhibitor), hepatorenal syndrome
- Decreased renal perfusion (bilateral renal artery stenosis, dissection)

Intrinsic process

- Acute tubular necrosis (ATN) from ischemia, drugs (aminoglycosides, IV contrast, vancomycin, amphotericin), myoglobinuria
- Acute interstitial nephritis (allergic, infectious), glomerulonephritis
- Small-vessel disease (cholesterol emboli, thrombotic microangiopathy)

Postrenal process
- Outflow obstruction (prostatic hypertrophy, neurogenic bladder, occluded Foley catheter)
- Ureteral obstruction (nephrolithiasis)
- Abdominal compartment syndrome

Preoperative risk factors
- Age >75 years, chronic renal insufficiency (CRI), hypertension, diabetes, peripheral vascular disease, preoperative diuretics

Intraoperative risk factors
- Cardiac, aortic surgery (cross-clamping)

Prevention of renal failure
- Adequate pre- and postoperative resuscitation (monitor ins and outs closely)
- Avoid nephrotoxic medications, especially in CRI (NSAIDs, angiotensin receptor blocker [ARB], ACE inhibitor, diuretics). Minimize use of IV contrast (premedicate with N-acetylcysteine and gentle hydration in patients with CRI).
- Avoid intraoperative and postoperative hypotension.
- Optimal cardiac function and intravascular volume (may use CVP, pulmonary artery catheter) are the most important factors in preventing renal failure.

Management of renal failure
- Identify and treat underlying etiology:
  - History and physical (medications, fluid status), electrolytes
  - Urinalysis, urine electrolytes and osmolality, FeNa (prerenal if <1%)
  - Renal ultrasound (rule out obstruction), serologies (glomerulonephritis), renal biopsy, creatine phosphokinase (CPK) levels, bladder pressure
- Avoid exacerbating renal insult (nephrotoxic medications) and/or adjust dosing and monitor levels of renally excreted medications.
- Optimize hemodynamic status (cardiac output, BP, fluid balance)
- Identify and aggressively treat sequelae from oliguric or anuric renal failure:
  - Fluid overload: limit fluids, follow oxygenation
  - Electrolyte disorders and acid base balance: monitor frequently, remove K^+ from all fluids, follow HCO_3.
  - Monitor mental status (uremic encephalopathy)
  - Adjust enteral and parenteral diet to renal formulation

Indications for dialysis
- Refractory fluid overload
- Refractory hyperkalemia (K^+ >6.5 meq/L) or rapidly rising levels
- Refractory metabolic acidosis (pH <7.1)
- Signs of uremia (encephalopathy, pericarditis)

Hyperkalemia

Hyperkalemia is due to excessive intake, decreased excretion (renal failure, hypoaldosteronism), or massive cellular release (acidosis, tissue necrosis, i.e., tumor lysis, rhabdomyolysis, ischemic bowel).

Clinical manifestations

- Weakness, nausea, paresthesias, acute hyperkalemia (K^+ >6.0) can cause life-threatening ventricular arrhythmias. ECG changes that herald myocardial dysfunction **are flattened P waves, wide QRS complexes, peaked T waves,** and sine wave (near-arrest).

Management

- Rule out pseudohyperkalemia (lab error, hemolyzed specimen, venipuncture above line infusing K^+).
- Treat the underlying cause.
- Treat the patient with ECG changes as an emergency:
  - Calcium gluconate 1–2 amps (stabilizes cell membrane)
  - Insulin (10 units) IV + 1–2 amps of D50W (drives K^+ into cells)
  - Bicarbonate 1–3 amps IV (drives K+ into cells in exchange for H^+)
  - β agonists (albuterol 10–20 mg inhaler or 0.5 mg IV (drives K^+ into cells)
  - Kayexalate 30–90 g po/pr (exchanges Na^+ for K^+ in gut)
  - Diuretics (furosemide 40 mg IV)
  - Hemodialysis for patients with refractory hyperkalemia despite these measures

Hypokalemia

Hypokalemia is due to excessive GI losses and associated with metabolic acidosis (diarrhea, laxative abuse, villous adenoma, vomiting or NGT drainage), renal losses (hyperaldosteronism, acidosis, diuretics), or cellular shifts (alkalosis, insulin).

Clinical manifestations

- Clinical manifestation: nausea, vomiting, weakness, muscle cramps. ECG changes include **U waves, ± increased QT interval, ventricular ectopy**

Management

- K^+ repletion po/IV, follow levels closely
- Treat the underlying cause.
- Educate patients on foods rich in potassium (bananas, prunes, apricots, tomatoes, orange juice).
- Adjust diuretic dose, change to K^+-sparing diuretics, and add oral K^+ supplements.

Acute urinary retention

This condition is common postoperatively, especially in elderly males, after abdominopelvic or anorectal surgery, or after anticholinergic therapy.

Clinical features
- Suprapubic discomfort, inability to initiate micturition, or dribbling
- History of prostatic disease or symptoms preoperatively
- Percussable bladder on examination

Prevention and management
- Minimize intra- and postoperative IV fluids
- Improve analgesia, treat constipation, mobilize, warm bath to encourage micturition, restart preoperative tamsulosin
- Insert a catheter (straight-catherize of indwelling) if conservative measures fail or the patient is in great discomfort, or if renal dysfunction is suspected.

Urinary tract infection (UTI)

UTIS are common in females and in patients catheterized for prolonged periods.

Clinical features
- Dysuria, frequency, dribbling, foul-smelling and cloudy urine, postoperative fever and leukocytosis
- Send for urinalysis (pH, ketones, protein, bilirubin, RBC and WBC numbers, leukocyte esterase and nitrites) and urine microscopy (RBC and WBC casts, crystals)
- Send specimen for microbiology to identify organism and sensitivities

Management
- Remove catheters as soon as possible.
- Encourage drinking or increase fluid infusion if it is safe to increase urine flow.
- Treat empirically with antibiotics (trimethoprim) until sensitivities are known.

Clinical pearls—physiology of diuretics

- **Osmotic diuretics**, e.g., mannitol, are not well reabsorbed in the distal tubules. Increased osmotic pressure reduces H_2O reabsorption.
- **Loop diuretics** inhibit $Na^+K^+Cl^-$ exchange in the ascending loop of Henle, decreasing osmolality in the medulla and water reabsorption.
- **Aldosterone antagonists**, e.g., spironalactone, and **sodium channel blockers**, e.g., amiloride, reduce Na^+ resorbtion and K^+ and H^+ secretion in the distal tubule.
- **Alcohol** inhibits antidiuretic hormone (ADH) release.

Wound emergencies

Infection

Causes

Most wound infections are acquired from the patient's own flora. The majority are skin organisms (e.g., *Staphylococcus aureus*, *Staphylococcus epidermidis*), followed by contamination from the GI tract (*Escherichia coli*) or biliary tree (*Pseudomonas*).

Risk factors

- Advanced age, obesity, perioperative hypothermia, malnutrition, diabetes, smoking, coexistent infections at a remote body site, colonization with microorganisms, immunosuppression

Signs and symptoms

- Pain, tenderness, localized erythema, induration, fluctuance or purulent drainage
- Malaise, anorexia, fever, tachycardia (systemic inflammatory features)

Complications

- Bacteremia, septicemia (rare unless organism is resistant or the patient is immunosuppressed)

Establish a diagnosis

- Send wound cultures for Gram stain and microbiology (culture and sensitivity)
- Send CBC and blood cultures (2 sets from different sites)

Treatment

- All infected wounds must be opened, drained, explored, irrigated, and debrided, and the integrity of the fascia must be assessed.
- Avoid opening the wound just partially. The wound must be opened sufficiently to allow evacuation of all the infection and to allow packing and dressing changes bid (wet to dry dressings).
- If fascia disruption is suspected, wound drainage should be performed in the operating room.
- If the wound is mild and superficial with no systemic signs of infection, drainage might be sufficient without adding antimicrobials.
- If systemic signs of infection present, start fluids and antibiotics (cover expected flora at the site of operation as well as gram-positive cocci from the skin).
- If the patient is immunosuppressed or septic, start broad-spectrum antibiotics and include anaerobic coverage.
- If there is real concern about MRSA infection, consult infectious diseases and consider adding vancomycin.

Dehiscence

Wound dehiscence may be superficial (including skin and subcutaneous tissue) or deeper (fascial). Fascial dehiscence can be partial or complete. Complete fascial dehiscence leads to the separation of all abdominal wall layers and may lead to evisceration (protrusion of abdominal viscera through the wound).

Causes

Most wound dehiscences are secondary to wound infection. Risk factors associated with increased risk of fascia disruption include conditions associated with poor healing and increased abdominal wall muscle tension overcoming suture strength. Common risk factors include the following:

- Advanced age, malnutrition, pulmonary disease, obesity, diabetes, radiation, immunosuppression, ascites.

Wound factors that contribute to fascial disruption include

- Poor surgical technique, fascial closure under tension, use of absorbable sutures, infection (wound infection or intra-abdominal process such as anastomotic leakage or abscess)

Signs and symptoms

Wound dehiscences are usually painless and present as an open wound with fluid drainage, with exposed subcutaneous tissues and fascia (superficial dehiscence), or with exposed viscera (fascial dehiscence).

- Occasionally associated organ dysfunction if involved by the accompanying wound infection (e.g., pericarditis or anterior mediastinitis in sternal dehiscence)

Treatment

Resuscitation

- Resuscitate with fluids.
- Reassure the patient, particularly if there is any degree of evisceration.
- If there are exposed viscera, cover these with saline-soaked dressings.
- Give IV antibiotics if there are features of wound infection (see above).
- If the dehiscence is superficial, ensure that the wound is open and any pus is fully drained; pack the wound with moist dressing.

Superficial dehiscence

- Wound care (dressing changes bid)
- For large defects, consider vacuum-assisted closure (VAC) dressing

Fascial dehiscence

- Reexplore the wound in the operating room.
- Debride the wound and fascia edges if necrotic or infected, drain collections, and aggressively wash out with saline.
- Close the fascia primarily if all infection is cleared and if fascial edges are easily apposed; otherwise use absorbable mesh (Vicryl®, Surgisis®, Alloderm®) or retention sutures.
- A late complication of fascial disruption is incisional hernia.

Gastrointestinal complications

Prolonged postoperative ileus (PPOI)

Ileus is defined as obstipation and intolerance of oral intake due to the cessation of GI tract motility. Physiologic POI is normally self-limited and resolves within 1–3 days. When prolonged, it is associated with malnutrition, prolonged hospital stay, increased susceptibility to infection, and increased hospital costs.

Causes
- Inflammation resulting from intestinal manipulation, peritonitis, and abdominal trauma (activation of inflammatory cells results in GI dysfunction)
- Electrolyte disturbances (most commonly hypokalemia, hypomagnesemia)
- Anticholinergics or opiates (interfere with enteric nervous system)
- Other: prolonged hypotension, hypoxia, immobilization, mediated by inhibitory neural reflexes and neurohumoral peptides (nitric oxide [NO], vasoactive inhibitory protein [VIP], corticotropin-releasing factor [CRF], substance P, and motilin)

Clinical features
- Nausea, vomiting, hiccups, obstipation
- Abdominal distension, bloating, absent bowel sounds
- Air/fluid-filled loops of small and/or large bowel on abdominal X-ray
- Inability to tolerate an oral diet

Prevention
- Epidural and local anesthesia, minimally invasive surgery, minimize intestinal manipulation and length of laparotomy, use opioid antagonists, substitute opioids, use fast-track programs (early feeding and mobilization)

Management
- Check and replete electrolytes.
- Reduce po intake (sips), continue IV fluids.
- Discontinue opiates, substitute with NSAIDs.
- NGT decompression should only be used to relieve severe vomiting and reduce the risk of aspiration.
- After 5–7 days, differentiate from small-bowel obstruction (SBO) by clinical exam ± radiologic studies (kidneys, ureter, bladder [KUB], CT scan, GI series) and address nutritional needs.

Postoperative mechanical small-bowel obstruction

Causes
- Early adhesions (usually self-limiting)
- Internal, parastomal, or wound herniation
- Intra-abdominal sepsis (usually later presentation)

Clinical features
- Nausea and vomiting, crampy abdominal pain
- Abdominal distension and tenderness, high-pitched bowel sounds

- Rule out incisional, stomal, or port-site hernias.
- Dilated loops of small bowel (relative paucity of gas in colon) on KUB, transition point on CT scan or GI series

Treatment
- Strict bowel rest, IV fluids, strict ins and outs
- Reoperation is rarely indicated as most early postoperative obstructive episodes resolve. Exceptions include obstruction due to hernias or adhesions that fail to resolve after several weeks of strict bowel rest and TPN. In the latter case wait a minimum of 6 weeks before reoperation.

Nausea and vomiting

These symptoms are very common. They predispose to aspiration pneumonia, malnutrition, poor absorption of oral medication, and metabolite imbalances. Causes include the following:
- Anesthetic agents (etomidate, ketamine, N_2O, opioids, spinal anesthesia)
- Postoperative ileus, bowel obstruction, constipation, gastric reflux, medications (antibiotics, opiates), pancreatitis, sepsis and hyponatremia

---

Box 1.9 Classification of antiemetics

Dopamine receptor antagonists
- Phenothiazines (prochlorperazine, chlorpromazine) for chemotherapy-induced emesis (CIE); side effects (SE): extrapyramidal reaction (dystonias, tardive dyskinesia, hypotension)
- Butyrophenones (droperidol, haloperidol); SE: same as above, sedation
- Benzamides (metoclopramide, domperidone, trimethobenzamide) also increases gastric emptying and LES tone; SE: dystonia, tardive dyskinesia

Antihistamines
- Diphenhydramine, cyclizine, dimenhydrinate, promethazine, used for motion sickness; SE: sedation

Anticholinergics
- M1-muscarinic receptor antagonist (scopolamine), used for motion sickness

Serotonin antagonists
- Odansetron, granisetron, dolasetron, palonosetron, lowest SE profile of all antiemetics, used primarily to prevent CIE

Corticosteroids
- Alone or in combination with serotonin antagonists for CIE

Constipation

Contributing factors: bed rest, poor nutrition, opiates, iron supplements, electrolyte imbalances. Treat with the following:

- Bulking agents (psyllium, methylcellulose)
- Stool softeners (sodium docusate)
- Osmotic laxative (lactulose, magnesium citrate, sodium phosphate)
- Stimulants laxative (senna, bisacodyl)
- Rectal enemas (phosphate, mineral oil, tap water, bisacodyl)

Diarrhea

Common causes in postoperative patients:

- Resolving ileus or obstruction
- Related to formulation of enteral nutrition
- Related to the type of surgery (ileal pouch, total colectomy)
- Antibiotic-related
- *Clostridium difficile* diarrhea (send stool for *C. difficile* cytoxin assay)

Neurological complications

Postoperative delirium

Delirium (acute confusional state) is common postoperatively, especially in older patients. Patients may become disoriented, uncooperative (pulling lines or catheters), or combative. Frequently it is more subtle, with lethargy, mental slowing, change in personality, and labile mood, usually noticed by relatives or nursing staff. Onset is acute and lasts for days to weeks. It often fluctuates in severity over the course of the day. It usually is multifactorial in etiology (see Box 1.10) but is often precipitated by exacerbating factors in the setting of postoperative state.

Box 1.10 Common risk factors for delirium

- Medications (particularly psychoactive medications including benzodiazepines, opiates, anticonvulsants, etc.), withdrawal (alcohol, sedatives)
- Stroke
- Hypoxia, hypercapnia
- Shock
- Infection and sepsis
- Metabolic disturbances (glucose, Na^+, Ca^{2+}, phosphate, magnesium)
- Preoperative dementia
- Immobility, restraints

Prevention
- Take a thorough history about alcohol and sedative consumption.
- Encourage early mobilization.
- Ensure that visual and hearing aids are provided to patients.
- Avoid sleep deprivation, provide orientation devices (clocks).

Management
- Identify delirium (Is the patient oriented in time, person, and place? Perform a quick mini mental-state examination if still unclear).
- Neurological examination, look for focal neurological deficit and consider head CT to exclude acute stroke
- Review recent history, labs, physical exam: identify precipitating factors (electrolyte disturbances, hypoxia, hypoglycemia, fever, arrhythmia, low perfusion state, medications).
- Use physical and/or chemical restraints to behavior that poses a physical danger to self or others. Otherwise, presence of a family member or companion is usually sufficient to keep patients calm.
- If sedation is needed, use low-dose haloperidol; avoid benzodiazepines unless you suspect alcohol withdrawal.
- Reassure patient and relatives: delirium is usually reversible.

Stroke

Stroke is most common in vascular and cardiac surgical patients (2%), but elderly patients undergoing any type of major surgery are at risk.

Risk factors for stroke
- Increasing age, diabetes
- Previous history of transient ischemic attack (TIA) or stroke
- Carotid artery atherosclerosis
- Perioperative hypotension
- Left-sided mural thrombus
- Mechanical heart valve
- Postoperative atrial fibrillation (AF)

Etiology
- **Ischemic** (embolic from carotid, cardiac thrombus from AF or paradoxical; thrombotic; or cerebral hypoperfusion—vasospasm, profound hypotension, raised [ICP], hypoxia)
- **Hemorrhagic** (intracerebral from AVM, postoperative anticoagulation, hypertension; subarachnoid bleed from ruptured aneurysm or trauma)
- **Cerebral hypoperfusion**: profound hypotension, raised ICP

Clinical features
Sudden neurologic deficit that resolves within 24 hr is a TIA. Clinical features of perioperative stroke include the following:
- Failure to regain consciousness once sedation has been weaned
- Hemiplegia (middle, anterior cerebral artery, total carotid artery occlusion)
- Initial areflexia becoming hyperreflexia and rigidity after a few days
- Aphasia, dysarthria, ataxia (gait or truncal), inadequate gag reflex
- Visual deficits, unilateral neglect, confusion, seizures
- Persistent severe hypertension
- Hypercapnia

Diagnosis
Establish a definitive diagnosis, a cause to guide appropriate secondary prevention, and a baseline of function to help plan long-term rehabilitation or withdrawal of therapy.
- Full neurological exam (cognitive function, cranial nerves, tone, power, reflexes, sensation in all four limbs)
- Non-contrast head CT (hemorrhagic vs. ischemic stroke ± MRI)

Initial management
- Assess airway, breathing, and circulation (intubate as needed).
- Monitor BP (hemorrhagic stroke: keep SBP <140 with labetolol unless risk of hypoperfusion; ischemic: do not lower unless >200 or MI/CHF)
- Full neurological examination if the patient is responsive
- Electrolytes, CBC, coagulation, lumbar puncture (if you suspect subarachnoid hemorrhage [SAH] not seen on CT)
- Urgent non-contrast head CT head (bleed), CT angiogram (assess cerebrovascular patency)
- Carotid and transcranial Doppler ultrasound (stenosis)
- ECG, cardiac monitor, Holter monitor (AF)
- Echocardiography with bubble study (cardiac thrombus, patent foramen ovale, valvular vegetations)

Definite management
- TIA: anticoagulation + antiplatelet therapy ± carotid revascularization
- Ischemic stroke: thrombolysis (intra-arterial or catheter-based with antiplatelet therapy)
- Hemorrhagic stroke: reverse coagulopathy ± surgical decompression or correction, calcium channel blocker (reduces vasospasm)

Hematological complications

Heparin-induced thrombocytopenia (HIT)

Type I (non-immune)
- Due to direct effect of heparin
- Incidence: 10%–20% after 1–4 days of exposure to heparin
- Characterized by fall in platelet count up to 50% of normal range (count usually >100,000/µL)
- Has no sequelae, heparin can usually be continued

Type II (immune)
- Results from formation of complement-mediated IgG antibodies against the heparin-platelet factor 4 complex
- Incidence: 1%–3% of patients exposed to heparin for more than 4 days
- Early-onset HIT: can occur after the first dose of heparin in patients with previous exposure to heparin within the last 3 months
- Delayed-onset HIT: can occur up to 9 days after stopping heparin
- Heparin-induced thrombocytopenia and thrombosis (HITT) occurs in 20%–30% of patients with HIT and is characterized by major thrombotic episodes and a mortality of about 30% (DVT, PE, limb gangrene, skin necrosis, cerebral sinus thrombosis).
- Rate hemorrhagic complications

Risk factors (type II)
- Longer duration of heparin therapy
- Use of unfractionated rather than LMWH
- Surgical > medical patients, females > males

Diagnosis (type II)
- Fall in platelet count by >30%–50% (count usually <100,000/µL)
- 14-C –serotonin release assay (sensitivity, specificity of >95%)
- Functional heparin-induced platelet aggregation (>90% specificity, low sensitivity)
- Heparin-PF4 ELISA assay (HIT antibodies, >90% sensitivity, low specificity)

Treatment (type II)
- Discontinue all heparin therapy, including heparinized saline flushes and LMWH.
- If ongoing anticoagulation is required (thrombosis), use lepirudin, argatroban, and danaparoid and bridge with warfarin (when platelets >100,000/µL)
- Platelet transfusion is not indicated in HIT unless there is active bleeding.

Disseminated intravascular coagulation (DIC)

Clinical features

DIC is characterized by widespread activation of coagulation with formation of intravascular fibrin, fibrin degradation products (FDPs), consumption of platelets and clotting factors, and, ultimately, thrombotic occlusion of the microvasculature, microangiopathic hemolytic anemia, and uncontrolled bleeding. Patients may present with bleeding from IV lines, wounds, and mucosal surfaces. If not reversed, DIC can result in life-threatening bleeding, end-organ damage (renal, hepatic, pulmonary, CNS dysfunction), and death.

Etiology
Septic shock, trauma, malignancy, and obstetrical complications

Diagnosis
There is no single diagnostic test. The following findings suggest DIC:
- Sudden fall in platelet count to <100,000/μL
- Bleeding and/or thrombotic complications
- Increased prothrombin time [PT], partial PT [PTT], INR, FDPs D-dimer, schistocytes
- Decreased fibrinogen and haptoglobin

Management
Treat the underlying disorder. Bleeding should be treated with FFP, platelets, blood, and cryoprecipitate as indicated by coagulation, Hct, and fibrinogen levels (keep fibrinogen >100 mg/dL). Low-dose and cautious heparinization can be considered in patients with predominantly thrombotic complications.

Excessive warfarinization

Warfarin inhibits carboxylation of vitamin K, therefore preventing synthesis of vitamin K–dependent factors (II, VII, IX, X, proteins C and S). Patients on warfarin frequently become excessively anticoagulated largely due to drug interactions (which interfere with absorption and metabolism) or diarrhea, liver failure, and vitamin K deficiency. The risk of bleeding increases with INR ≥5.0, but can occur at lower values in the setting of surgical trauma. Management depends on INR level and evidence of active bleeding.
- INR <5.0, no bleeding: lower daily dose OR skip ≥1 dose, check INR qd, restart warfarin when INR within therapeutic range
- INR >5.0, no bleeding: skip ≥1 dose ± vitamin K (1–2.5 mg) po
- INR >9.0, no bleeding: hold warfarin, vitamin K (5–10 mg) po and repeat prn, follow INR, restart warfarin at lower dose when INR is therapeutic
- If bleeding (regardless of INR): hold warfarin, give vitamin K (10 mg) IV and repeat prn, FFP ± recombinant human factor VIIa
- In patients with mechanical valves, the risk of thromboembolic events when anticoagulation is reversed is <0.1% per day. Anticoagulation with heparin or warfarin should be restarted within 1–2 weeks once bleeding is resolved.

Clinical pearls—physiology of hemostasis

- **Vascular phase**—vasospasm, local edema, and hematoma
- **Platelet phase**—adherence of platelets activated by ADP, collagen, and von Willebrand factor and mediated by IIb/IIIa, fibrinogen, 5-HT, thromboxane A_2
- **Clotting phase**:
  - **Intrinsic** (kallikrein, XII, XI, and IX)
  - **Extrinsic** (thromboplastin, VII) pathways converge on common pathway (X, thrombin, fibrinogen)
- **Fibrinolysis** depends on plasmin, antithrombin III, proteins C and S, tissue factor pathway inhibitor

Deep venous thrombosis and pulmonary embolism

Deep vein thrombosis (DVT) involves popliteal, femoral, or iliac veins. DVT is common in patients over 40 years of age who are undergoing major surgery. The combination of (1) blood stasis, (2) endothelial injury, and (3) thrombophilia (inherited disorders and acquired) contribute to thrombosis (Virchow's triad). Predisposing factors include the following:

Acquired disorders
- Trauma, major surgery, pelvic or hip surgery, previous history of DVT or pulmonary embolus (PE)
- Malignancy, inflammatory bowel disease, smoking
- Oral contraceptives, pregnancy, hormone replacement therapy, tamoxifen
- Immobilization, extended air travel, indwelling central venous catheter
- Myeloproliferative disorders, hyperviscosity, congestive heart failure, obesity

Inherited disorders
- Deficiency in protein C or S or antithrombin
- Gene mutations in factor V Leiden and prothrombin
- Hyperhomocysteinemia

Diagnosis

Clinical features
- Fever, calf pain, leg swelling, edema, erythema, warmth, tenderness, pain on dorsiflexion (Homan's sign), palpable cord
- May present as PE or, rarely, with acute lower limb ischemia or gangrene with extensive iliofemoral thrombosis (phlegmasia cerulean dolens)

Investigations
- Compression ultrasonography: sensitivity and specificity >95%, but iliac vein and femoral vein DVT are difficult to detect
- Impedance plethysmography: sensitivity, specificity >90%, cumbersome
- Contrast venography: most sensitive and specific but invasive
- D-dimer: with other negative noninvasive tests, can help exclude DVT

Treatment

Idiopathic DVT/PE should prompt a workup for thromboembolic risk factors (malignancy, hypercoagulable state). The goal is to prevent clot progression, prevent PE, and reduce the risk of recurrence and sequelae (postphlebitic syndrome, chronic venous insufficiency).
- Symptomatic isolated distal DVT (calf vein): anticoagulate with heparin (unfractionated or LMWH; see Box 1.11) followed by warfarin for 3 months
- Symptomatic proximal lower extremity or calf vein DVT extending to proximal vein:
  - First idiopathic DVT or PE: warfarin for 6–12 months
  - First DVT or PE in patients with nonreversible risk factors (malignancy, paralysis, protein C deficiency) for minimum of 6–12 months

- - DVT or PE with reversible risk factor (surgery): warfarin for
    3–6 months
  - Recurrent idiopathic DVT/ PE or recurrent DVT/PE in patients with
    nonreversible risk factors: long-term warfarin therapy
- Upper-extremity DVT with indwelling catheter: remove catheter,
  anticoagulate
- Thrombolysis (tPA, streptokinase) or thrombectomy may be required
  for extensive DVT (phlegmasia cerulean dolens).

Pulmonary embolism

Without treatment, PE is associated with a 30% mortality rate. Risk factors
are the same as for DVT. Some 50% of patients with symptomatic DVT
have asymptomatic PE, and 60% of patients with PE have DVT.

Clinical features

- Dyspnea, pleuritic chest pain, tachypnea, tachycardia, crackles, fever,
  cyanosis, loud P2 heart sound. Massive PE is associated with acute right
  ventricular failure, syncope, hypotension, and pulmonary
  endarterectomy (PEA).

Investigations

- Chest X-ray (effusion, atelectasis), ECG (sinus tachycardia, signs of
  right ventricular strain, right bundle branch block), ABG (hypoxemia,
  hypocapnea, respiratory alkalosis, increased A-a gradient), D-dimer
  (elevated)
- CT angiography (most useful, sensitivity and specificity >90%–95%), VQ
  lung scan (low diagnostic accuracy: 15%–86%), pulmonary angiography
  (gold standard, but 5% morbidity)

Treatment

Massive proximal PE, hemodynamic instability, right ventricular dysfunction

- Surgical thrombectomy/embolectomy
- Thrombolysis (except if high risk of bleeding, i.e., surgery in previous
  30days)

Relative hemodynamic stability, small PE

- Sit the patient up, use 100% O_2, non-rebreathing face mask (NRFM),
  may require intubation
- IV access, start anticoagulation with heparin (unfractionated or
  LMWH) followed by warfarin
- IVC filter: indicated if anticoagulation is contraindicated or results in
  complications (active bleeding), if recurrent PE during adequate antico-
  agulation, or in bilateral ileofemoral DVT to prevent PE
- Workup for PE/DVT

Box 1.11 Anticoagulation

Acute
- IV unfractionated heparin: 80 units/kg bolus, then 18 units/kg/hr, titrate to goal PTT 60–85 sec
- Low molecular weight heparin (LMWH): enoxaparin 1 mg/kg SC bid or dalteparin 200 IU/kg SC qd

Long-term
- Warfarin: start when PTT therapeutic or after first dose of LMWH, overlap for 5 days with heparin, goal INR 2–3

Thrombolysis
- Tissue plasminogen activator (tPA) over 2 hr or 0.6 mg/kg over 3–15 min

Risk scoring

Scoring systems that quantify the severity of illness have been developed to objectively evaluate clinical outcomes in response to various interventions and compare outcomes across institutions. In addition, scoring systems can help predict prognosis more accurately.

Examples of risk scoring systems

- Predict the risk of dying in hospital (APACHE III)
- Quantify morbidity (ASA score, Apgar score)
- Quantify symptoms (NYHA angina classification)
- Predict operative mortality (EUROscore, Parsonnet score in cardiac surgery, POSSUM)
- Predict risk of dying on waiting list (New Zealand score in cardiac surgery)
- Predicting risk of dying for specific illnesses (Ranson criteria in pancreatitis, MELD score in end-stage liver disease)

APACHE III (Acute Physiology and Chronic Health Evaluation) scoring system

This predicts a patient's risk of dying in the hospital. Twenty-seven patient variables (physiological variables, such as core temperature, heart rate, BP, creatinine, age, and chronic illness variables) are entered into a program that gives a score, which can be compared against previous performance to give a risk of dying in the hospital. There are approximately 60 hospitals worldwide where the APACHE III methodology is used to generate reports that compare their actual average ICU outcomes with those predicted by the APACHE III methodology.

EuroSCORE (European System for Cardiac Risk Evaluation)

This is a weighted additive score, based on a European sample of cardiac surgical patients. Variables such as age, renal function, and comorbidity are given points that add up to an approximate percentage of predicted perioperative mortality. Scoring systems like this are useful when consenting patients for surgery, and in risk-stratifying operative outcomes so that surgeons and hospitals can be compared with each other.

POSSUM (Physiologic and Operative Severity Score for the enUmeration of Mortality and morbidity)

This is a weighted additive score. Eighteen variables are combined to produce a physiological score and an operative score, which in turn are combined to produce an estimate of the percentage risk of defined morbidity and mortality. (Variants exist for vascular, orthopedic, and colorectal surgery).

Hypotension in the recovery room

Evaluation

- Treat like a trauma case, assess ABCs, and complete primary and secondary survey.
- Assess the airway and breathing; if the patient is on a ventilator, check for bilateral breath sounds and check tube connections.
- Repeat BP in both arms, check pulses, check the cardiac monitor for heart rate and rhythm, check for evidence of ischemia, review all ins and outs.
- Review recent infusions (blood, anti-arrhythmics, BP medications, antibiotics).
- Physical exam: Is the patient cold and clammy (hypovolemic shock) or warm and flushed (anaphylactic shock)? Is there evidence of pulmonary edema and JVD (cardiogenic shock)?
- Check all wounds for bleeding or hematoma, and check output and effluent from all drains.
- Order chest X-ray, 12-lead ECG, ABG, CBC, electrolytes, coagulation, cardiac enzymes.
- Bolus with crystalloids, unless cardiogenic shock is suspected
- If fluid status and etiology of hypotension are still unclear, place central line and pulmonary artery catheter.

Differential diagnosis

- Hypovolemia, postoperative bleeding
- Cardiogenic shock (myocardial infarction, cardiac tamponade, arrhythmia)
- Pneumothorax, aspiration, ventilator failure
- Infection (sepsis)
- Blood transfusion reaction
- Malignant hyperthermia
- Acute adrenal failure (Addisonian crisis)
- Air/fat/pulmonary embolism

Treatment

Treatment should be directed to specific causes.

- Aggressive fluid resuscitation, blood transfusion, reverse coagulopathy, reexploration
- Echocardiogram, pericardiocentesis, antiplatelet agents, fluid restriction, inotropic support, anti-arrhymics, cardioversion
- Chest tube placement, intubation, change ventilator
- Blood cultures, broad-spectrum antibiotics
- Stop blood transfusion, provide supportive care
- Dantrolene, aggressive fluid resuscitation, cooling, supportive care
- Stress-dose steroids, aggressive fluid resuscitation
- Anticoagulation, supportive care

ICU admission

Recognizing the critically ill surgical patient

Intubated patients and patients requiring inotropic support or dialysis require ICU admission. The goal is to identify hemodynamically unstable patients early and stabilize them before they become critical or avoid delays in transfer to the ICU.

Signs that a patient might be in critical condition

- **History**. "I feel like I'm going to die." *Timor mortis* (fear of dying) may accompany MI, hypovolemic shock, and respiratory failure. Evaluate the patient promptly.
- **Nurses**. "Mr Smith just doesn't look right." Experienced nurses quickly recognize the patterns of critical illness, take them seriously, and evaluate the patient promptly.
- **General**. Hypothermia or high fevers, rigors, acute change in drain output and/or character, profuse bleeding from wounds
- **Cardiovascular**. Chest pain, drop in BP, persistent tachycardia, new arrhythmias
- **Respiratory**. Tachypnea, hypoxia
- **Renal**. Oliguria, anuria
- **Gastrointestinal**. GI bleed, new-onset nausea and vomiting, hiccup, peritoneal signs
- **Neurological**. Acute confusion, agitation or drowsiness, seizures

Immediate management

Identify and treat potentially life-threatening conditions (cardiac or respiratory failure, severe hypotension, arrhythmia with hemodynamic compromise). Once stabilized, reassess the patient's condition (critical, guarded, fair), and make a plan regarding further need for cardiac monitoring, diagnostic tests, and therapeutic interventions.

- Quickly assess airway, breathing, and circulation. Follow advanced life support (ALS) algorithm, manage seizure, hemorrhage, and shock.
- Intubate the patient or place on NRFM and high-flow O_2.
- Secure IV access, place Foley catheter, send labs including arterial blood gas, 12-lead ECG, and chest X-ray.
- Resuscitate the patient unless you suspect pump failure and fluid overload.
- Review medications, recent vital sign trends, fluid balance, radiologic studies, blood cultures, and labs.
- Focused history and examination: Are there recent symptoms? Change in diet or medications? Recent procedure, removal or insertion of drains?
- Evaluate condition: does the patient need to go to the operating room, or be transferred to a surgical, cardiac, or neurology ICU or to a step-down bed? Make the appropriate arrangements.
- If additional diagnostic tests are needed (CT scan), is the patient stable enough for transport and the procedure?

Step-down unit (SDU)
The SDU allows a level of care between ICU and the regular floor. Vital signs are monitored frequently with cardiac monitors and invasive monitoring (arterial line, CVP tracing). Vasoconstrictors (pressors) are routine but ventilation, dialysis, and inotropic support are not. The nurse-to-patient ratio is higher. Patients in guarded condition who require aggressive pulmonary toilet, frequent ins and outs, cardiac monitoring, aggressive wound care, and close observation should be admitted to the SDU.

Intensive care unit
The ICU offers advanced ventilatory, inotropic support, renal replacement therapy, full invasive monitoring, and more aggressive nursing care (see Box 1.12).

Box 1.12 Guidelines for admission to the ICU

- Need for mechanical ventilation
- Failure of two or more organ systems
- Need for advanced monitoring (pulmonary artery catheter)
- Need for inotropic support and more invasive cardiac support (intra-aortic balloon pump, external pacer)
- Consultant involvement is essential (cardiology, infectious disease, gastroenterology, etc.)
- Patient's advanced directives should be reviewed from records.

The surgical team should consider ICU admission for both elective and emergency surgical patients
- Anticipate whether patients undergoing elective procedures will require ICU admission postoperatively (high-risk patients, high-risk procedure, i.e., Whipple, lobectomy, vascular bypass).
- Anticipate patients with low pulmonary reserve preoperatively in whom you anticipate difficulty weaning from the ventilator postoperatively.
- Plan transfer postoperatively if a surgical procedure was complicated by significant bleeding, coagulopathy, or hemodynamic instability.
- Plan ICU transfer for emergency cases due to anticipated massive fluid shifts and hemodynamic instability (trauma, ruptured AAA).

Common ICU terminology

Cardiac function—see cardiothoracic surgery
Hemodynamic status—see invasive monitoring and circulatory support

Oxygenation and ventilation

$PaCO_2$

- *Ventilation*, the movement of air in and out of the lungs, is described in terms of minute volume (respiratory rate × tidal volume), and assessed by measuring the partial pressure of CO_2 in arterial blood ($PaCO_2$).

PaO_2

- *Oxygenation*, the amount of oxygen in arterial blood, is described in terms of the partial pressure of oxygen in arterial blood (PaO_2).
- Oxygenation is dependent on minute volumes until they are very low.
- In postoperative patients the primary cause of hypoxia is atelectasis, which must be reversed before the patient can benefit from increasing the fraction of oxygen in inspired air (FiO_2).
- Positive end expiratory pressure (PEEP) and continuous positive airway pressure (CPAP) treat and prevent atelectasis and improve PaO_2.
- In patients on the ventilator, hypoxemia can be improved by increasing FiO_2 and/or PEEP.

SvO_2

- Oxygen consumption is assessed indirectly by measuring the percentage saturation of mixed venous hemoglobin with oxygen (SvO_2). SvO_2 varies inversely with the amount of oxygen extracted from peripheral tissues. SvO_2 can be measured from blood drawn from the distal port of the pulmonary artery (PA) catheter (PA or mixed venous blood).

Lung volumes

- Pulmonary ventilation is described in terms of four "volumes"—*tidal volume* (TV), *inspiratory reserve volume* (IRV), *expiratory reserve volume* (ERV), and *residual volume* (RV)—that may be combined to give four "capacities": *inspiratory capacity* (IC), *functional residual capacity* (FRC), *vital capacity* (VC), and *total lung capacity* (TLC). Loss of FRC through atelectasis, supine position, lobar consolidation and collapse, effusions, and obesity results in hypoxia. CPAP, PEEP, and physiotherapy are aimed at limiting this loss.

Hemodynamic monitoring

Central venous pressure (CVP)

- Central venous pressure is recorded from the proximal port of the PA catheter located in the superior vena cava or right atrium.

Pulmonary capillary wedge pressure (PCWP)

- When the pulmonary artery (PA) catheter is in proper position, inflation of the balloon at the tip of the catheter causes pulsatile PA pressure to disappear, which is considered to be the pressure in the pulmonary microcirculation, or PCWP. This pressure is often used as a reflection of left-ventricular filling during diastole (ventricular preload). Assuming normal compliance of the ventricle and absence of aortic insufficiency, PCWP is the most accurate reflection of left ventricular preload, left atrial pressure, and left-ventricular end-diastolic pressure (PCWP = LAP = LVEDP).

Invasive monitoring

Invasive monitoring is used in the ICU. It provides accurate and sensitive real-time measurements, access for frequent blood draws, and administration of medications.

Arterial monitoring

The radial artery is a favored site for arterial cannulation (it is most superficial, accessible, and easy to keep clean). Additional sites include the ulnar, brachial, and femoral arteries.

Indications

- Precise BP measurement and arterial blood gas sampling

Contraindications

- **Absolute**. Infection at the site of insertion, distal limb ischemia
- **Relative**. Coagulopathy, proximal arterial obstruction, surgical considerations, radial artery contraindicated if positive Allen test (inadequate collateral flow through the ulnar artery if the radial artery is occluded)

Complications

- Arterial occlusion, digital ischemia, hematoma, infection

Central venous pressure lines

The subclavian vein is the most commonly used central venous access, followed by the internal jugular vein and femoral vein.

Indications

- Continual right atrial pressure measurements in patients requiring circulatory support
- Infusion port for some drugs that cannot be administered peripherally
- Insertion PA catheter or transvenous pacing wires
- Infusion port for TPN

Contraindications

- **Absolute**. SVC syndrome, infection at the site of insertion
- **Relative**. Coagulopathy, undrained contralateral pneumothorax, uncooperative patient. DVT of the head and neck vessels may make cannulation difficult. Patients with septal defects are at risk of cardiovascular accident (CVA) from air emboli caused by poor technique

Complications

- Accidental puncture or cannulation of the carotid artery, laceration, thrombosis, pneumothorax, hemopneumothorax, venous air embolism, infection

Pulmonary artery catheter

The PA catheter is 7 French in diameter, 110 cm long, and has two internal channels, one that opens at the distal tip (distal port, in the PA) and the other that opens 30 cm from the tip (proximal port, in the right atrium). The tip of the catheter has a balloon and a transducer device that senses changes in temperature on the outer surface of the catheter, 4 cm from the catheter tip (thermistor). By measuring the flow rate of cold fluid injected through the proximal port, calculation of the cardiac output (CO) can be calculated.

Indications

A PA catheter is indicated in patients with refractory hypotension, heart failure, and shock in whom accurate determination of intravascular volume and cardiac function is required. Parameters measured directly from the PA catheter (see common terminology in ICU) include the following:

- CVP, PCWP, CO, right arterial pressure (RAP), right ventricular pressure (RVP), pulmonary artery pressure (PAP), SvO_2
- Several parameters of cardiovascular performance are expressed in relation to body surface area (BSA) and are called *index*.

Parameters derived from the PA catheter:

- CI (cardiac index = CO/BSA)
- SVRI (systemic vascular resistance index = (MAP − RAP) x 80/CI
- SVI (stroke volume index = CI/heart rate)
- DO_2 (arterial O_2 delivery = CI x 13.4 x Hb x SaO_2)
- Oxygen uptake (VO_2 = CI x 13.4 x Hb x (SaO_2 − SvO_2))

Contraindications

Contraindications are as for central venous catheters. Those specific to PA catheterization include tricuspid or pulmonic valvular stenosis, RA and RV masses that may embolize, tetralogy of Fallot, severe arrhythmias, and coagulopathy.

Complications

Complications of insertion are the same as for CVP lines, with specific complications related to the pulmonary catheter, including atrial and ventricular arrhythmias, and PA infarction or perforation

Waveforms (Fig. 1.7)

Arterial waveform

Fast upstroke, slower downstroke with a notch that represents aortic valve closure.

Central venous pressure waveform

Three upstrokes (the *a*, *c*, and *v* waves) and two descents (the *x* and *y* descent). The *a* wave—atrial systole; *v* wave—venous return filling the right atrium; *c* wave—bulging of the closed tricuspid valve cusps into the right atrium. The *x* descent occurs in atrial diastole. The *y* descent occurs in ventricular diastole

Pulmonary artery pressure waveform

Waveform progression during correct insertion of the PA catheter shows the following:

1. Oscillations in the pressure recordings (catheter tip advanced from the vena cava to the right atrium, pressure 1–6 mm Hg). The balloon should be fully inflated ("balloon up") and the catheter slowly advanced.

2. A sudden increase in systolic pressure as the catheter crosses the tricuspid valve into the right ventricle with pulsatile waveform (systolic pressure 15–30 mmHg, diastolic pressure is the same as the RAP)

3. As the catheter crosses the pulmonary valve into the PA, the diastolic pressure increases while the systolic pressure remains unchanged (diastolic pressure 6–12 mmHg).

4. As the catheter is advanced along the PA, the systolic component of the waveform abruptly disappears ("wedging"), leaving the PCWP, which is the same as the PA diastolic pressure. At this point, the catheter should no longer be advanced and the balloon should be deflated ("balloon down"). The pulsatile PA pressure will reappear.

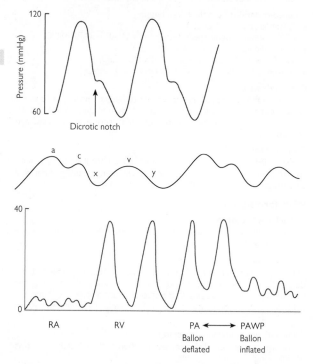

Fig. 1.7 (a) Arterial waveform. (b) Central venous pressure waveform, and responses to fluid boluses. (c) Pulmonary artery pressure waveform.

Ventilatory support

Invasive methods

Indications

- Apnea, improve gas exchange (oxygenation and alveolar ventilation)
- Relieve respiratory distress (decrease work of breathing and respiratory muscle fatigue)
- Protect the airway, aggressive pulmonary toilet

Positive end-expiratory pressure (PEEP)

Instead of allowing airway pressures to fall to zero at the end of expiration, a small positive airway pressure is maintained throughout expiration (PEEP), preventing collapse of small airways and alveoli at the end of expiration.

- FRC, intrapulmonary shunts, lung compliance, and PaO_2 are improved, and the work of breathing is reduced.
- High levels of PEEP (>15 cm H_2O) may be necessary to reverse established atelectasis but raise intrathoracic pressure, and reduce venous return and cardiac output, which may in turn reduce PaO_2. High PEEP is associated with a risk of barotrauma (pneumothorax).
- PEEP as low as 5 cm H_2O may cause hemodynamic compromise in the setting of poor LV function.
- Physiological PEEP is provided by an intact glottis: patients with COPD purse their lips during expiration to increase physiological PEEP.

Ventilator modes

Assist control ventilation (ACV)

In this volume-cycled ventilation, the machine breathes at a pre-selected rate and inflation volume is provided. The patient can initiate a breath that will trigger a fully assisted machine breath. It is the preferred mode for patients in the OR with respiratory muscle weakness. Disadvantages include the potential to overventilate and decreased time for exhalation, leading to hyperinflation.

Intermittent mandatory ventilation (IMV)

In this volume-cycled ventilation, machine-initiated breaths are given at a preselected rate and volume but spontaneous breathing is allowed. In synchronized IMV (SIMV), positive airway pressure may be synchronized with patient-initiated breaths but each spontaneous breath does not always trigger a machine breath, which reduces the risk of hyperinflation. Machine-initiated breaths are given if no spontaneous breaths occur in a preset time. This mode is the preferred setting for patients who are spontaneously breathing (awake). Disadvantages include increased work of breathing during spontaneous breaths to overcome the resistance of breathing through ventilator circuits.

Pressure-controlled ventilation (PCV)

PCV is pressure-cycled ventilation where the patient can initiate each mechanical breath, but when this is not possible, machine breaths at a preselected pressure are administered. Inspiratory flow decreases during lung inflation to reduce peak airway pressures and improve gas exchange. Disadvantages include the variability of inflation volumes.

Inverse-ratio ventilation (IRV)

In this pressure-cycled ventilation, PCV is combined with prolonged inflation time. During conventional volume-cycled ventilation, the inspiratory-to-expiratory duration ratio of 1:2 or 1:4 is reversed to 2:1 in IRV. Prolonged inflation time helps prevent alveolar collapse. Disadvantages include potential inadequate emptying of the lung, leading to hyperinflation and auto-PEEP. It is the preferred mode for patients with ARDS with refractory hypoxemia or hypercapnea during conventional modes of mechanical ventilation.

Pressure support ventilation (PSV)

Patient-initiated breaths can be supported with a preset inspiratory pressure. The ventilator detects the drop in airway pressures as the patient begins inspiration and assists air inflow with a positive airway pressure (5–10 cm H_2O). This is a mode of partial ventilation, since it does not provide full ventilatory support. It is used to augment inflation volumes during spontaneous breathing to overcome the resistance of breathing through ventilator circuits.

Other ventilator settings

After choosing a ventilator mode, other settings that need to be set include respiratory rate, tidal volume, FiO_2 (fraction of inspired air that is O_2), PEEP, inspiratory time (I:E usually 1:2 or 1:4 except in IRV), inspiratory flow rate, peak inspiratory pressure (PIP), and plateau pressure.

Noninvasive methods

Continuous positive airway pressure (CPAP)

In CPAP, positive pressure is maintained throughout the respiratory cycle. The patient does not have to generate a negative airway pressure to receive the inhaled gas, which eliminates the work of inhaling. 100% O_2 can be administered. CPAP is delivered through specialized tight-fitting face masks or nasal masks. It is used in extubated cooperative patients with COPD and obstructive sleep-apnea. CPAP is used primarily for hypoxemia

Biphasic positive pressure ventilation (BiPAP)

BiPAP is a solution to the problem of air trapping, particularly for those with COPD on CPAP. Airway pressure (inspiratory and expiratory) is cycled at preset rates between high and low levels. BiPAP is used primarily for hypoventilation.

Face masks

- The Venturi face mask has a valve that draws in an amount of air through calibrated inlets which is mixed with O_2 before entering the mask. The maximum FiO_2 that can be delivered by a Venturi mask is about 60%.
- The low-flow face mask has a set rate of O_2 flowing into the mask which is diluted by air drawn into the mask. The maximum FiO_2 that can reliably be delivered is about 30%. Use of a non-rebreathing mask and reservoir bag, into which high-flow O_2 is drawn during expiration and then inhaled, increases FiO_2 to up to 60%.

Nasal prongs

- These are less obtrusive, allowing the patient to expectorate and eat. They increase tracheal FiO_2 to slightly more than room air levels, particularly if the patient breathes through their mouth.

Circulatory support

Principles

Improvement of cardiac function and end-organ perfusion involves
- Careful fluid balance to optimize preload or "filling"
- Use of vasoconstrictors and vasodilators to optimize afterload
- Use of inotropes and chronotropes to improve cardiac output
- Mechanical support in selected cases

Vasopressors (cause vasoconstriction)

- α_1-adrenergic stimulation causes vasoconstriction and increases SVR and PVR.
- Some agents also have β_1- and β_2-adrenergic effects.

Phenylephrine 10–300 μg/min

Synthetic adrenergic agonist
- Action: direct α_1 agonist
- Indication: hypotension due to low SVR
- Does not act on heart directly

Norepinephrine (noradrenaline) 1–40 μg/min

Catecholamine produced by the adrenal medulla
- Action: direct α_1 agonist, which predominates over β_1-agonist effect
- Indication: hypotension due to septic or cardiogenic shock, primarily acts to increase SVR
- Can be associated with end-organ ischemia

Vasopressin 0.01–1.0 U/min

- Action: acts on vasopressin receptor to cause vasoconstriction
- Indication: hypotension due to low SVR
- Can be associated with end-organ ischemia

Epinephrine 2–20 μg/min or bolus in cardiac arrest

Catecholamine produced by the adrenal medulla
- Action: Direct agonist at α_1, α_2, β_1, β_2 receptors
- Indications: (1) cardiac arrest (asystole, VF, PEA), (2) anaphylaxis (SQ dosage different from dosage used during cardiac arrest), (3) shock
- Not first-line agent for shock because of narrow therapeutic window and risk of adverse effects, including arrhythmia, coronary ischemia

Dopamine 0.5–>10 μg/kg/min

Endogenous catecholamine
- Action: at lower doses (0.5–3 μg/kg/min), preferential activation of dopamine receptors in renal, mesenteric, and cerebral circulation to increase blood flow to these tissues. At intermediate doses (3–7.5 μg/kg/min), activates β_1 and β_2 receptors in heart and peripheral circulation, increasing cardiac output. At higher doses (>7.5 μg/kg/min), activates α-receptors, causing vasoconstriction
- Indications: (1) low dose for oliguric renal failure, (2) cardiogenic shock, (3) septic shock
- Continued administration is associated with tachyphylaxis. Dopamine can cause supraventricular and ventricular arrhythmia. The most serious complication is limb ischemia.

Inotropes (increase contractility)

- β_1 stimulation leads to increased contractility, heart rate, and conduction.
- β_2 stimulation causes peripheral dilatation and bronchodilation.
- Dopamine stimulation causes coronary, renal, and mesenteric vasodilatation.
- The β_2 effect can cause hypotension if the vasodilatory effect outweighs the β_1 effect

Milrinone 0.375–0.75 μg/kg/min

Phosphodiesterase inhibitor

- Action: potent inotropic and vasodilator effects. Does not stimulate adrenergic receptors
- Indication: low cardiac output state in the setting of increased SVR
- Dose adjustment is needed in renal dysfunction. Can cause supraventricular and ventricular arrhythmia

Dobutamine 2–20 μg/kg/min

Synthetic catecholamine

- Action: potent inotrope via β_1 effects. Also has milder β_2-agonist effects, which can cause vasodilatation
- Indication: low cardiac output state in the setting of increased SVR
- Can cause supraventricular and ventricular arrhythmia

Chronotropes (increase heart rate)

- β_1 stimulation leads to increased contractility, heart rate, and conduction.
- Muscarinic cholinergic activity is predominantly parasympathetic.

Atropine (0.5–1 mg IV bolus)

Atropine is a belladonna alkaloid.

- Action: a competitive antagonist at muscarinic cholinergic receptors, reducing parasympathetic tone to "reveal" underlying sympathetic tone
- Indication: bradyarrhythmias, reduction of oral secretions
- Can be given down endotracheal (ET) tube if there is no IV access

Isoproterenol (0.1–10 μg/min)

Synthetic catecholamine

- Action: direct β_1 and β_2 agonist effects. No α activity
- Indication: bradycardia unresponsive to atropine

Mechanical support

Intra-aortic balloon counterpulsation

The intra-aortic balloon pump (IABP) is a polyethylene balloon filled with helium, ranging from 2 to 50 cm^3 in size, that sits in the descending aorta just distal to the left subclavian artery. The balloon inflates in early diastole, improving coronary perfusion, and deflates just before systole, reducing afterload. The myocardial oxygen supply:demand ratio is improved. Cardiac output may be increased by up to 40%.

The IABP is indicated for weaning from cardiopulmonary bypass, refractory ischemia, and cardiogenic shock. It is contraindicated in aortic regurgitation (balloon inflation during diastole will worsen AR) and aortic dissection.

Ventricular assist devices (VADs)

VADs are pumps that are anastomosed to the great vessels and cardiac chambers to support failing the right, left, or both ventricles. They can be used as a "bridge" to transplantation or as "destination" therapy for patients who are not transplant candidates.

Dialysis

Indications for dialysis

- Refractory fluid overload
- Refractory hyperkalemia (K^+>6.5 meq/L) or rapidly rising levels
- Refractory metabolic acidosis (pH <7.1)
- Signs of uremia (encephalopathy, pericarditis)
- Drug toxicity

There are three types of dialysis: hemodialysis (HD), hemofiltration (HF), and peritoneal dialysis (PD).

Hemodialysis and hemofiltration

Hemodialysis and hemofiltration are the two main techniques of renal replacement therapy used in intensive care units. In both techniques access to the circulation is required and blood passes through an extra-corporeal circuit that includes either a dialyser or a hemofilter

Hemodialysis

In hemodialysis, blood flows along one side of a *semipermeable* membrane as the dialysate flows on the other side of the membrane. Fluid is removed via transmembrane pressure gradient and solute via transmembrane concentration gradient. Solute removal is inversely proportional to size: molecules move from high to low concentration, and smaller molecules move faster (effective for removal of K, urea, and Cr but not phosphate). The amount of solute removed depends on its concentration in the dialysis fluid and on the size of the molecule. Larger-size molecules are not effectively removed.

Hemofiltration

In hemofiltration, blood under pressure passes down one side of a *highly permeable* membrane. Fluid and solutes are removed via transmembrane gradient. The filtrate fluid is discarded and replacement fluid is infused. All molecules are removed at a similar rate, including large molecules. Replacement fluid has a solute concentration similar to plasma except for K^+, urea, creatinine, and phosphate.

Types of hemofiltration

Hemofiltration has become an increasingly popular form of renal-replacement therapy for acute renal failure postoperatively, even though it is more expensive than dialysis. This is because the continuous nature of the process avoids the large fluctuations in fluid balance and electrolytes associated with hemodialysis. Hemofiltration is associated with less hypotension than dialysis and allows the removal of inflammatory mediators. There are several variants.

Continuous arteriovenous hemofiltration (CAVH)

This is the original and simplest form of filtration. The femoral artery and vein are cannulated, and blood passes through the hemofilter under arterial pressure alone. It is therefore less appropriate for patients with low cardiac output states. The rate of solute clearance is relatively low. Prolonged arterial cannulation carries complications.

Continuous arteriovenous hemodialysis with filtration

Because of the low solute clearance rates with CAVH, a dialysis circuit is added to the equipment, improving clearance rates at considerable cost.

Continuous venovenous hemofiltration (CVVH)

An occlusive extracorporeal blood pump is incorporated into the circuit to drive blood so that venous cannulation is all that is required. This also allows control of blood flow and filtration rate. Clearance of up to 100 mL/min can be achieved. This is the most commonly used system in ICUs.

Continuous venovenous hemodialysis with filtration

Some systems add hemodialysis to the CVVH circuit for additional fine control.

Management of the hemofiltered patient

- A double-lumen catheter (Vascath) is inserted into a central vein (subclavian, internal jugular, or femoral vein).
- Anticoagulation with heparin is required to maintain the patency of the extracorporeal circuit.
- Complications include hypotension, bleeding, clotting of the dialyser, access-related difficulties, and electrolyte and fluid imbalance.

Peritoneal dialysis

The peritoneum acts as a membrane. Fluid balance is controlled by glucose concentration in the dialysate. PD can be performed intermittently or continuously, manually or with an automated device.

Relative to HD and HF, PD has several advantages:

- It is relatively easy to perform with easy peritoneal access, especially in children.
- Large amounts of fluid can be removed with gradual correction of acid–base and metabolite imbalances in hemodynamically unstable patients.
- Arterial and venous access and anticoagulation are not required.

PD is contraindicated in patients with recent abdominal surgery, intra-abdominal infection, severe respiratory failure, and severe fluid overload of hyperkalemia (fluid and K^+ are not removed as quickly as other methods). Complications include hyperglycemia and peritonitis.

Enteral and parenteral support

Also see Nutrition in surgical patients.

Enteral nutrition

Depletion of nutrients in the bowel lumen is accompanied by degenerative changes in the bowel mucosa and translocation of enteric pathogens across the bowel mucosa with subsequent risk of sepsis. Enteral nutrition is the preferred method of feeding and should be initiated when nutrient intake has been inadequate for 7–10 days.

Routes and methods for supplemented enteral nutrition
- Nasogastric/Duotube
- Percutaneous endoscopic gastrostomy (PEG) and jejunostomy (PEJ)
- Open surgical gastrostomy or jejunostomy

Examples of enteral feeds

- Standard feeds: Osmolite®, Isocal®, Enrich®, Ensure®, Ultracal®
- Fiber enriched: Jevity®, Nutren® 1.0 with fiber, Ultracal®, Fibersource®, Glucerna®, Profiber®
- High energy: Ensure® plus, Deliver® 2.0, Isocal®

Standard feeds provide approximately 1 kcal/mL based on carbohydrate content. They also contain 35–40 g of protein/L (intact proteins). Fiber-enriched feeds contain soy polysaccharides that remain undigested in the colon, where they are fermented by bacteria to produce short-chain fatty acids promoting absorption of sodium and water and reducing diarrhea. They are also probiotic. High-energy feeds provide 1.5 to 2 kcal/mL and are used in patients with high daily energy needs requiring reduced fluid input. The lipid content of most feeds is 30% of total calories.
- Patients with renal failure require high-energy, low-volume, and electrolyte feeds. Nepro® provides 2 kcal/mL and high protein content.
- Patients with respiratory failure require high lipids. Pulmocare® uses lipids that provide 55% of total calories (to reduce CO_2 production).
- Patients with impaired intestinal absorption (diarrhea, inflammatory bowel disease) require formulas rich in small peptides rather than intact protein to facilitate absorption (Peptamen®).

Indications for supplementary enteral feeding
- Inadequate oral intake due to anorexia, dysphagia, altered mental status, induced nausea, chronic ventilatory support
- Hypercatabolism exceeding normal intake (e.g., chronic major sepsis, malignancy, trauma, burns)
- Gut intact but absorption impaired by excessive losses, chronic diarrhea, high-output stoma or fistula

Contraindications to enteral feeding
- Patients in circulatory shock
- Intestinal ischemia
- Partial or complete mechanical bowel obstruction or ileus

Complications of supplementary enteral feeding

- **Complications of feeding tube**. Malposition, blockage (wound infection around jejunostomy tubes)
- **Complications of administration**. Aspiration (the risk of aspiration of gastric feeds is the same as that for duodenal feeds), diarrhea, bloating, nausea, cramps
- **Complications of contents**. Vitamin and trace mineral deficiencies, electrolyte imbalances, drug interactions

Diarrhea is the most common complication of enteral feeding. Reducing the osmotic load is effective (using half-strength feed or slowing the infusion). Omeprazole, Lomotil®, and erythromycin may be tried. It is mandatory to exclude other causes of diarrhea, especially infectious causes (Clostridium difficile).

Parenteral feeding (TPN and PPN)

TPN consists of specially formulated feed given IV. Because TPN solutions have high osmolality, they cause thrombophlebitis if infused into peripheral veins. TPN is given via central lines (subclavian or internal jugular), which may be tunneled for long-term use. PPN osmolarity is much lower than that of TPN.

- Final TPN formulation consists in a dextrose–amino acid mixture (needed to deliver estimated daily protein and calorie requirements), lipids, electrolyte mixture, multivitamins, and trace elements (chromium, copper, manganese, zinc, selenium). A standard TPN mixture is made of 10% amino acid and 50% dextrose, and 10% lipid emulsion.
- To prevent osmotic damage to peripheral vessels, PPN must be delivered with dilute amino acid and dextrose solutions, and since lipids are isotonic, they can be used to provide a significant proportion of non-protein calories. A standard mixture is made of 3% amino acids, 20% dextrose, and 10% lipids.

Indications of parenteral feeding

- Failure of bowel to absorb food (radiation damage, severe acute enteritis, or malabsorption syndromes) or contraindications to enteral feeding
- Failure of adequate length of bowel for absorption (short-bowel syndrome)
- GI tract not accessible for enteral route (acute severe pancreatitis, esophagogastric surgery, or disease in which tube feeding is not possible)
- Failure of enteral feeding to meet nutritional needs

Complications of parenteral feeding

- Complications of central venous catheter insertion
- Intestinal mucosal atrophy (predisposes to translocation of enteric pathogens across bowel mucosa and subsequent septicemia)
- Acalculous cholecystitis
- Late complications: line sepsis, migration, erosion, DVT, occlusion
- Metabolic complications (hyperglycemia, hypophosphotemia, fatty liver, hypercapnea from CO_2 retention)

Sepsis, SIRS, MODS, and ALI

Systemic inflammatory response syndrome (SIRS) is a pro-inflammatory state that does not include a documented source of infection. It may lead to multiple-organ dysfunction syndrome (MODS).

Box 1.13 Definitions of SIRS, sepsis, MODS, ALI, & ARDS

SIRS
- Any two or more of the four following signs:
  - Heart rate >90 beats/min
  - Tachypnea >20 breaths/min
  - Temperature >38°C or <36°C
  - White blood count >12 × 10⁹/L (or <4 × 10⁹/L)
- *Without* identifiable bacteremia or need for organ support *and* in the setting of a known cause of endothelial inflammation, such as:
  - Suspected infection
  - Pancreatitis
  - Ischemia
  - Multiple trauma and tissue injury
  - Hemorrhagic shock
  - Immune-mediated organ injury

Sepsis
- SIRS with a suspected or proven infection

Multiple-organ dysfunction syndrome (MODS)
- Presence of altered organ function in an acutely ill patient such that homeostasis cannot be maintained without intervention

Acute lung injury (ALI)
- Acute onset
- $PaO_2/FiO_2 \leq 300$
- Bilateral infiltrates on chest X-ray
- Pulmonary artery wedge pressure <18 mmHg or no clinical evidence of raised left atrial pressure

Acute/adult respiratory distress syndrome (ARDS)
- As for ALI, except PaO_2/FiO_2 <200

Pathophysiology

The pathophysiology entails systems involved in inflammation, immunity, ischemia, and homeostasis, including complement, clotting and cytokine cascades, cell-mediated immunity, and humoral immunity.
- Metabolic acidosis is a frequent accompaniment to SIRS and is principally due to lactate.
- SIRS may affect all organ systems and may lead to MODS.
- Cell-signaling molecules involved include interleukins IL-1, IL-5, and IL-6, chemokines, and tumor necrosis factor (TNF).

- Theories on SIRS development include
  - Immunologically mediated inflammation
  - Increased intestinal permeability and colonization with gram-negative anaerobes that produce endotoxins that migrate across the mucosa to drive the inflammatory and immune response

ALI and ARDS

These conditions can be the result of direct lung injury (pneumonia, aspiration, inhalation injury, lung contusion, near drowning) or indirect injury (sepsis, shock, DIC, pancreatitis, trauma, transfusion). ARDS is one end of the continuum of ALI.

Management of ALI/ARDS and SIRS/sepsis

- Management of ALI is supportive, including low tidal-volume ventilation ($V_T \leq 6$ mL/kg), minimizing barotrauma ($P_{plat} \leq 30$ cm H_2O), and PEEP to prevent alveolar collapse. Steroids are of no clear benefit and may be harmful. Experimental treatment includes inhaled nitric oxide, prone ventilation, and extracorporeal membrane oxygenation (ECMO).
- Management of sepsis involves identification and treatment of the underlying cause. Early goal-directed therapy (EGDT) involves supplemental oxygen and mechanical ventilation, administration of fluids to a target CVP of 8–12, use of vasoactive agents for MAP <65 mmHg, transfusion of red blood cells, and use of inotropic agents when SvO_2 <70%.

Surgical statistics

Summarizing simple data

This pattern of results (see Table 1.5) is called a **normal** or **Gaussian distribution**: the curve is a symmetrical **bell-shaped curve**. Height, weight, age, serum sodium, and BP are other examples of normally distributed data.

- The **mean** is the same as the **average**: add up every result and divide by the number of results. The average Hb here is 11.1 g/dL.
- The **standard deviation** (SD) is a measure of how spread out the values are: result − mean = its deviation.

  $\sqrt{(\text{sum of deviations}^2/(\text{sample size} - 1))}$ = SD. Here SD = 1.6 g/dL.

- With normally distributed data the mean   1 SD includes 68% of observations;   2 SD includes 95%;   3 SD includes 99%.

This pattern of results (see Table 1.6) is called a **skewed** distribution. Postoperative blood loss, length of stay, and survival all show skewed distributions.

- Don't use mean and standard deviations to summarize skewed data.
- The mean blood requirement is skewed to 8 units of blood because of one outlier (*).
- The best summary statistic for skewed data is the **median** (2 units of blood, which is the value exactly halfway through the sample).
- The **interquartile range** is what the middle 50% of observations were (1–2 units here) and should be used instead of standard deviations when summarizing skewed data.

Table 1.5 Auditing preoperative Hb in 100 patients

Hb (g/dL)	No. patients	Hb (g/dL)	No. patients
7–7.9	1	11–11.9	36
8–8.9	3	12–12.9	9
9–9.9	9	13–13.9	4
10–10.9	37	14–14.9	2

Table 1.6 Auditing postoperative blood transfusions in 100 patients

Units of blood	No. patients	Units of blood	No. patients
0	1	4	5
1	34	5–10	1
2	41	10–20	0
3	17	20–30	1*

* Outlier

Tests

	Disease present	No disease
Test is positive:	a	b
Test is negative:	c	d

Sensitivity (a/(a+c)). A measure of how good the test is at correctly identifying a positive result (>98% is very sensitive). If a very **sen**sitive test is negative it rules the condition **out**.

Specificity (d/(b+d)). A measure of how good the test is at correctly identifying a negative result (>98% is very sensitive). If a very specific test is negative it rules the condition in.

Likelihood ratio This is the chance that a person testing positive has the disease, divided by the chance that a person testing positive doesn't have the disease, or **sensitivity/(1 – specificity)**. A likelihood ratio >10 is large and represents an almost conclusive increase in the likelihood of disease, <0.1 is an almost conclusive decrease, and 1 signifies no change.

Treatments and hazards

	Outcome event	No outcome event
Exposure	a	b
No exposure (control)	c	d

Absolute risk reduction (ARR) a/(a + b) – c/(c + d). The difference in the event rate between the control and the exposed group. It reflects the prevalence of a disease, and the potency of a treatment or hazard.

Relative risk or risk ratio (RR) a/(a + b)/c/(c + d). The event rate in the exposed group divided by the event rate in the control group. Used in RCT and cohort studies. It is not affected by the prevalence of a disease.

Relative risk reduction (RRR) (a/(a + b) – c/(c + d))/(c/c + d). Absolute risk reduction divided by the control event rate. Reflects disease prevalence.

Number needed to treat (NNT) 1/**ARR**. The number of people that must be treated to prevent one event.

Odds ratio This is the odds of an exposed person having the condition divided by the odds of the control group having the condition. If the event is rare, it approximates to relative risk. Odds ratios are less intuitive than relative risk but they are used because they are
- usually larger;
- mathematically versatile;
- always used in case–control studies and appear in meta-analyses of case–control studies;
- the basis of logistic regression analysis.

Statistical significance

Studies are designed to disprove the **null hypothesis** that findings are due to chance.

- The **p value** is the probability of a study rejecting the null hypothesis if it was true (a **type I error**), i.e., finding a difference where none exists.
- **Statistical significance** is commonly taken as a less than 1 in 20 chance of this happening, i.e., $p < 0.05$.
- **Power** is the probability of detecting an association if one exists. Underpowered trials contain too few patients and may make **type II errors**: accepting the null hypothesis when it is false, i.e., finding no difference where one does exist.
- **95% confidence intervals**, derived from the mean and standard deviation, are the range of results predicted if the study were repeated 95 times.

Other useful terms

Censored data: essentially incomplete data, usually due to variable length of follow-up. This is common in surgical studies because 1) some patients will have been lost to follow-up and 2) patients will have shorter follow-up when they had operations more recently in a study.

Actuarial and Kaplan–Meier survival: two methods used to calculate the percentage of study patients that survive a specified time after an operation when a study provides **censored data**

Survival curves: usually not curves. A linear graph, with percentage survival (or freedom from a complication) on the x-axis and time on the y-axis, which drops as each study patient dies (or gets the complication). If there are thousands of patients in the study, the curve is smooth. If there are very few, it is possible to see individual deaths or events as steps in the graph. Ideally these graphs should have **confidence intervals**.

Confidence intervals: these reflect the precision of the study results. Narrow confidence intervals are better than wide ones, because the confidence interval provides a range of values for the percentage survival (or odds ratio, or other proportion) that has a specified probability (usually 95%) of containing the true value for the entire population from whom the study patients were recruited. Always look for confidence intervals: they give you a "best-case and worst-case" snapshot.

Regression analysis: essentially looking back from a group of patients with a known outcome (e.g., dead/alive) to see whether there were any predictors (e.g., age, recent MI). **Univariate analysis** looks at single variables in turn. **Mulitvariate analysis** looks at a group of variables together: it is used to identify **independent risk factors** for an outcome. For example, age may be found to be a risk factor for postoperative death in univariate analysis, but that is because elderly patients are more likely to have other risk factors for postoperative death (e.g., recent MI). If age is not found to be an independent risk factor in multivariate analysis, it suggests that elderly people without other risk factors (e.g., recent MI) are not at higher risk of postoperative death.

Critical appraisal

Types of study
Studies appraising treatments can take several forms.

Randomized controlled trial (RCT) Prospective study in which participants are allocated to control or treatment groups on a random basis. The RCT is the gold standard for assessing treatment efficacy, but time consuming and expensive to run.

Cohort study Partly prospective study in which two cohorts of patients are identified, one of which was exposed to the treatment and one of which is the control group. They are followed over time to see outcome. Cohort studies are cheaper and quicker than RCT, and suitable for looking at prognosis, but prone to bias or false associations.

Case–control study Retrospective study in which patients with the outcome of interest are identified and paired with patients without the outcome of interest, and the exposure rates are compared. This is the cheapest and quickest way of looking for causation. Bias arises when patients are misclassified as cases or controls.

Case series A collection of anecdotes or case reports

Systematic review Differs from the traditional literature review by applying explicit, systematic, and reproducible methods to retrieve and appraise literature to answer a clearly formulated question. Large amounts of data are summarized and conclusions are more accurate.

Meta-analysis A mathematical synthesis of the results of two or more primary studies increasing the statistical significance of positive overall results. However, it reduces the ability of studies to demonstrate local effects.

Levels of evidence
Studies of treatment/hazard can be arranged in order of decreasing statistical validity:
- Level 1a. Systematic review of RCTs
- Level 1b. High-quality RCT with narrow confidence intervals
- Level 1c. All-or-none case series (either *all* patients died before treatment became available but some now survive *or* some used to die but now with treatment *all* survive)
- Level 2a. Systematic review with homogeneity of cohort studies
- Level 2b. Cohort study or low-quality RCT
- Level 2c. "Outcomes" research
- Level 3a. Systematic review with homogeneity of case–control studies
- Level 3b. Individual case–control study
- Level 4. Case series, and poor-quality cohort and case–control studies
- Level 5. Expert opinion without explicit critical appraisal, or based on physiology, bench research, or first principles

How to appraise a paper

Answer these questions systematically. This information should all be stated explicitly within the manuscript.

How relevant is the paper?

- Does the paper address a clearly focused, important, and answerable clinical question that is relevant to my patients?

How valid are the findings?

- Was the paper published in an independent, peer-reviewed journal?
- Does the paper define the condition to be treated, the patients to be included, the interventions to be compared, and the outcomes to be examined?
- Was a power calculation performed and is the power adequate?
- Were all clinically relevant outcomes reported?
- Was follow-up adequate?
- Were all patients accounted for at the end of the study?
- Was the appropriate study type selected, and was design appropriate?
- Were the statistical methods described and were they appropriate?
- Were the sources of error discussed?

Systematic reviews

- Is the clinical question clearly defined and an acceptable basis for including or excluding papers?
- Was the literature search thorough and were other potentially important sources explored?
- Were trials appropriately included and excluded?
- Was methodological quality assessed and were trials appropriately weighted?

RCTs

- Were patients properly randomized?
- Were patients treated equally apart from the intervention being studied?
- Was analysis on an intention-to-treat basis?
- Are confidence intervals narrow and not overlapping?

Case–control studies

- Were patients correctly classified as case or control?
- Were all patients accounted for at the end of the study?

How important are the results?

- Were the results statistically significant?
- Were the results expressed in terms of numbers needed to treat, and are they clinically important?

How applicable are the findings?

- Were the study patients similar to mine?
- Is the treatment feasible within my practice: is information on safety, tolerability, efficacy, and price presented?

Chapter 2

Surgical pathology

Rubin Rodriguez, MD

Cellular injury

Causative agents

Cellular injury is caused by the following:
- Trauma
- Thermal injury
- Chemicals, including drugs
- Infectious organisms
- Ionizing radiation

Mechanisms of injury

These causative agents cause cell damage via a number of mechanisms.
- **Mechanical disruption**: trauma, freezing, osmotic imbalance
- **Failure of membrane integrity**: failure of ion pumps, cytolysis, trauma
- **Blockage of metabolic pathways**: cellular respiration (e.g., cyanide), protein synthesis (e.g., streptomycin), DNA damage or loss (e.g., X-rays)
- **Deficiency of essential metabolites**: O_2 (ischemia), glucose (diabetic ketoacidosis), hormones (trophic hormones result in apoptosis)
- **Free radicals**: toxins, ischemia–reperfusion injury, intracellular killing of bacteria

Necrosis

Necrosis is death of tissue or cells.

Coagulative necrosis

This is the most common form of necrosis and occurs in all organs. Cells retain their shape as cell proteins coagulate and metabolic activity stops. Digestion by macrophages may cause the tissue to become soft. Histologically there is progressive loss of staining. The presence of necrotic material normally provokes an inflammatory response.

Colliquative necrosis

This occurs in the brain because of the lack of tissue architecture provided by substantial surrounding stroma.

Caseous necrosis

Dead tissue lacks any structure and is characterized by a white, soft, or liquid "cheesy" appearance. This is common in TB.

Gangrene

Gangrene is necrosis with desication or putrefaction.

Fibrinoid necrosis

In malignant hypertension, necrosis of smooth-muscle vessel walls allows seepage of plasma into the media and deposition of fibrin.

Fat necrosis

- Direct trauma: release of extracellular fat produces an inflammatory response, fibrosis, and, eventually, in some cases a palpable mass.
- Acute pancreatitis: fat is digested by pancreatic lipase to produce fatty acids that precipitate with calcium in the process of saponification.

Apoptosis

Apoptosis (programmed cell death) is the cell-mediated, controlled elimination of individual cells.

Apoptosis, an energy-dependent physiological process, is the normal means of maintaining the size of an organ in the face of continuing cell turnover or a reduction in size during atrophy. It is mediated by endogenous endonucleases. The cell shrinks and fragments into apoptotic bodies. Examples include the following:

- Physiological
  - Epithelium of GI tract
  - Bone marrow
  - Clonal selection in immune system
  - Targets of cytotoxic T cells
- Pathological
  - After exposure to ionizing radiation, chemotherapy
  - Smooth muscle cells around atherosclerotic plaque
  - Viral hepatitis

Inflammation

Inflammation is the local physiological response to tissue injury. It can be acute or chronic.

Acute inflammation

This is the initial tissue reaction to a wide range of agents, with accumulation of neutrophil polymorphs in extracellular space being diagnostic. Acute inflammation lasts hours to days. Usually it is described with the suffix -*itis*.

Causes
- Physical and chemical, e.g., mechanical trauma, X-rays, acid, alkali
- Infection: bacteria, viruses, parasites, fungi, or protozoa
- Ischemia
- Hypersensitivity

Macroscopic appearance
Calor, rubor, tumor, dolor, and functio laesa (heat, redness, swelling, pain, and impaired function). Special macroscopic appearances include the following:
- **Serous** inflammation + abundant fluid rich exudates, e.g., peritonitis
- **Catarrhal** inflammation + mucus hypersecretion, e.g., common cold
- **Hemorrhagic** inflammation + vascular injury, e.g., pancreatitis
- **Suppurative** inflammation + pus produced to form abscess or empyema
- **Fibrinous**: exudates contain fibrin, which forms coating, e.g., pericarditis
- **Membranous**: coating of fibrin and epithelial cells, e.g., laryngitis
- **Pseudomembranous**: superficial mucosal ulceration with slough, e.g., pseudomembranous colitis secondary to *Clostridium difficile*
- **Necrotizing (gangrenous)** inflammation + tissue necrosis

Microscopic changes
Such changes are mediated by endogenous chemicals released by cells (histamine, pro-staglandins, leukotrienes, serotonin, and lymphokines) and plasma factors (complement, kinin, coagulation, and fibrinolytic cascades). Changes are as follows.
- Changes in vessel caliber and flow
  - Immediate and transient smooth muscle vasoconstriction
  - Vasodilation (active hyperemia) lasting 15 min to hours
  - Capillaries, then arterioles, dilate to increase blood flow.
- Increased vascular permeability and fluid exudate
  - Capillary hydrostatic pressure is increased.
  - Endothelial cells contract, creating gaps.
  - Plasma proteins escape into extracellular space.
  - An increase in colloid osmotic pressure draws more fluid.
- Formation of cellular exudates
  - Accumulation of neutrophil polymorphs in extracellular space
  - Begins with margination of neutrophils (flow next to vessel walls)
  - Neutrophils then adhere to vessel walls: mechanism is unknown.

- Migrate by ameboid movement through gaps between cells
- Neutrophil polymorphs phagocytose debris and kill microbes intracellularly using oxygen-dependent (H_2O_2 and hydroxyl radicals) and independent (lysosymes) means.

Sequelae of acute inflammation

- Resolution. Restoration of tissue to normal. This is likely if there is minimal tissue damage, rapid destruction of causal agent, rapid removal of exudates by good vascular drainage, and an organ with restorative capacity, e.g., liver.
- Suppuration: formation of pus
- Organization: replacement by granulation tissue
- Chronic inflammation

Chronic inflammation

This is an inflammation in which lymphocytes, plasma cells, and macrophages predominate. Granulation tissue often accompanies it.

Causes

- Resistance of infective agent to phagocytosis (TB, viral infections)
- Foreign body (endogenous, e.g., urate, or exogenous, e.g., asbestos)
- Autoimmune (e.g., contact hypersensitivity, rheumatoid arthritis [RA], organ-specific)
- Primary granulomatous disease (e.g., Crohn's disease, sarcoidosis)
- Unknown etiology (e.g., ulcerative colitis)

Macroscopic appearances

- Chronic ulcer, e.g., peptic ulcer
- Chronic abscess cavity, e.g., empyema
- Thickening of wall of hollow viscus, e.g., Crohn's disease
- Granulomatous inflammation, e.g., TB
- Fibrosis, e.g., chronic cholecystitis

Microscopic changes

Lymphocytes, plasma cells, and macrophages predominate; neutrophil polymorphs are scarce; eosinophil polymorphs are present. Fluid exudate is not prominent.

Granuloma

A **granuloma** is an aggregate of epithelioid histiocytes.

Causes

- Specific infections: TB, fungi, parasites, syphilis
- Foreign bodies
  - Endogenous: necrotic bone or fat, keratin, urate
  - Exogenous: talc, silicone, asbestos, sutures
- Drugs: sulfonamides, allopurinol
- Unknown: Crohn's disease, sarcoidosis, Wegener's granulomatosis

Wound healing

Classification of wounds

- **Clean**: non-traumatic wounds with no break in surgical technique, no septic focus, and no viscus opened (e.g., hernia repair)
- **Clean-contaminated**: non-traumatic wounds with contaminated entry into a viscus but with minimal spillage (e.g., elective cholecystectomy)
- **Contaminated**: clean traumatic wounds, or significant spillage from a viscus, or acute inflammation (e.g., emergency appendectomy)
- **Dirty**: traumatic wounds from a dirty source, or when significant bacterial contamination or release of pus is encountered

General principles of healing

Tissue healing in any organ follows some basic principles (see Box 2.1).

- Cells may be **labile** (good capacity to regenerate, e.g., surface epithelial cells), **stable** (capacity to regenerate slowly, e.g., hepatocytes), or **permanent** (no capacity to regenerate, e.g., nerve and striated muscle cells).
- Tissue architecture is important: complex arrangements cannot be reconstructed if destroyed, e.g., renal glomeruli.
- **Complete restitution** occurs when part of a labile population of cells is damaged, e.g., a minor skin abrasion.

Box 2.1 The four stages of wound healing

When specialized tissue is destroyed it cannot be replaced, and a stereotyped response called **repair** then follows in four stages.

- **Hemostasis**: immediate. In response to exposed collagen, platelets aggregate at the wound and degranulate, releasing inflammatory mediators. Clotting and complement cascades are activated. Thrombus formation and reactive vasospasm achieve hemostasis.
- **Inflammation**: 0–3 days. Vasodilatation and increased capillary permeability allow inflammatory cells to enter the wound, and cause swelling. Neutrophils amplify the inflammatory response by release of cytokines, reduce infection by bacterial killing, and debride damaged tissue. Macrophages follow and secrete cytokines, growth factors, and collagenases. They phagocytose bacteria and dead tissue and orchestrate fibroblast migration, proliferation, and collagen production.
- **Proliferation**: 3 days to 3 weeks. Fibroblasts migrate into the wound and synthesize collagen. Specialized myofibroblasts containing actin cause wound contraction. Angiogenesis is stimulated by hypoxia and cytokines and granulation tissue forms.
- **Remodeling**: 3 weeks to 1 year. Re-orientation and maturation of collagen fibers increase wound strength.

- **Granulation tissue** is the combination of capillary loops and myofibroblasts. This is unrelated to a granuloma.
- **Organization** is the process in which specialized tissues are repaired by formation of mature connective tissue, e.g., pneumonia or infarcts.
- **Wound contraction**, mediated by myofibroblasts, can reduce the tissue defect by up to 80%, but can lead to problems, e.g., burns, contractures.
- Scar is formed by the simultaneous secretion of collagen.

Factors affecting wound healing

- Impaired arterial supply or venous drainage (global or local)
- Excessive movement, local distension, or distal obstruction
- Infection, malignancy, foreign body, necrotic tissue, smoking
- Malnutrition: obesity, recent weight loss, nutrient deficiency
- Immunosuppression: cancer, steroids, immunosuppressants, HIV
- Anticancer therapies: radiotherapy and chemotherapy
- Metabolic: diabetes, jaundice, uremia, musculoskeletal diseases, age

Wound healing in specific tissues

Skin: primary intention healing

This takes place where there is close apposition of clean wound edges.

- Thrombosis in cut blood vessels prevents hematoma formation.
- Coagulated blood forms a surface scab that keeps the wound clean.
- Fibrin precipitates to form a weak framework between the two edges.
- Capillaries proliferate to bridge the gap.
- Fibroblasts secrete collagen into the fibrin network.
- Basal epidermal cells bridge the gap and are eventually resorbed.
- The elastic network in the dermis cannot be replaced.

Skin: secondary intention healing

This takes place in wounds where skin edges are not cleanly apposed.

- There is phagocytosis to remove debris.
- Granulation tissue fills in defects.
- Epithelial regeneration covers the surface.

Gastrointestinal tract

- **Erosion** is loss of part of the thickness of the mucosa.
  - Adjacent epithelial cells proliferate to regenerate the mucosa.
  - Healing may take place this way in a matter of hours.
- **Ulceration** is loss of the full thickness of the mucosa.
  - Mucosa is replaced from the margins.
  - Muscularis propria cannot be regenerated; it is replaced by scar.
  - Damaged blood vessels bleed; fibrin covers the raw surfaces.
  - Macrophages migrate in and phagocytose dead tissue.
  - Granulation tissue is produced in the base.
  - If the cause persists, the ulcer becomes chronic.
  - Fibrous scar tissue may result in contractions or stricture.

Ulcers

An **ulcer** is a breach in an epithelial surface.

Classification: Venous, arterial, diabetic, neuropathic, malignant, traumatic.

Features to note on examination

- *Site*. Neck, groin, and axilla (TB); legs and feet (vascular); anywhere (malignant)
- *Surface*. Usually depressed. Elevated in malignancy, vascular granulations
- *Size*. Measure the ulcer. Is it large by comparison to the length of history?
- *Shape*. Oval, circular, serpiginous, or straight edges
- *Edge*. Eroded (actively spreading), shelved (healing), punched out (syphilitic), or rolled or everted (malignant)
- *Base*. is the ulcer fixed to underlying structures? Mobile? Indurated? Penetrating?
- *Discharge*. Purulent (infection), watery (TB), or bleeding (granulation or malignancy)
- *Pain* usually occurs during the extension phase of nonspecific ulcers. In diabetic patients ulcers are relatively painless.
- *Number*. Widespread locally (local infection such as cellulitis), or widespread generally (constitutional upset)
- *Progress*. Short history (pyogenic), or chronic (vascular or trophic, e.g., post-phlebitic syndrome, decubitus ulceration of paraplegia)
- *Lymph nodes* in the region of an ulcer may indicate secondary infection or malignant change.

Natural history

- *Extension*. There is discharge, a thickened base, and inflamed margin. Slough and exudates cover the surface.
- *Transition*. Slough separates and the base becomes clean. The discharge becomes scanty, the margins less inflamed.
- *Repair*. Granulation becomes fibrous tissue and forms a scar after re-epithelialization.

Chronic leg ulcers

Their etiology is diverse, but they can usually be diagnosed clinically.

Venous ulcers

These are part of post-phlebitic limb syndrome in which there may be a history of past DVT. The ulcer is associated with edema, lipodermato-sclerosis (woody thickening of soft tissues around the calf), and venous congestion with secondary calf perforators and varicose veins. The ulcer is usually over the medial malleolus but can be large, involving the whole of the lower leg and foot.

- If pulses are absent in the foot, there may be an arterial element, which can be excluded by measurement of the ankle–brachial pressure index (ABI).
- If any doubt persists, a vascular referral for arterial reconstruction should be considered, and compression bandaging must be avoided when there is arterial insufficiency.

Arterial ulcers

These are often multiple and occur distally over and between the toes or at pressure points, such as heels or malleoli. They may occur elsewhere on the leg, usually when there is an associated diabetic or venous element. There is usually a history of arterial disease, particularly peripheral vascular disease with claudication.

- Unlike venous ulcers, where bacterial colonization is common, the presence of organisms suggests infection, particularly when there is moisture around the ulcers: wet gangrene (caused by staphylococci and streptococci, not clostridia; see below) may ensue with cellulitis.
- If the leg is kept dry, infection is minimized and a line of demarcation may aid in decision-making for the level of amputation.
- Arterial reconstruction should be considered before this stage.

Diabetic ulcers

These commonly occur in conjunction with arterial disease. They represent large- and small-vessel disease with an impaired ability to heal and increased susceptibility to infection. Ulcers may occur in the arterial distribution, particularly at pressure points, and involve deep tissue infections (such as plantar abscesses) and osteomyelitis. The associated diabetic neuropathy with Charcot's joints presents with deformed feet and joints that are susceptible to ulceration.

- Management involves good diabetic and ulcer care, which includes orthotics help with shoes and gait.
- Surgical aims: avoidance of major amputation. Debridement of necrotic tissue, drainage of abscesses, and excision of dead tissue, often involving bone as "ray" excisions of toes, are required.

Other causes

These include pressure, vasculitic, lymphatic, infectious, and artefactual causes. Leg ulcer clinics have emphasized the value of a multidisciplinary approach.

Cysts, sinuses, and fistulas

Cysts

A **cyst** is a collection of fluid in a sac lined by endothelium or epithelium, which usually secretes the fluid.
- True cysts are lined by endo- or epithelium.
- False cysts are the result of exudation or degeneration, e.g., pseudocyst of pancreas, cystic degeneration in a tumor.

Classification
Congenital

- Sequestration dermoid. Due to displacement of epithelium along embryonic fissures during closure, e.g., skin. Sites include outer and inner borders of orbit, midline of the body, anterior triangle of neck (brachial cyst; e.g., implantation dermoid due to skin implantation from injury).
- Tubulodermoid/tubuloembryonic. Abnormal budding of tubular structures, e.g., enteric cysts, postanal dermoid, thyroglossal cyst.
- Dilatation of vestigial remnants, e.g., urachal, vitello-intestinal, paradental, and branchial cleft cysts; hydatid of Morgagni; Rathke's pouch

Acquired

- Retention cysts. Due to blocking of a glandular or excretory duct, e.g., sebaceous cyst (sweat gland), ranula (salivary gland), and cysts of the pancreas, gallbladder, parotid, breast, epididymis, Bartholin's glands, hydronephrosis, hydrosalpinx
- Distension cysts. Due to distension of closed cavities as a result of exudation or secretion, e.g., thyroid or ovarian cysts, hygroma (lymphatic cysts), hydrocele, ganglia, bursas (false cysts)
- Cystic tumors, e.g., cystadenoma, cystadenocarcinoma of ovary
- Parasitic cysts, e.g., hydatid cysts (*Taenia echinococcus*)
- Pseudocysts. Due to necrosis of hemorrhage with liquefaction and encapsulation, e.g., necrotic tumors, cerebral softening, or coalescence of inflammatory fluid collections, e.g., pseudocyst of pancreas

Clinical features
Subcutaneous and superficial

Cysts are smooth, spherical, soft, and fluctuant when palpated in two planes with the fingers at right angles to each other. If tense, they may produce pain. If the fluid is clear, the swelling will transilluminate. Ultrasound and aspiration of contents are methods of determining whether a given swelling is cystic and may differentiate a cyst from a lipoma. They may compress surrounding tissues. They may produce pain if complications supervene. Cysts are also subject to infection, torsion if on a pedicle, hemorrhage, and calcification.

Treatment
- Excision—only if symptomatic, cosmetic, or concern over diagnosis
- Marsupialization (deroofing and suture of the lining to skin)—if chronic or infected
- Drainage (deep site)—if symptomatic or complicated. Not if there is concern over malignancy

Sinuses/fistulas

- A **sinus** is a blind epithelial track, lined by granulation tissue that extends from a free surface into the tissues, e.g., pilonidal sinus.
- A **fistula** is an abnormal communication between two epithelial surfaces. It is lined by granulation tissue and colonized by bacteria. Examples are fistula-in-ano, pancreaticocutaneous, colovesical, and vesicovaginal fistulas.

Causes
- Specific disease, e.g., Crohn's disease
- Abscess formation and spontaneous drainage, e.g., diverticular abscess discharging into vagina with fistula formation
- Penetrating wounds
- Iatrogenic (e.g., anastomotic leak discharging via wound)
- Neoplastic

Persistence of a fistula is due to the following
- Presence of foreign material, e.g., suture or bone in a sinus
- Distal obstruction of the viscus of origin
- Continuing active sepsis, e.g., TB, actinomycosis
- Epithelialization of the track
- Chronic inflammation, e.g., Crohn's disease
- Malignancy in the track

Investigation
Establish the extent by sinography or fistulogram. MRI is often helpful.

Treatment
Principles of sinus treatment
- Ensure adequate drainage—lay it open and remove granulations.
- Remove infected material, foreign bodies.
- Biopsy sinus wall if there is concern about the underlying diagnosis.
Principles of fistula treatment
- Treat any sepsis, fluid imbalances, and poor nutrition if associated.
- Ensure good drainage to prevent fistula extension.
- Identify the anatomy—use examination under anesthetic (EUA) or imaging if required.
- Biopsy the fistula if there is concern over the underlying diagnosis.
- Definitive treatment requires
  - Excision of the organ of origin or closure of the site of origin
  - Removal of the chronic fistula track and surrounding inflamed tissue
  - Closure of the "recipient" organ if internal or drainage of external site if to skin

Cellulitis and abscesses

Definitions

- *Cellulitis:* the presence of actively dividing infectious bacteria within the tissues of the skin
- *Abscess:* a (semi) liquid collection of pus lined by granulation tissue (if acute) or granulation tissue and fibrosis (if chronic)
- *Lymphangitis:* the presence of actively dividing infectious bacteria in the lymphatic vessels of an area of the body

Cellulitis
Pathological features
- Skin entry by pathogenic bacteria (e.g., scratch, ulcer, hair follicle)
- Gram-positive cocci (e.g., *Strep. pyogenes, Staph. aureus*)
- Usually heals by resolution if treated promptly
- Spread may result in **lymphangitis**; suppuration results in a **furuncle** (skin gland), **carbuncle** (upper dermis), or **abscess** (deep skin tissues).

Clinical features
- Skin widely involved—warm, red, swollen, and exquisitely painful
- Crepitus indicates the development of gas forming tissue necrosis.

Treatment
- IV antibiotics
- Always assess with Gram stain and culture of tissue fluid.

Abscess
Pathological features
- Contain polymorphic neutrophils (PMNs) macrophages, lymphocytes (live and dead), bacteria (dead and viable), and liquefied tissue substances
- May lead to rupture ("pointing"), discharge into another organ (fistula formation), or opening onto an epithelial surface (sinus)
- Incomplete treatment due to resistant organisms (mycobacterium) or poor treatment may lead to a chronic abscess.
- Complete elimination of the organisms in a chronic abscess without drainage can lead to a "sterile" abscess ("anti-bioma").

Typical causes
- Suppuration of tissue infection (e.g., renal abscess from pyelonephritis)
- Contained infected collections (e.g., subphrenic abscesses)
- Hematogenous spread during bacteremias (e.g., cerebral abscesses)

Diagnosis

Deep abscesses are characterized by fever, rigors, and high WBC. Untreated they lead to catabolism, weight loss, and a falling serum albumin. Ultrasound, CT, MRI, or isotope studies may be necessary to confirm the diagnosis.

Treatment
- Drain the pus with, e.g., incision and drainage (perianal abscess), radiologically guided drain (renal abscess), closed surgical drainage (chest empyema), or surgical drainage and debridement (intra-abdominal abscess).
- Give IV antibiotics (course may be prolonged).

Atherosclerosis

Atherosclerosis is a degenerative disease of large- and medium-sized arteries characterized by lipid deposition and fibrosis.

Etiology

Reversible risk factors include smoking, hypercholesterolemia, obesity, and hypertension. Irreversible risk factors include diabetes, male sex, age, and family history.

Pathological features

- There are three stages of atheromatous lesion. Fatty streaks are linear lesions on the artery lumen, composed of lipid-filled macrophages, which progress to fibrolipid plaques, and finally complex lesions.
- In sites predisposed to atherosclerosis (sites of vessel bifurcation, turbulent flow, post-stenotic areas, and areas denuded of endothelial cells) lipid-laden macrophages enter the vessel wall via gaps between endothelial cells.
- A fibrolipid plaque contains a mixture of macrophages and smooth muscle cells, which migrate into the plaque, capped by a layer of fibrous tissue.
- Growth factors, particularly platelet-derived growth factor (PDGF), stimulate the proliferation of intimal smooth muscle cells and the synthesis of collagen, elastin, and mucopolysaccharide.
- Lipid accumulates within the plaque extracellularly and in the myocytes, ultimately producing foam cells.
- Cell death eventually ensues with the release of intracellular lipids, calcification, and a chronic inflammatory reaction.
- High levels of circulating LDL-cholesterol are thought to lead to atherosclerosis by damaging endothelium, both directly by increasing membrane viscosity and indirectly through free-radical formation and by inducing secretion of PDGF.
- In larger vessels such as the aorta, atherosclerotic plaques may release atheroemboli and mural thrombus, or impinge on the vessel media, causing tissue atrophy resulting in aneurysm formation or dissection.
- Acute MI is caused by three processes in coronary vessels: progressive atherosclerosis, disruption of unstable plaque with acute thrombosis, and acute hemorrhage into the intima around the plaque.

Clot and thrombus: ischemia and infarction

Thrombus

A **thrombus** is a solid mass of blood constituents formed within the vascular system.

The formation, structure, and appearance of thrombus and clot are completely different.

The three types of risk factors for thrombus are called Virchow's triad (Box 2.2). Not all three are needed: any one of them may result in thrombus formation in arteries or veins. Arterial thrombus is most commonly associated with **atheroma**; venous thrombus, with **stasis**.

Box 2.2 Virchow's triad

- Disruption in the blood vessel endothelium
  - Atheromatous plaque, e.g., acute myocardial infarction
  - Thrombophlebitis, e.g., deep venous thrombosis
  - Trauma, e.g., from pressure, surgery, fractures, previous thrombus
- Disruption in the pattern of blood flow
  - Stasis, e.g., immobilization, surgery, low cardiac output states
  - Turbulence, e.g., post-stenotic, atherosclerotic plaques
- Changes in blood constituents
  - Age
  - Smoking
  - Malignancy
  - DIC, HITT
- Pregnancy, oral contraceptive pill

Thrombus formation

Wherever thrombus forms, the principal mechanisms are similar.
- Initial trigger is one or more of Virchow's triad
- Fibrin deposition on vessel wall and formation of platelet layer
- Red cells trapped in fibrin meshwork on top of platelet layer
- Mass projects into lumen, causing turbulent blood flow
- Thrombus grows in direction of blood flow: **propagation**
- In veins, alternating patterns of white platelets and red blood cells may be seen: **lines of Zahn**
- **Thrombophlebitis** is inflammation of veins secondary to thrombus.
- **Phlebothrombosis** is thrombus formation secondary to phlebitis.
- **Phlegmasia alba dolens** (white painful leg) occurs after slow thrombosis formation in the ileofemoral veins and is a chronic condition.
- **Phlegmasia caerulean dolens** (blue painful leg) is due to acute massive ileofemoral venous thrombosis, and can result in shock and gangrene.
- **Thrombophlebitis migrans** are transient thromboses in previously healthy veins anywhere in the body, suggesting visceral cancer.

Embolism

An **embolism** is a mobile mass of material in the vascular system that is capable of blocking its lumen.

The **etiology** is very different, depending on the cause of embolism. The clinical effects depend on territory supplied by the vessel that is blocked. Emboli can be divided into
- systemic emboli; and
- pulmonary emboli

Both of these can be further classified according to substance involved.
- Thrombus. Most emboli are derived from thrombi.
- Gas. Injection or entraining of air, decompression sickness
- Fat. Long-bone fractures, severe burns, extensive soft-tissue trauma
- Amniotic fluid. Increased intrauterine pressure forces fluid into uterine veins.
- Septic emboli. Vegetations from heart valves
- Atheromatous plaque. Peripheral vascular disease, iatrogenic
- Tumor. Common route of metastasis
- Foreign bodies. IV drug users, medically inserted catheters

Clot

A **clot** is a solid collection of blood cells within a fibrin network.

Clot forms in vessels after death, or outside the body as part of the response to trauma. Activation of the clotting cascade results in formation of fibrin from fibrinogen, resulting in the formation of fibrin meshwork that enmeshes cells in a solid, elastic clot.

Ischemia and infarction

Ischemia is a tissue *effect* due to insufficient oxygen delivery.
Infarction is tissue *death* due to insufficient oxygen delivery.

Oxygen supply–demand mismatch is caused by the following:
- Vascular narrowing (atherosclerosis, thrombus, embolus, spasm)
- Global hypoperfusion (shock, cardiopulmonary bypass)
- Hypoxemia (anemia, hypoxia)
- Vascular compression (ventricular distension, venous occlusion)
- Increased oxygen demand (exercise, pregnancy, and hyperthyroidism)

The shape of the infarct depends on the territory and perfusion of the occluded vessel.
- Seconds. Change from aerobic to anaerobic metabolism
- Minutes. Decreased contractility of muscle; cell and mitochondrial swelling
- Hours. Myocyte death; coagulation necrosis; muscle is pale, edematous
- Days. Inflammatory exudates with polymorphonuclear leukocytes, then fibroblast infiltration beginning scar formation. Macroscopically the infarcted area appears yellow and rubbery with hemorrhagic border.
- Weeks. Neovascularization and margins
- Months. Scar maturation—tough, white, contracted area

Gangrene and capillary ischemia

Gangrene

> **Gangrene** is ischemic tissue necrosis with desiccation (dry gangrene) or putrefaction (wet gangrene).

Etiology
- **Thrombosis**, e.g., appendiceal artery secondary to inflammation
- **Embolus**, e.g., atherosclerotic emboli in peripheral vascular disease
- **Extrinsic compression**, e.g., fracture, organ torsion, tourniquet

Clinical appearances
Dry gangrene
The affected limb, digit, or organ is black (because of breakdown of hemoglobin), dry, and shriveled. Dry gangrene shows little or no tendency to spread. A zone of demarcation appears between the dead and viable tissue and separation begins to take place by aseptic ulceration in a few days.

Wet gangrene
Veins and arteries are blocked. Pain is initially severe but lessens as the patient becomes more septic. There is always infection. The skin and superficial tissues become blistered. There is a broad zone of ulceration that separates it from normal tissue. Proximal spread is a feature leading to septicemia and death.

Gas gangrene
Gangrene is complicated by infection with gas-producing anaerobic bacteria, e.g., *Clostridium perfringens*. Gases elaborated from putrefaction lead to surgical emphysema and crepitus.

Principles of treatment
- Systemic treatment
  - Aggressive fluid resuscitation is often necessary.
  - Pain relief (IV morphine 5–10 mg)
  - IV antibiotics—broad-spectrum
- Conservative treatment is only possible for nonvital organs affected by dry gangrene (e.g., toes, forefoot). The aim is to let the affected areas mummify and spontaneously separate.
- *Surgical salvage procedures.* Conservative excision, possibly combined with reconstruction or restoration of blood supply (e.g., foot amputation and bypass surgery for distal lower limb gangrene)
- *Radical surgical excision* is only possible when the affected organ is completely resectable (e.g., limbs, perineal tissues)—excision must be radical in treating spreading or gas gangrene. Make sure that all pus is released and all affected tissue (not just the necrosed area) is excised back to bleeding healthy tissue. Multiple operations are often required to ensure adequate excision of infected tissue.
- *Palliative care.* Consider for unresectable gangrene (e.g., retroperitoneal gangrene, very extensive intestinal gangrene) or for elderly sick patients in whom surgery is inappropriate.

Capillary ischemia

This is ischemia mediated by injury to capillaries.

- **Frostbite**. Exposure to cold with freezing results in fixed capillary contraction, ischemia, and infarction.
- **Trenchfoot**. Exposure to cold without freezing results in capillary contraction followed by fixed dilatation.
- Disseminated intravascular coagulation
- Cryoglobulinemia, sickle cell, parasites

Tumors

Definitions

- **Metaplasia** is the reversible transformation of one type of terminally differentiated cell into another fully differentiated cell type.
- **Dysplasia** is a potentially premalignant condition characterized by increased cell growth, atypical morphology, and altered differentiation.
- **Neoplasia** is autonomous abnormal growth of cells that persists after the initiating stimulus has been removed.
- A **tumor** or **neoplasm** is a lesion resulting from neoplasia.

Metaplasia

This represents an adaptive response of a tissue to environmental stress, mediated by changes in expression of genes involved in cellular differentiation. It does not progress to malignancy. However, if the environmental changes persist, dysplasia may result and progress to malignancy. Examples of metaplasia:

- Change from ciliated to squamous cells in the respiratory epithelium of the trachea and bronchi in smokers
- Change from squamous to columnar cells in the esophageal epithelium of patients with gastroesophageal reflux disease

Dysplasia

Potentially a premalignant condition, dysplasia may be a response to chronic inflammation or exposure to carcinogens. Early forms may be reversible; severe dysplasia has a high risk of progression to malignancy:

- Dysplasia arising in colonic epithelium due to chronic ulcerative colitis
- Squamous dysplasia in the bronchi of smokers (sputum cytology)

Classification of tumors

Use the following classification to give a differential diagnosis for any neoplasm (see Table 2.1):

- Tissue of origin. Organ and tissue type
- Behavior: benign or malignant
- Primary or secondary

Benign tumors

These tumors are slow growing and usually encapsulated. They do not metastasize, do not recur if completely excised, and rarely endanger life. Their effects are due to size and site. Histology is well differentiated with a low mitotic rate; it resembles tissue of origin.

Malignant tumors

These tumors expand and infiltrate locally. Encapsulation is rare. They metastasize to other organs via blood, lymphatics, or body spaces and endanger life if untreated. Histology is varying degrees of differentiation from tissue of origin, pleomorphic (variable cell shapes), with a high mitotic rate.

Table 2.1 Structural classification of tumors

Tissue of origin	Tumor types
Epithelium	**Benign**: papilloma, adenoma (glandular epithelium)
	Malignant: carcinoma (adenocarcinoma, squamous cell carcinoma—indicate cell types)
Connective tissue	**Benign**: fibroma (fibrous tissue), lipoma (fat), chondroma (cartilage), osteoma (bone), leiomyoma (smooth muscle), rhabdomyoma (striated muscle)
	Malignant: sarcoma. E.g., fibrosarcoma, osteosarcoma, etc. (if well differentiated). Spindle cell sarcoma, etc. (if poorly differentiated)
Neural tissue	These arise from nerve cells, nerve sheaths, and supporting tissues, e.g., astrocytoma, medulloblastoma, neurilemmoma, neuroma
Hemopoietic	The leukemias, Hodgkin's disease, multiple myeloma, lymphosarcoma, reticulosarcoma
Melanocytes	Melanoma
Mixed origins	E.g., fibroadenoma, nephroblastoma, teratoma (all 3 germ layers), choriocarcinoma
Developmental blastomas	E.g., neuroblastoma (adrenal medulla), nephroblastoma (kidney), retinoblastoma (eye)

Invasion

Invasion is the most important single criterion for malignancy, and is also responsible for clinical signs and prognosis, as well as dictating surgical management. Factors that enable tumors to invade tissues:

- Increased cellular motility
- Loss of contact inhibition of migration and growth
- Secretion of proteolytic enzymes such as collagenase, which weakens normal connective tissue bonds
- Decreased cellular adhesion

Metastasis

Metastasis, a consequence of these invasive properties, is the process by which malignant tumors spread from their site of origin (primary tumor) to form secondary tumors at distant sites. Carcinomatosis denotes extensive metastatic disease. The routes of metastasis are as follows:

- Hematogenous: via the bloodstream
  - Five tumors—breast, bronchus, kidney, thyroid, prostate—classically metastasize via hematogenous spread to bone.
  - Lung, liver, and brain are common sites for secondary tumors.
- Lymphatic—to local, regional, and systemic nodes
- Implantation—during surgery or along biopsy tracks

Carcinogenesis

Carcinogenesis is the process that results in malignant neoplasm formation (see Table 2.2). Usually more than one carcinogen is necessary to produce a tumor, a process that may occur in several steps, considered the multistep hypothesis.

- **Initiators** produce a permanent change in the cells but they do not cause cancer, e.g., ionizing radiation. This change may be in the form of gene mutation.
- **Promoters** stimulate clonal proliferation of initiated cells, e.g., dietary factors and hormones. They are not mutagenic.
- **Latency** is the time between exposure to carcinogen and clinical recognition of tumor due to
  - Time taken for clonal proliferation to produce a significant cell mass
  - Time taken for exposure to multiple necessary carcinogens
- **Persistence** is when clonal proliferation no longer requires the presence of initiators or promoters and the tumor cells exhibit autonomous growth.

Tumor growth

Tumor doubling time depends on **cell cycle time, growth function,** and **cell loss fraction**. In tumors such as leukemias, the doubling time remains remarkably constant: the cell mass increases proportionally with time. This is **exponential growth**. In solid tumors doubling time slows as size increases. This is referred to as **Gompertzian growth**.

Genetic abnormalities in tumors

Two genetic mechanisms of carcinogenesis are proposed:
- **Oncogenes**: enhanced expression of stimulatory dominant genes
- **Tumor suppressor genes**: inactivation of recessive inhibitory genes

Oncogenes

At least 60 oncogenes have been identified. They can be classified according to the function of the gene product (e.g., growth factors, cell signaling agents). The proteins produced (oncoproteins) can be produced in abnormal quantities or be abnormally active forms, and cause
- Independence from extrinsic growth factors
- Production of tumors in immunotolerant animals
- Production of proteases to assist in invasion of normal tissues
- Reduced cell cohesiveness assisting metastasis
- Growth to higher cell densities and abnormal cellular orientation

Examples include *BRCA1*, *p53*, *k-ras*, *APC*, and *DCC*.

Table 2.2 Common risk factors for cancer

Known carcinogen	Type of cancer
Chemicals	
Polyaromatic hydrocarbons	Lung cancer (smoking), skin cancers
Aromatic amines	Bladder cancer (rubber & dye workers)
Alkylating agents	Leukemia
Viruses	
HIV	Kaposi's sarcoma, lymphoma
Epstein–Barr virus	Burkitt's lymphoma, nasopharyngeal cancer
Human papillomavirus	Squamous papilloma (wart), cervical cancer
Hepatitis B virus	Liver cell carcinoma
Radiation	
UV light (UVB > UVA)	Malignant melanoma, basal cell carcinoma
Ionizing radiation	Particularly breast, bone, thyroid, marrow
Biological agents	
Hormones, e.g., estrogens	Breast and endometrial cancer
Mycotoxins, e.g., aflatoxins	Liver cell carcinoma
Parasites, e.g., schistoma	Bladder cancer
Miscellaneous	
Asbestos	Mesothelioma and lung cancer
Nickel	Nasal and lung cancer

Host factors	Type of cancer
Race: Caucasians	Malignant melanoma, stomach cancer
Diet	
High dietary fat	Breast, colorectal cancer
Alcohol	Breast cancer
Gender, inherited risks	
Female gender	Breast cancer
Familial polyposis coli	Colorectal cancer
Multiple endocrine neoplasia	Pheo, parathyroid, medullary cancer thyroid
BRCA1–17q21	Breast, ovarian, and prostate cancer
Premalignant lesions and conditions	
Adenomatous rectal polyp	Colorectal adenocarcinoma
Mammary ductal hyperplasia	Breast carcinoma
Ulcerative colitis	Colorectal adenocarcinoma
Transplacental exposure	
Diethylstilboestrol	Vaginal adenocarcinoma

Screening

Screening is the testing of any population for a disease.

The aim is reduction in morbidity and mortality from screened diseases.

Requirements for successful screening
- The screening **test** must be
  - Sensitive
  - Specific
  - Safe
  - Inexpensive
  - Acceptable
- The **population** screened must be easily identified, contactable, and compliant.
- The **disease** screened must be
  - Detectable in a treatable, premalignant form, or earlier stage
  - Preventable or more amenable to successful or curative treatment
  - A sufficient burden on the population to justify cost of screening
  - Chronic or of suitable evolution for sporadic testing to detect it

Disadvantages of screening
- Cost (time and resources)
- The benefit may be small.
- False-positive tests may be physically or psychologically detrimental.

Examples of screening programs
Breast cancer
A meta-analysis of 13 breast cancer screening trials concluded that screening mammography significantly reduced breast cancer mortality in women aged 50–74. A *BMJ* (*British Medical Journal*) analysis reached the following conclusions:
- For every 1000 women screened over 10 years, around 200 (depending on age) are recalled because of an abnormal result, and of these
  - ~60 will have at least one biopsy
  - ~15 will have invasive cancer, and 5 will have ductal carcinoma in situ (DCIS)
- Approximately 0.5, 2, 3, and 2 fewer deaths from breast cancer occur over 10 years per 1000 women aged 40, 50, 60, and 70 years, respectively, who choose to be screened.
- 10% of invasive carcinoma is not radiologically detectable.
- Risk of a false-positive screen is approximately 25% over 10 years.
- Studies suggest up to a 30% reduction in mortality from screen-detected early breast cancer.
- Features looked for on screening mammography include spiculated calcification and microcalcification.

Prostate cancer

A third of men >50 years have evidence of prostate cancer at post-mortem, but <1% of these have clinically active disease. Screening is controversial.

- Prostate-specific antigen (PSA), rectal examination, and transrectal ultrasound have low specificity and sensitivity alone or in combination.
- Treatment of prostate cancer is controversial.
- No randomized trial has shown a survival benefit in screened populations: screening may cause more harm than good.

Grading and staging

Staging is the process of assessing the extent of local and systemic spread of a malignant tumor or the identification of features that are risk factors for spread.

Grading is the process of assessing the degree of differentiation of a malignant tumor.

The objectives of staging and grading a tumor are
- to plan appropriate (treatment) for the individual patient;
- to give an estimate of the prognosis; and
- to compare similar cases when assessing outcomes or designing clinical trials.

Staging and grading methods

Staging

The most useful system is the internationally agreed-upon TNM classification (see Table 2.3). It is not appropriate for leukemia, lymphomas, or myeloma. A four-stage classification (I, II, III, IV) is also often used and is compatible with TNM. Specific staging systems also exist for some tumor sites (e.g., Duke's stage in colorectal cancer).

Staging may be either radiological or pathological.
- **Radiological** (often performed preoperatively) is indicated by the prefix r before the letter (e.g., rT3, rM1). If different radiological modalities are used, separate prefixes can be used, e.g., u for ultrasound (uT2). Radiological staging is used to plan treatment (e.g., neoadjuvant therapy, selection for surgery, planning of surgery).
- **Pathological** (performed on surgical specimens) is indicated by the prefix p before the letter (e.g., pT3, pN2, pM1). If there has been preoperative radiotherapy, the prefix y is used to denote that the pathological stage may have been modified by this, e.g., ypT2. Pathological staging is used to plan adjuvant treatment (chemotherapy or radiotherapy) and for informing prognosis.

An example of lung cancer staging:
- Stage I (T1 N0, T2 N0): 85% 5-year survival with surgery
- Stage II (T1 N1, T2N1, T3N0): 60% 5-year survival with surgery
- Stage IIIa (T3 N1 or any N2): 20% 5-year survival with surgery
- Stage IIIb (any T4, any N3): <20% 5-year survival; no benefit with surgery
- Stage IV M1: <10% 5-year survival; no benefit with surgery

Other pathological features may be included with the TNM system for some tumors, for example:
- Presence of vascular invasion V0 or V1
- Presence of lymphatic invasion Ly0 or Ly1
- Presence of viable tumor cells at or within 1 mm of the surgical margin of excision R0, R1 (microscopic), R2 (macroscopic)

Histological grading

This gives a guide to the behavior of a cancer by describing the degree of differentiation of the tumor (e.g., breast cancer).

- *Grade 1* represents the least malignant tumors.
- *Grade 2*: 25%–50% of the cells are undifferentiated
- *Grade 3*: 50%–75% of the cells are undifferentiated
- *Grade 4*: more than 75% of the cells are undifferentiated

Other methods of describing tumors

- Depth of invasion (e.g., Breslow thickness in malignant melanoma)
- Tumor type (e.g., small-cell versus non-small-cell lung cancer)

Table 2.3 Basic form of TNM classification*

Classification	Interpretation
Primary tumor (T)	
TX	Primary tumor cannot be evaluated
T0	No evidence of primary tumor
Tis	Tumor-in-situ
T1, T2, T3, T4	Size and extent of primary tumor
Regional lymph nodes (N)	
NX	Regional lymph nodes cannot be evaluated
N0	No regional lymph node involvement
N1, N2, N3	Number and location of involved lymph nodes
Distant metastasis (M)	
MX	Distant metastasis cannot be evaluated
M0	No distant metastasis
M1	Distant metastasis

* Additional codes used with TNM classification: pul, pulmonary; hep, hepatic; V, vascular; Ly, lymphatic vessels; R, radial margin. Prefixes used with TNM: u, ultrasound; r, radiological; p, pathological.

Tumor markers

Tumor markers (see Table 2.4) are proteins or complex molecules that can be detected by a variety of techniques including chemical, immunological, or bioactivity testing.

Most markers are molecules produced by normal cells in small amounts but which may be produced in increased amounts by tumor cells due to changes in cellular function (e.g., increased production, increased gene expression, decreased degradation, increased release).

Non-tumor-related elevations in tumor marker levels may occur because of the following:

- Increased production or release by pathological processes such as inflammation, infection, trauma, or surgery
- Decreased removal or destruction (e.g., renal failure, liver disease)

Testing is most commonly in vitro and may be via serum measurement or testing of tissue specimens.

Common uses include

- Screening (detection of subclinical disease)
- Diagnosis (including differentiation of tumor origin in metastatic disease)
- Monitoring response to treatment
- Monitoring during follow-up for development of recurrence

Abbreviations for some tumor markers

- AFP, α-fetoprotein
- B-hCG, β-human chorionic gonadotropin
- PAP, placental alkaline phosphatase
- CEA, carcinoembryonic antigen
- LDH, lactic dehydrogenase
- PSA, prostate-specific antigen.

Table 2.4 Commonly used tumor markers

Marker	Useful in	Notes/use
AFP	Hepatoma; teratoma (75% of cases); pancreatic carcinoma some patients	Elevated in liver disease, e.g., hepatitis, cirrhosis, and pregnancy
B-hCG	Choriocarcinoma (almost all cases); testicular tumors/teratoma (75%); other germ cell tumors	Measured both in blood and urine
PAP	Seminoma; ovarian adenocarcinoma	
CEA	Colonic adenocarcinoma; ovarian adenocarcinoma; advanced breast cancer; pancreatic cancer	Not useful for diagnosis or screening. Used to monitor response to treatment and identify relapse in tumors showing raised CEA at diagnosis. May be elevated in pancreatitis, ulcerative colitis, gastritis, and heavy smokers
CA-19–9	Pancreatic cancer (80%); advanced colorectal cancer (75%)	A polysialated antigen (Lewis blood group antigen). Ratio of CA19:9:CEA most sensitive for pancreatic cancer diagnosis
LDH	Lymphoma	
Thyroglobulin	Thyroid cancer	Used to monitor and identify relapse after treatment
Calcitonin	Medullary carcinoma of the thyroid	Used to monitor and identify relapse after treatment
PSA	Prostatic cancer	May be measured in serum and tissue by IHC. Serum level closely relates to disease status
Alkaline phosphatase	Osteosarcoma	Also raised in bony metastases, osteitis, Paget's disease

Surgical microbiology

Sources of surgical infection

Nosocomial infections are acquired in the hospital.
Community-acquired infections are acquired outside the hospital.

Three-quarters of nosocomial infections occur in surgical patients, who account for 40% of hospital inpatients. Sources of infection include the following:

- Patient's own body flora
  - Failure of correct aseptic technique
  - Contaminated surgery
- Indirect contact
  - Contact from hands of doctors, nursing staff, patients, visitors
  - Contaminated surfaces, e.g., door handles, cups
- Direct inoculation
  - Surgeon or environmental flora through failure of aseptic technique
  - Contaminated instruments or dressings
  - Colonization of indwelling drains, catheters, IV lines
- Airborne contamination
  - Skin and clothing of staff, patients, and visitors
  - Air flow in operating room or floor
- Hematogenous spread
  - IV and intra-arterial lines
  - Contaminated infusions
  - Sepsis at other anatomical sites
- Food- and water-borne
- Fecal–oral
- Insect-borne

Risk factors for wound infection

- General
  - Age
  - Malnutrition
  - Immunosuppression, including steroid therapy, chemotherapy
  - Endocrine and metabolic disorders, e.g., diabetes, jaundice, uremia
  - Malignancy
  - Obesity
  - Hypoxia and anemia
- Local
  - Type of surgery (see Table 2.5)
  - Lengthy procedures
  - Necrotic tissue
  - Residual local malignancy
  - Foreign bodies, including prosthetic implants
  - Ischemia
  - Hematoma

- Microbiology
  - Lack of antibiotic prophylaxis
  - Type and virulence or organism
  - Size of inoculate

Modes of occupational infections of health-care workers

- Direct percutaneous inoculation of infected blood (e.g., needle-stick injury, scalpel wounds)
- Entry of infection through minute skin abrasions after contact with spilled infectious bodily fluids (e.g., blood, saliva, semen, urine, feces)
- Entry of infection via mucosal surfaces after exposure to contaminated infectious bodily fluids (e.g., eye splashes, fecal–oral route)
- Transfer of infection by fomites (e.g., via contaminated equipment—prions transferred by neurosurgical equipment)

Procedures designed to minimize transmission

- Identify infected (infectious) patients by serology.
- Identify potentially infected (infectious) patients by risk factors (e.g., IV drug users at risk from hepatitis B carriage).
- Specific procedures for the care of infected (infectious) patients (e.g., barrier nursing for *Clostridium difficile* diarrhea)
- Careful disposal of disposable items related to patient care
- Specific treatment and sterilization of nondisposable equipment
- Universal precautions
  - Make all procedures "safe" procedures by having the highest standards of safety and care when using instruments and sharps—remember *all* patients may be infected or infectious.
  - Wear plastic aprons in procedures with expected soiling from urine, feces, or ascites.
  - Wear two pairs of gloves to reduce the risk of skin exposure when gloves tear.
  - Wear reinforced gloves for procedures with a high risk of penetrating injury (e.g., fragmented fractures).
  - Wear glasses, goggles, or visors for eye protection.
  - Handle all sharps using a transfer container—never pass them hand to hand.
  - Don't allow unnecessary blood or fluid spillage.

Table 2.5 Expected wound infection rates after surgical procedures

Type of surgery	Rate of postoperative infection (%)
Clean (no viscus opened), e.g., hernia repair	<2
Clean contaminated (viscus opened, minimal spillage), e.g., cholecystectomy	<10
Contaminated (open viscus with spillage or inflammatory disease), e.g., simple appendectomy	15–20
Dirty (pus or perforation or incision through abscess), e.g., perforated appendectomy	>40

Surgically important microorganisms

Normal body flora

These are usually involved in infections in surgical patients and include the following.

Staphylococci

- Normal flora of skin, oropharynx, and nasopharynx
- *S. aureus* is an important pathogen in many surgical infections.
- *S. aureus* is the only staphylococcus that can coagulate plasma.
- **Coagulase-negative** effectively means non–*S. aureus* staphylococcus, e.g., *S. epidermis*. They are usually dismissed as contaminants, but they are an increasingly common cause of line and prosthesis infections, particularly in immunocompromised patients.
- **Antibiotic sensitivities**. Cephalosporins, especially cefuroxime, gentamicin, fusidic acid, vancomycin, rifampicin, and teicoplanin
- **Antiseptic sensitivities**. Chlorhexidine, povidone–iodine
- Methicillin-resistant *S. aureus* (MRSA) is resistant to all cephalosporins.

Streptococci

- Normal flora of skin, oropharynx, and nasopharynx
- α-hemolytic streptococci hemolyze blood agar, e.g., *S. pyogenes*.
- β-hemolytic streptococci also hemolyze erythrocytes, e.g., *S. viridens*.
- Pneumococci and enterococci are subtypes of streptococci.
- *S. pyogenes* has been called "the most important human pathogen." It causes strep throat, a range of skin infections, septicemia, necrotizing fasciitis, toxic-shock syndrome, and valvular disease in rheumatic fever.
- **Antibiotic sensitivities**. Penicillin, erythromycin, cephalosporins, clindamycin, fusidic acid, mupirocin
- **Antiseptic sensitivities**. Chlorhexidine, povidone–iodine

Enterococci

- Normal flora of large intestine
- These are an increasingly important cause of nosocomial infections.
- They are involved in wound infections, intra-abdominal sepsis, UTI, intravascular line infections, and dialysis-related infections.
- **Antibiotic sensitivities**. Enterococci are intrinsically resistant to many antibiotics, including all cephalosporins, and must usually be treated by a combination drug regime, e.g., ampicillin plus glycoside.
- Vancomycin-resistant *Enterococcus* (VRE) is resistant to all cephalosporins and vancomycin, and sometimes teicoplanin.

The gram-negative rods

- Normal flora of large intestine
- Gram-negative bacilli (also known as *coliforms*) include *Escherichia coli*, *Salmonella*, *Klebsiella*, *Enterobacter*, and *Proteus*.
- *Pseudomonas* and *Actinobacter* are non-coliform Gram-negatives.

- **Antibiotic sensitivities**. Most are intrinsically resistant to penicillin, and there is increasing resistance to amoxicillin and ampicillin. Cephalosporins are the most common first-line treatment for nonresistant forms. "Extended-range" penicillins (e.g., piperacillin/tazobactam) and aminoglycosides (e.g., gentamicin, streptomycin, amikacin, tobramycin), alone or in combination with cephalosporins, offer good bactericidal action.

Anaerobes

- Normal flora of skin, oropharynx, large bowel, terminal ileum, and genitourinary tract
- Include *Bacteroides* and clostridia (bowel)
- *C. difficile* causes pseudomembranous colitis (📖 p. 339).
- Cause anaerobic infections, including cellulitis, gas gangrene, and empyemas, and colonize diabetic foot ulcers
- Act usually with aerobes to produce "synergistic" necrotizing infections of skin, fascia, and muscle spontaneously or after trauma or surgery
- **Antibiotic sensitivities**. Metronidazole is only active against anaerobes and resistance is rare. Most anaerobes are also sensitive to penicillins, cephalosporins, clindamycin, erythromycin, and co-trimoxazole.

Specific infections

Gas gangrene

Gas gangrene is caused by *C. perfringens*, a gram-positive bacillus found in soil or feces. Injury may be trivial. It is more common in immunocompromised patients. There is exudate and gas in the tissues; skeletal muscle is affected. Edema, spreading gangrene, and systemic signs follow. Aggressive debridement and fasciotomies are required, with resuscitation, organ support, and penicillin (2 g 4 hourly IV) and metronidazole.

Synergistic spreading gangrene (Meleney's or Fournier's gangrene)

This is also known as *necrotizing fasciitis*. The organisms involved are not clostridial, but rather aerobes and synergistic microaerophilic/anaerobes. Patients may be immunocompromised. The initial wound might have been minor or an uneventful operation. Severe wound pain and gas in the tissues (crepitus) may be seen; the extent of subdermal gangrene may not be apparent. Systemic support and antibiotics are required, with excision of involved tissues.

Tetanus

Although a rare infection it is common in many parts of the world, with a mortality rate of about 60%. The causal organism, *C. tetani*, produces a powerful exotoxin that is neurotoxic. It enters the spinal cord via peripheral nerves, where it blocks inhibitory spinal reflexes. It is found widely: infection often follows a trivial puncture wound. Treatment is benzylpenicillin 1 g q6hr IV, metronidazole, and human anti-tetanus immunoglobulin 30 U/kg IM. If a wound is present, it is excised and left open to heal by secondary intention. Immunization with 10-yearly boosters is protective.

Blood-borne viruses and surgery

Viral hepatitis

- Most common liver disease in the world
- May cause acute liver failure or chronic active hepatitis

Hepatitis A

- Formerly known as infectious hepatitis. This is the most common form of jaundice in children and young adults.
- Spread is by the fecal–oral route. The incubation period is 1 month.
- The antibody to the virus is anti-HAV.
- There is no vaccine, and health-care workers do not have to be tested.

Hepatitis B

- Double-shelled DNA virus: 10% of adults fail to clear the virus after infection. Up to 5% people worldwide are carriers.
- Infection is largely blood-borne and is transmitted by blood transfusion, inoculation, sharing syringes (drug addicts), sexual intercourse during menstruation (with an infected partner), and anal intercourse.
- Transmission from a contaminated hollow-bore needle approaches 30%.
- Antigens appear in the serum: **HBsAg** the surface antigen; **HBcAg**, the hepatitis core antigen; **HBeAg**, the 'e' antigen; the Dane particle; double-stranded DNA; and DNA polymerase activity.
- Antibodies formed against these antigens (anti-HBs, anti-HBe) can be detected in the peripheral blood.
  - **HBsAg positive**: failure to clear infection, residual infectivity
  - **HBsAb positive**: protection marker from immunization or infection
  - **HBeAg positive**: close correlation of infectivity
- Hospital staff is routinely offered vaccination for hepatitis B.
  - Infectious carriers may not perform exposure-prone procedures.
  - Vaccination against hepatitis B is not compulsory: the alternatives are frequent testing to check infectivity or limited clinical practice.

Treatment

Any health-care worker who remains HBeAg positive may undergo antiviral therapy:
- Immunomodulation with interferon
- Viral suppression with nucleoside analogues

Hepatitis C

This RNA virus causes cirrhosis of the liver and primary liver cancer. There is no vaccination. It is detected in 1 in 150 screened blood donations. Transmission from a contaminated sharps injury is 2%–3%.

Human immunodeficiency virus (HIV)

This double-stranded RNA retrovirus is transmitted by passage of infected body fluids from one person to another via several methods: anal and vaginal sexual intercourse; peripartum; sharps; and infected blood products.
- HIV infection results in widespread immunological dysfunction, manifested by a fall in CD4-positive lymphocytes, monocytes, and antigen-presenting cells (APCs).
- There is usually a 3-month asymptomatic but infective viremia.

- During this period, ELISA tests for HIV antibodies are negative.
- At seroconversion an acute illness can occur.
- This is followed by generalized lymphadenopathy.
- Acquired immunodeficiency syndrome (AIDS) develops in 5–10 years.
- Median survival with untreated AIDS is 2 years; with treatment it is >15 years.

High-risk procedures

Always use universal precautions. High-risk procedures include

- Any invasive procedure
- Biopsies for the diagnosis of opportunistic infection or suspected HIV
- Procedures to deal with malignancies, e.g., Kaposi's sarcoma, B-cell and non-Hodgkin's lymphoma, squamous oral carcinoma

---

Box 2.3 Precautions and post-exposure prophylaxis (PEP)

- The HIV risk from an HIV-contaminated hollow needle is 0.3%.
- The risk from splashes on broken skin or mucous membranes is 0.1%.

For PEP, go to the occupational health or emergency room. PEP reduces the risk of seroconversion by over 80% **if started within 1 hr of exposure**; PEP is continued for 4 weeks. Side effects include diarrhea and vomiting.

Universal precautions are designed to protect workers from exposure to diseases spread by blood and body fluids. *All* patients are assumed to be infectious for blood-borne diseases, including HIV.

- Universal precautions apply to blood; amniotic, synovial, pleural, peritoneal, and pericardial fluid; semen; vaginal secretions; and cerebrospinal fluid (CSF).
- They do not apply to feces, sputum, urine, vomit, or saliva.
- Universal precautions include the following:
  - Use of protective clothing, e.g., gloves, gowns, masks, eye-guards
  - Removing hazards from the workplace, e.g., sharps bins, ventilation
  - Work practice, e.g., hand-washing, handling of sharps, transport of soiled goods, reduction in unnecessary procedures
  - Single-use, disposable injection equipment
  - Hospital policy for all sharps injuries: squeeze, wash, and report

Disorders of bleeding and coagulation

Hemostasis

This is the physiological process by which bleeding is controlled. It has four components:

- **Vessel wall response**. Primarily, vasoconstriction due to smooth-muscle contraction is the first response.
- **Platelet activity** results in formation of a platelet plug.
  - Platelets adhere to exposed endothelial collagen, a process that requires von Willebrand factor (factor VIII).
  - Release of ADP, arachidonic acid, prostaglandin, and thromboxane A2 promotes **platelet aggregation**.
  - Aggregated platelets react with thrombin and fibrin, forming a **plug**.
  - Aspirin irreversibly inhibits cyclooxygenase-mediated formation of prostaglandin, lasting for the life of the platelet (7–10 days). Clopidogrel irreversibly inhibits ADP-mediated aggregation (7–10 days).
- The **coagulation cascade** converts prothrombin to thrombin to produce a fibrin clot: two interacting pathways are involved.
  - The **intrinsic pathway** involves only normal blood components and starts when factor XII (Hageman factor) is activated by binding to a damaged vessel, resulting in the sequential activation of factors XI, IX, VIII, and X.
  - The **extrinsic pathway** requires thromboplastin (a tissue phospholipid), which forms a complex with calcium and factor VII, which activates factor X.
  - Both of these pathways converge at the activation of factor X, which converts **prothrombin** to **thrombin**: thrombin converts soluble **fibrinogen** to **fibrin** to produce a stable clot.
  - All of the soluble factors are manufactured by the liver except for factor VIII (made by endothelium).
  - **Warfarin** inhibits the manufacture of vitamin K–dependent clotting factors (prothrombin, VII, IX, and X), taking 3–4 days to have effect.
- The **fibrinolytic system** terminates thrombus propagation to maintain circulating blood in a fluid state: it depends on four proteins.
  - **Plasmin**, a serine protease that is produced by the action of thrombin on plasminogen and attacks unstable bonds between fibrin molecules to generate fibrin degradation products
  - **Antithrombin III**, which deactivates thrombin, XIIa, IXa, and Xa
  - **Proteins C and S**, which prevent thrombin generation by binding factors Va and VIIIa. **Tissue factor pathway inhibitor**, produced by platelets, inhibits factors Xa and VIIa.
  - **Heparin** potentiates antithrombin III with immediate effect. Protamine binds heparin, reversing its effect almost immediately.

Disorders of hemostasis

These can be thought of in terms of the following four components:

- **Vessel wall abnormalities**, e.g., Henoch–Schönlein purpura, Cushing's syndrome, steroid use, vitamin C deficiency (scurvy)
- Platelet abnormalities
  - **Thrombocytopenia** ($<100 \times 10^9/L^3$) caused by reduced production (bone marrow failure, radiotherapy, chemotherapy, infiltrative disease, e.g., neoplasia, leukemia); faulty maturation (e.g., folate and B_{12} deficiency); abnormal distribution (splenomegaly); increased destruction (autoimmune disorders, drugs, DIC, hemorrhage); and dilutional thrombocytopenia in massive banked blood transfusion
  - **Abnormal function**, e.g., von Willebrand's disease, uremia, idiopathic causes, drug effects, especially aspirin and clopidogrel.
- Coagulation abnormalities
  - Congenital, e.g., hemophilia A (↓ factor VIII), hemophilia B or Christmas disease (↓ factor IX), von Willebrand's disease (↓ vWF).
  - Acquired, e.g., DIC (📖 p. 112); ↓ vitamin K (which is produced by gut flora) secondary to poor nutrition, antibiotic therapy, obstructive jaundice; liver disease; exogenous anticoagulants

Preoperative evaluation of hemostasis

- Routine testing is not recommended unless the patient is ASA 3 as a result of renal disease.
- For at-risk patients undergoing major + cardiac surgery or neurosurgery, testing may be considered.

History and examination

- Ask about bleeding problems, e.g., menorrhagia, bruising, family history of bleeding, and medication. Specifically, aspirin, clopidogrel, and warfarin should all be stopped 5 days before elective surgery.
- Look for petechia and purpura, jaundice, and hepatosplenomegaly.

Laboratory tests

- **Platelet count.** Normally $200–400 \times 10^9/L$. $70 \times 10^9/L$ is needed for surgical hemostasis; $<20 \times 10^9/L$ results in spontaneous bleeding.
- **Blood film.** Estimate of platelet count and indicates morphology
- **Bleeding time.** Useful, as normal bleeding time indicates normal platelets, normal function, and normal vascular response to injury, but uncommonly used as a screening test
- **PT.** Reflects the extrinsic pathway (I, II, V, VII, X)
- **PTT.** Reflects the intrinsic pathway (all factors except VII)
- **Individual clotting factor assays**
- **Thrombin time** (TT). Rate of conversion from fibrin to fibrinogen
- **Fibrin degradation products.** These are released by the action of plasmin and are raised in DIC.

Principles of management

- Indications for FFP, platelets, and anti-fibrinolytics are listed on 📖 p. 80.
- IV heparin may be reversed with protamine and/or FFP.
- Warfarin may be reversed over 12–24 hr with 1 mg vitamin K SC or acutely with FFP.

Anemia and polycythemia

Anemia

This is a reduction in Hb concentration below normal (~13–16 g/dL in men, 11.5–15 g/dL in females), classified as follows.

- Decreased red cell production
  - Hematinic deficiency (↓ Fe, B$_{12}$, folic acid)
  - Bone marrow failure (congenital, chemotherapy, radiotherapy, infiltrative disease)
- Abnormal red cell maturation
  - Myelodysplasia
  - Sideroblastic anemia
- Increased red cell destruction—hemolytic anemias
  - Inherited (e.g., sickle cell, thalassemia)
  - Acquired (e.g., autoimmune, DIC—📖 p. 112)
- Chronic disease—common cause of anemia in surgical patients
  - Renal failure (↓ production erythropoietin)
  - Endocrine, liver disease

Iron deficiency anemia

This is the most common cause of anemia in surgical patients. Causes include the following:

- Menstruation (in 15% of females)
- GI losses (peptic ulcer, esophagitis, gastric carcinoma, colorectal carcinoma
- Reduced iron uptake—poor diet, celiac disease, malabsorption

Sickle cell anemia

A single base substitution gene defect causes an amino acid substitution in hemoglobin, making HbS instead of HbA. Deoxygenated HbS polymerizes and causes red blood cells to sickle, resulting in occlusion of small blood vessels and infarction. This condition is common in people of African descent. Homozygotes have high levels of HbS and are prone to crises. Heterozygotes ("sickle trait") are only symptomatic in hypoxic conditions, e.g., unpressurized aircraft, limb ischemia.

- Most patients are diagnosed: screening for sickle cell is widespread.
- The patient typically has an Hb of 6–8 g/dL, reticulocytes 10%–20%.
- There are three types of sickle-cell crisis:
  - Thrombotic crises: precipitated by cold, dehydration, infection, ischemia; may mimic acute abdomen or pneumonia, priapism
  - Aplastic crises: due to parvoviruses and require urgent transfusion
  - Sequestration crises: spleen and liver enlarge rapidly from trapped erythrocytes, resulting in RUQ pain, ↑ INR, ↑ LFT, ↓↓ Hb.
- Treatment: remove causes and decrease percentage of HbS.
  - Keep warm and well hydrated—if necessary with IV fluids.
  - Give O$_2$.
  - Give opiate analgesia.
  - Give empirical antibiotics if there is any evidence of sepsis.
  - If Hb <6 g/L, give blood; if Hgb >9 g/dL, exchange transfusion.
- Exchange transfusion to maintain HbA >60% before cardiac surgery.

Thalassemia

Thalassemias are genetic diseases of Hb synthesis resulting in underproduction of one chain, which results in destruction of red cells while they are still in the bone marrow. α-Thalassemia leads to ↓ α-chain production with unbalanced β-chain production, and β-thalassemia leads to

- β chain production. Common in Mediterranean to Far East
- Severity correlates with the genetic deficit
- Death may result by 1 year of age without transfusion.
- Symptoms of iron overload after 10 years: endocrine failure, liver disease, and cardiac toxicity
- Death at 20–30 years due to cardiac siderosis

Preoperative screening of anemia

- CBC should be considered for all surgery in adults >60 years of age.
- CBC is recommended for intermediate surgery (e.g., primary repair of inguinal hernia, varicose vein surgery) in adults >60 years of age.
- CBC is recommended in any adult undergoing major surgery.
- Sickle-cell screening is recommended in any patient of African descent undergoing a general anesthetic: **consent** should be obtained.

Preoperative evaluation of anemia

↓ Mean cell volume (MCV) or microcytic anemia

- Iron deficiency (blood loss, dietary): ↓ serum ferritin and iron, ↑ total iron binding capacity (TIBC)
- Thalassemia (↑ serum iron and ferritin, ↓ TIBC)
- Hyperthyroidism

↑ MCV or macrocytic anemia

- B$_{12}$ or folate deficiency (dietary, pernicious anemia, anti-folate drugs)
- Alcohol
- Liver disease
- Myelodysplasia and bone marrow infiltration
- Hypothyroidism

Normal MCV or normocytic anemia

- Anemia of chronic disease, renal failure, bone marrow failure, hemolysis, pregnancy, dilutional

Management of anemia

- Elective patients should be investigated and treated appropriately.
- Blood transfusion (📖 p. 82) is indicated in patients with Hb <8 g/dL undergoing emergency or elective surgery.
- Evidence suggests that maintaining Hb at 7–9 g/dL has a better outcome than maintaining Hb at 10–12 g/dL, except in patients with unstable angina.

Polycythemia

- **Relative** (↓ plasma volume): dehydration from alcohol or diuretics
- **Absolute** (↑ red cell mass)
  - Primary (polycythemia rubra vera)
  - Secondary (altitude, smoking, COPD, tumors, e.g., fibroids)
- Treat underlying cause; consider venesection.

Practical procedures

Denise Gee, MD

Endotracheal intubation

This procedure is indicated in cardiac arrest, serious head injury, certain acute respiratory and trauma settings, and prior to many surgical operations.

- ▶ Effective bag and mask ventilation is better than multiple attempts at endotracheal intubation in the arrest setting.
- ▶ Except in a dire emergency, endotracheal intubation should not be performed without expert supervision.

Equipment

- 10 mL syringe
- Endotracheal tube (ET; size 6–7 for females and 7–8 for males)
- Laryngoscope
- Ribbon to secure tube; lubricating jelly

Preparation

- Pre-oxygenate the patient.
- Ensure that the laryngoscope and ET cuff are functioning.
- Remove any dentures, and suction excess saliva and secretions.
- Extend the neck.
- Insert the laryngoscope, pushing the tongue to the left (see Fig. 3.1).
- Advance the scope anterior to the epiglottis and pull gently but firmly upward to expose the vocal cords. Take care not to lever on the upper teeth.
- Insert the lubricated ET tube between the cords into the trachea.
- Confirm correct positioning of the tube by observing chest movements, and listening over lung bases and stomach.
- Progressively inflate the cuff and attach ventilation equipment.
- Confirm correct cuff inflation by listening for whistling or bubbling in the larynx suggesting air leak and secure the tube in place with ribbon.
- ▶ Patients not in cardiac arrest or who maintain a gag reflex will need anesthesia prior to oropharyngeal intubation, i.e., administration of inducing agent plus muscle relaxant.
- ▶ The best setting in which to learn intubation is preoperatively under controlled conditions and good supervision.

Clinical pearls—anatomy of the lower pharynx and larynx

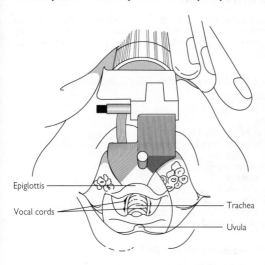

Epiglottis

Vocal cords

Trachea

Uvula

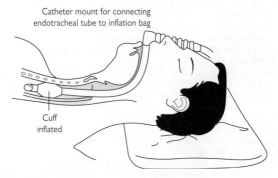

Catheter mount for connecting endotracheal tube to inflation bag

Cuff inflated

Fig. 3.1 Annotated diagram of larynx as seen at intubation.

DC cardioversion

Synchronized direct current (DC) cardioversion is the treatment of choice for tachyarrhythmias compromising cardiac output, such as atrial fibrillation (AF) and supraventricular tachycardia (SVT), and for AF refractory to chemical cardioversion (see Box 3.1).

> **Box 3.1 Checklist for elective DC cardioversion**
>
> - Is it indicated?
>   - Is the patient still in AF?
> - Is it safe?
>   - Either AF has lasted less than 24 hr
>   - or the patient must have had at least 4–6 weeks of formal anticoagulation
>   - or an echocardiogram excluding intracardiac thrombus.
> - Is the patient ready?
>   - The potassium should be 4.5–5.0 mmol/L.
>   - The INR if anticoagulated should be >2.0.
>   - The patient should have a valid consent form.
>   - The patient should be NPO for 6 hr.

DC cardioversion for AF and SVT

- The patient should be anesthetized.
- Use adhesive external defibrillator pads (remain fixed to the patient until procedure is completed), or handheld paddles and gel pads.
- Expose the chest.
- Place pads on chest in the position shown in Fig. 3.2: the aim is to direct as much of the current as possible through the heart.
- Place three ECG electrodes on the patient as shown, and connect to the fibrillator so that an ECG trace is visible.
- Switch defibrillator on and turn dial on to appropriate power setting (100J, 200J, 360J).
- ▶ Press the SYNC button, and ensure that each R wave is accented on the ECG. Failure to do this can mean that a DC shock is delivered while the myocardium is repolarizing, resulting in ventricular fibrillation (VF). Check that the SYNC button is on before every shock for AF.
- If you are using handheld paddles, hold them firmly on the gel pads.
- Perform a visual sweep to check that no one is in contact with the patient at the same time as saying clearly, "Charging. Stand clear."
- Press the charge button.
- Press the shock button when the machine is charged.
- If the shock has been delivered successfully, the patient's muscles will contract violently: anyone in contact with the patient will experience a large electric shock.
- Check the rhythm.
- If there is still AF, press the charge button and repeat the sequence.

Complications of DC cardioversion
- Complications of general anesthesia
- Systemic embolization
- Failure to cardiovert
- Burns from incorrect application of gel pads
- Muscle pain from involuntary contraction
- Arrhythmias, including asystole and VF

Common pitfalls
Failure to deliver a shock
Check that the defibrillator is switched on and adequately charged. Check that the correct power setting has been selected. Change the machine.

Failure to cardiovert
Check that the latest available serum potassium was 4.5–5.0. Check that the correct power setting has been selected. Replace gel pads with fresh ones. Reposition the patient on their side and the pads as shown and try two further shocks at 200J (Fig. 3.2). Do not start at too low a power setting, as each shock leaves the myocardium less sensitive to further shocks. There is some evidence that 360J as the first power setting results in less myocardial damage and a better conversion rate than multiple shocks at lower power settings.

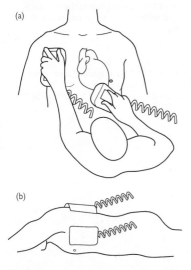

Fig. 3.2 Using defibrillators. (a) Correct positioning for defibrillation and cardioversion. (b) Alternative positioning for synchronized DC cardioversion.

Defibrillation

Defibrillation is the treatment of choice for VF and pulseless VT.

Defibrillation for VF and pulseless VT

Do not delay defibrillation for maneuvers such as intubation, cardiac massage, or administration of drugs.

- Expose the chest.
- Place gel pads on chest in the position shown in Fig. 3.2 (📖 p. 189): the aim is to direct as much of the current as possible through the heart.
- Switch defibrillator on and turn dial on to appropriate power setting (100J, 200J, 360J).
- Press charge button.
- If you are using handheld paddles instead of adhesive external defibrillator pads, place them firmly on gel electrodes and hold.
- Perform a visual sweep to check that no one is in contact with the patient at the same time as saying clearly, "Charging. Stand clear."
- Press the shock button.
- If the shock has been delivered successfully, the patient's muscles will contract violently: anyone in contact with the patient will experience a large electric shock.
- Check the rhythm.
- If there is still VF, press the charge button and repeat the sequence.
- If the rhythm changes to one compatible with an output, check the pulse before proceeding further.

Common pitfalls

Failure to deliver a shock

- Check that the defibrillator is switched on and adequately charged.
- Check that the correct power setting has been selected.
- Check that the SYNC button is **off** if you are trying to defibrillate VF.
- Change the machine and paddles.

Failure to defibrillate

- Exclude causes of intractable VF.

Venopuncture

This is a mandatory skill to learn for all doctors, but many patients will have "difficult" veins, thus regular practice is needed.

Indications   Obtaining venous blood samples for laboratory analysis.

Equipment
- Tourniquet
- 23G or 21G needle
- Vacuum tube system
- Alcohol swabs
- Appropriate laboratory sample tubes
- Cotton-wool ball and tape

Preparation   Apply tourniquet above the elbow and inspect the arm for suitable engorged veins.

Method
- Clean the skin thoroughly at the site of access.
- Tether the skin distal to the site.
- Pass the needle obliquely through the skin at a point ~1 cm distal to the point of planned entry to the vein.
- Advance the needle slowly until a "give" is felt as the vein is entered and a "flashback" is seen in the tubing.
- Attach a blood sample tube to the vacuum tube system and it will fill automatically.
- Release the tourniquet *before* gently withdrawing the needle.
- Apply pressure to the site to arrest any bleeding. Do not assume that the patient, e.g., stroke patients, can help with this.

Tips and problems
- *Poor veins*. If the patient is cold and the samples are non-urgent, use heat packs—this may aid venodilatation. Veins on the dorsum of the hand may be the only ones readily available—try using a smaller or butterfly needle to obtain samples.
- *Obese patients*. Try the dorsum of the hand or the radial aspect of the wrist; access may be easier here.
- *Failed attempts*. Repeated failed attempts will distress the patient and demoralize the doctor! Ask someone to help. If the samples are extremely urgent, a femoral approach may be the best option for obtaining blood samples, e.g., during cardiac arrest.
- *IV cannula*. If blood samples and IV access are needed, a sample can be taken immediately after inserting the cannula (see Table 3.1). However, do not use a peripheral cannula for routine samples, as they can be hemolyzed, contaminated by IV fluids, and unreliable.

- *Sample bottles and request forms.* Ensure that these are labeled correctly and that the appropriate tests are ordered. If in doubt about a particular test, seek advice from the laboratory.
- *Blood cultures.* Ensure that the skin is swabbed thoroughly. Do not touch the skin again unless wearing sterile gloves. Once the sample is taken, change the needle before transferring the sample to the appropriate culture bottle.

Clinical pearls—venous drainage of the upper limb

- Superficial venous system
  - **Cephalic vein.** Commences from the lateral end of the dorsal venous network overlying the **anatomical snuffbox**, ascending the lateral and anterolateral aspect of the arm to the **deltopectoral groove**, piercing the clavipectoral fascia to join the **axillary vein**
  - **Basilic vein.** Commences from the medial end of the dorsal venous network, ascending along medial and anteromedial aspect of forearm, piercing the deep fascia to join the **venae comitantes of the brachial artery**, which eventually join the **axillary vein**
  - **Median cubital vein.** Connects these two veins in the cubital fossa
- Deep system
  - Venae comitantes of ulnar, radial, and brachial artery, which flow into the axillary vein
- Most common sites for **phlebotomy** and IV insertion are
  - Dorsal venous network
  - Median cubital vein
  - Cephalic vein in the forearm

Intravenous cannulation

This skill is similar to that of simple venopuncture but needs plenty of practice for the clinician to become competent.

Indications Venous access for administration of IV fluids, blood, or IV drugs.

Equipment
- Tourniquet
- Cannula: 20G or 18G (see Table 3.1)
- Adhesive dressing or tape
- Alcohol swabs
- 5 mL syringe containing 0.9% saline or heparinized saline
- IV fluid bag with giving set, if necessary

Preparation Apply tourniquet above or below the elbow and inspect the arm for suitable engorged veins.

Method
- Clean the skin thoroughly at the site of access.
- Identify a suitable vein.
- Tether the skin distal to the proposed site of puncture.
- Pass the cannula obliquely through the skin at a point ~1 cm distal to the point at which you wish to enter the vein.
- Advance the cannula smoothly until the vein is entered: a "give" will be felt and a "flashback" seen in the hub of the cannula.
- Hold the hub of the needle with one hand and advance the cannula into the vein while maintaining skin fixation until the cannula is well into the vein.
- Remove the tourniquet and press on the vein proximal to the cannula as the needle is removed. Apply the screw cap to the end of the cannula.
- Secure the cannula in place with a dressing.
- If the cannula is not going to be used immediately, flush with heparinized saline.

Tips and problems
- *Agitated or fitting patients.* Try not to place the cannula over a joint, as these tend to become easily dislodged or "tissued."
- *Secure the cannula.* Cannulas are all too easily dislodged because of poor fixation to the skin. Use of two cannula dressings (one placed above and one below) and a bandage is often needed.
- *Hairy arm.* Shaving the skin at the planned cannula site seems tedious but will allow the cannula to be secured adequately.
- *Non-dominant hand.* Placing the cannula in the non-dominant hand, if possible, will allow the patient a little bit more freedom and may prevent the cannula from becoming dislodged easily.

- *Fragile veins.* This tends to be a problem in elderly or debilitated patients. Try using a smaller cannula: the dorsum of the hand is often an ideal site.
- *Poor peripheral access.* In some patients with multiple collapsed or damaged veins, alternative cannula sites may have to be considered, e.g., feet. If peripheral cannulation becomes impossible, a central line will have to be considered.
- *Blood transfusion.* If blood is being given IV, then an 18G or 16G cannula will be needed.

Complete failure to cannulate

- Is a cannula necessary?
  - Can IV medication or fluids be omitted until an elective central- or long-line insertion is possible?
  - Can medication or fluids be given orally or via NGT?
  - Discuss with microbiology if antibiotics are involved: changing route of administration often requires appropriate changes in antibiotic.
  - Fluid and insulin regimes can be modified to be given SC if desperate.
  - Many painkillers and antiemetics can be given PR or IM.
- Ask another member of your team to try: sometimes a fresh pair of hands is all that is needed.
- If peripheral access is impossible or required for a long time (e.g., IV antibiotic regimes for infected prostheses) consider the following:
  - Elective PICC line insertion (long-term line inserted electively by specialist nurse into basilic vein)
  - Elective central line insertion (📖 p. 198)
  - Femoral line insertion (this is less ideal as this location limits patient mobility)

Table 3.1 Size and function of different cannula

Size	Flow mL/min	Use
22G	3–10	Small, fragile veins; pediatrics
20G	55	IV drugs and fluid, slow transfusion
18G	90	IV fluids, drugs
17G	135	
16G	170	Rapid IV fluids, in emergencies
14G	265	

Insertion of arterial cannula

Indications and contraindications See 📖 p. 122.

Equipment
- Two 20G arterial cannulas with guidewire
- Connectors and three-way tap
- 2 mL 1% lidocaine
- 5 mL syringe and 25 gauge needle
- 10 mL saline
- Skin prep
- Gauze swabs

Preparation
- Explain the procedure to the patient, if appropriate.
- It is good practice to perform Allen's test (see next page) to demonstrate that the ulnar arterial supply to the hand arcades is intact.
- For radial artery cannula insertion, place the forearm on a pillow so that the wrist is dorsiflexed; for femoral artery insertion abduct and flex the hip slightly.

Landmarks
- **Radial artery** lies between tendon of the flexor carpi radialis and head of radius.
- **Femoral artery** lies midway between the anterior superior iliac spine and the symphisis pubis.

Technique
- Prepare and check equipment and prep the skin.
- Infiltrate local anesthetic in the skin but avoid distorting the anatomy.
- Palpate pulse between two fingers for 2–3 cm.
- Pass cannula at 45° into the skin.
- Once the cannula is in situ, aspirate and flush via the three-way tap.

Transfixion technique
The cannula is passed through both artery walls, the needle completely withdrawn, and the cannula then withdrawn slowly until flashback occurs, at which point it is advanced into the artery (see Fig. 3.3).

Partial transfixion technique
The cannula is advanced until flashback stops, and the needle withdrawn while holding the cannula steady, which is then advanced into the artery.

Artery not transfixed
The cannula is advanced carefully in 0.5-mm increments until flashback is seen, at which point the catheter is carefully slid off the needle in the artery.

Guidewire
A guidewire is useful where it is possible to get flashback, but difficult to advance the catheter up the artery.

Complications

These include ischemia, thrombosis, bleeding, and damage to radial and median nerves, and inadvertent intra-arterial injection of drugs.

Allen's test

This test is used to demonstrate a patent palmar collateral circulation: the patient clenches their fist to exclude blood from the palm, and the doctor firmly compresses both ulnar and radial pulses while the patient opens the palm, which should be blanched. The doctor releases the ulnar compression while still occluding the radial pulse; the palm becomes pink in less than 5 sec if there is good collateral supply from the ulnar artery. About 3% of people do not have a collateral palmar supply, and hand ischemia is a real risk if the radial artery is cannulated. Pressure readings are more accurate from proximal arteries: brachial, axillary, and femoral.

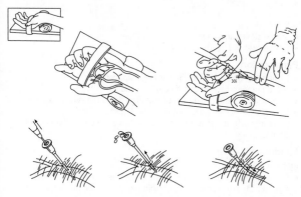

Fig. 3.3 Transfixion technique of arterial cannula insertion.

Insertion of central venous catheter

Indications and contraindications See 📖 p. 122. Cannulas can be single- or multilumen sheaths (for insertion of PA catheters and pacing wires), tunneled, or long lines.

Equipment

- Appropriate central venous catheter
- Ultrasound probe if this is to be used
- Enough three-way taps for all individual lumens
- 10 mL 1% lidocaine
- 10 mL syringe
- 21 gauge and 18 gauge needles
- 20 mL saline
- 2 or 3/0 silk suture
- 11 blade scalpel
- Skin prep
- Sterile drape
- Sterile gloves and gown
- Gauze swabs

Preparation

- Explain the procedure to the patient, if appropriate.
- Ask a nurse to be available if help is needed.
- Patient's ECG and pulse oximetry should be continually monitored.
- Ensure that there is adequate light and a space behind the bed where you can work, and that it is possible to place the bed in Trendelenburg position.

Landmarks

Internal jugular vein

- **Central approach.** The apex of the triangle is formed by clavicular and sternal heads of sternocleidomastoid muscle, aiming the needle toward the opposite nipple.
- **Posterior approach.** Point where the line is drawn horizontally from the cricoid cartilage to the lateral border of the clavicular head of sternocleidomastoid, aiming the needle toward the sternal notch.
- **Anterior.** Medial border of the sternal head of sternocleidomastoid. Aim needle toward the ipsilateral nipple.

Subclavian vein

- Advance the needle at 45° to the junction of the outer and middle third of the clavicle 1–2 cm, then direct needle toward the sternal groove.

Technique

There are numerous techniques. Only one technique is described below.

- Prep the patient.
- Drape so that all landmarks are exposed.
- Palpate the carotid pulse.
- Infiltrate local anesthetic around the planned puncture site.
- Spend 2–3 min laying out the equipment in the order of use; secure three-way taps to central line and turn to closed position.

- Place the bed in 10°–20° of Trendelenburg position.
- Using aseptic technique and a 21 gauge needle on a 10 mL syringe, enter the skin at 45° as described in Landmarks.
- On aspirating venous blood, remove the syringe but leave the needle in situ as an exact marker of position, depth, and direction.
- Take the large-bore hollow needle attached to the 10 mL syringe and, using the 21 gauge needle as a guide, cannulate the internal jugular vein.
- Aspirate 3–5 mL blood when there is flashback and then remove the syringe, leaving the wide-bore needle in situ.
- Pass the guidewire down the wide-bore needle, **keeping hold of the guidewire at all times**.
- Once an adequate length of wire is in place, remove the needle over the wire, and apply pressure to the vein.
- Make a 3-mm nick in the skin over the wire with a scalpel.
- Pass the dilators over the wire through the skin but not into the vein.
- Remove the dilators, apply pressure, and pass the central venous cannula over the wire into the vein up to an appropriate length.
- The wire normally protrudes through the brown (proximal) lumen of a triple lumen line, which should, therefore, be left open.
- Remove the guidewire.
- Aspirate, flush, and close all lumens and suture the catheter to the skin.
- Check that there is a satisfactory pressure trace if a transducer is used.
- Get a chest X-ray to rule out pneumothorax and ensure proper location of the catheter tip.

Complications

- **Immediate**: damage to nearby structures (carotid artery puncture, pneumothorax, hemothorax, chylothorax, brachial plexus injury, arrhythmias), air embolism, loss of guidewire into right side of heart.
- **Late**: sepsis, thromboembolism, AV fistula formation.

Clinical pearls–anatomy of the internal jugular vein

- In the upper neck, the internal jugluar vein may be cannulated as it lies within the carotid sheath. The important relations here are the following:
  - The sheath is just anterior to the anterior border of sternocleidomastoid (SCM).
  - The carotid artery is anteromedial.
  - The vagus nerve lies between the two.
- In the lower neck, the internal jugular vein may be cannulated as it lies behind SCM. The important relations are as follows:
  - The vein lies 45° lateral and 45° inferior to the junction of the sternal and clavicular heads of SCM.
  - The pleura lies inferomedial to the vein.
  - The subclavian artery lies lateral to the vein.
- The internal jugular drains into the brachiocephalic vein; on the right, this is shorter and drains more vertically into the superior vena cava (SVC), making a jugular cannula easier to pass into the SVC.

Insertion of chest tube

Indications
- Pneumothorax
  - In any patient if it is causing respiratory compromise
  - In any ventilated patient
  - Tension pneumothorax
- Malignant pleural effusion
- Empyema and complicated parapneumonic pleural effusion
- Traumatic hemopneumothorax
- Postoperative, e.g., thoracotomy, esophagectomy, cardiac surgery

Equipment
- 28 gauge intercostal drain
- Underwater seal containing water up to mark
- Connection tubing and compatible connectors
- Line clamp
- 2 Kelly clamps for blunt dissection
- 20 mL 1% lidoocaine
- 10 mL syringe
- 21 gauge and 18 gauge needles
- 20 mL saline
- 2 or 3/0 silk suture
- 11 blade scalpel
- Skin prep materials
- Sterile drape
- Sterile gloves and gown
- Gauze

Preparation
- Explain the procedure to the patient, if appropriate.
- Ensure continual monitoring of pulse oximetry.
- Position the patient at 45° with the arm abducted.

Technique
- Usual insertion site is the **5th intercostal space in the anterior axillary line** (see Fig. 3.4).
- Prep and drape the skin.
- Infiltrate site for tube insertion with local anesthetic, ensuring anesthesia at all layers down to and including the parietal pleura, and the periosteum of the ribs posterior to the line of the incision.
- A 2-cm transverse skin incision is made and the intercostal space is dissected bluntly.
- Firmly and carefully pass a blunt-ended clamp over the lower rib through the pleura, and spread to widen the hole.
- If necessary, place a finger into the pleural space to ensure that there are no adhesions.
- Pass a chest tube into the pleural space, guiding it superiorly for a pneumothorax and basally for a hemothorax.
- Secure drain with at least one strong suture, and connect immediately to an underwater seal.

Complications

- Misplacement: subcutaneous, intraparenchymal
- Trauma to other structures: diaphragm, **spleen, liver, heart, aorta, lung parenchyma, intercostal arteries** (entry sites too low, posterior, or trocar used instead of blunt dissection)
- Surgical emphysema
- Wound infection, empyema
- Pain

Pigtail insertion

A 14G pigtail inserted by Seldinger technique is a safe and effective way to drain an uncomplicated pneumothorax and effusions. Use the same landmarks and technique as described for a chest drain but do not make the 2-cm incision.

- Take the large-bore needle on the set and pass it carefully onto the 4th or 5th rib, then "walk" it over the rib into the pleural space.
- Holding the needle with one hand, pass the guidewire gently down the needle—the wire should move without resistance.
- Remove the needle, holding the guidewire in place.
- Make a 3-mm nick in the skin over the guidewire and pass the dilator over the guidewire.
- Remove the dilator and pass the pigtail over the guidewire—this may be a bit difficult, as the pigtail tends to want to curl.
- Connect to a water seal, secure with suture, and obtain a chest X-ray.

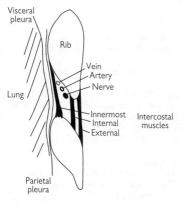

Fig. 3.4 Anatomy of the intercostal space.

Pericardiocentesis

Indications
This procedure is rarely used to relieve acute pericardial tamponade. Surgical pericardiocentesis is carried out under direct vision usually via a subxiphoid incision or sternotomy.

Equipment
- Pericardiocentesis needle or catheter
- 10 mL 1% lidocaine
- 10 mL syringe
- 21 G needle and 18G needle
- 20 mL saline
- 2 or 3/0 silk suture
- 11 blade scalpel
- Skin prep materials
- Sterile drape
- Sterile gloves and gown
- Gauze

Preparation
- Explain the procedure to the patient, if appropriate.
- Ensure that patient has continual ECG monitoring.

Landmarks These are 0.5 cm below and to the left of the xiphoid, aiming at 45° to skin, pointing at the left shoulder or nipple.

Technique (see Fig. 3.5)
- Prep and drape the skin.
- Infiltrate 5 mL 1% SC lidocaine and make a nick in the skin.
- To begin, identify the needle entry site 0.5 cm immediately to the left of the xiphoid tip.
- Insert the needle, applying continuous aspiration in the direction described above.
- After needle entry into the skin and subcutaneous tissue, watch the ECG monitor (or transthoracic echo/screening monitor if available) as the needle is slowly advanced. If there is ectopy or change in the ST segments, stop and withdraw the needle a few millimeters.
- When in contact with the pericardium, advance the needle a few millimeters into the pericardial space.
- If ST segment elevation is present, this indicates contact with the myocardium and the needle should be withdrawn slightly into the pericardial space, where no ST segment elevation should be seen.
- When in the pericardial space, aspirate fluid.
- If the tamponade is successfully reduced, right atrial pressures should be decreased, cardiac output should increase, and pulsus paradoxus should disappear.

Complications
- Cardiac puncture
- Laceration of a coronary artery
- Air emboli
- Cardiac arrhythmias
- Hemothorax.
- Pneumothorax
- Infection

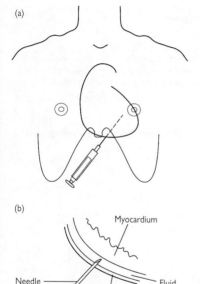

Fig. 3.5 Technique of pericardiocentesis. (a) Landmarks for needle periocardiocentesis; (b) pericardiocentesis.

Cricothyroidotomy

Indications
- Emergency need for a surgical airway
  - Major maxillofacial injury
  - Oral burns
  - Fractured larynx
- Need for tracheal toilet in the extubated patient (tracheostomy is usually preferred)

Needle cricothyroidotomy
- Patient in peri-arrest
- Use the landmarks described below.
- Omit local anesthetic infiltration, cut-down, and dissection.
- Pass a 12G (or larger) needle directly though the cricoid membrane.
- Oxygenate using jet insufflation until a formal airway can be established.

Equipment
- Minitracheostomy, size 6.0 ET tube or 12G cannula in emergencies
- Artery forceps
- 10 mL 1% lidocaine
- 10 mL syringe
- 21G and 18G needle
- 20 mL saline
- 2 or 3/0 silk suture
- 11 blade scalpel
- Skin prep materials
- Sterile drape
- Sterile gloves and gown
- Gauze

Preparation
- Explain procedure to the patient, if appropriate.
- The trauma patient's C-spine should be immobilized in the neutral position.

Landmarks The cricoid membrane is a small, diamond-shaped membrane palpable just below the prominence of the thyroid cartilage.

Technique (see Fig. 3.6)
- Prep and drape.
- If the patient is conscious and maintaining their own airway, infiltrate local anesthetic using an aseptic technique.
- Stabilize the thyroid cartilage with the left hand.
- With your right hand make a 2-cm transverse incision (smaller for minitracheostomy) through the skin overlying the cricothyroid membrane, and then straight through the cricothyroid membrane.
- Now turn the scalpel blade 90° within the airway so that it acts as a temporary retractor.

- Place an artery forceps through the incision and open it. Remove the scalpel and insert a size 6.0 ET tube.
- Suction the tube, secure, and connect to a source of oxygen.
- Some minitracheostomy kits use the Seldinger technique: aspirating air freely is a sign that the needle is in the trachea and that a guidewire can be gently passed down the lumen.

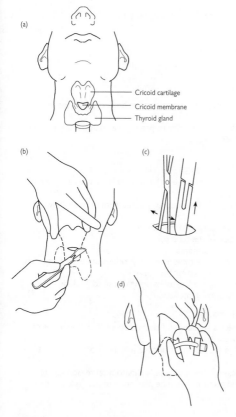

(a)

Cricoid cartilage
Cricoid membrane
Thyroid gland

(b)

(c)

(d)

Fig. 3.6 Technique of cricothyroidotomy. (a) Structures involved. (b) Incision. (c) Keeping cricothyroidotomy patent. (d) Inserting minitracheostomy.

Nasogastric tube insertion

Indications
- Intestinal obstruction
- Paralytic ileus
- Perioperative gastric decompression
- Enteral feeding adjunct (fine-bore tube)

Equipment
- Nasogastric tube (NGT; sizes 10–12 French)
- Gloves
- Lubricating gel
- Benzocaine throat spray
- Stethoscope
- Tape

Preparation
- Position the patient, preferably in a sitting position, with the head tilted slightly forward.
- Chilling NGT in the fridge prior to passing may help stiffen the tube and make it easier to pass.

Method
- Lubricate the tip of the NGT with gel.
- Pass the tube **horizontally** along the floor of the nasal cavity, aiming toward the occiput.
- As the tube engages in the pharynx, ask the patient to swallow: the tube should pass into the esophagus.
- Advance the tube approximately 60 cm.
- Check the position of the tube by
  - Aspirating gastric contents
  - Blowing air down the tube. This will produce bubbling that can be heard on auscultation over the stomach.
  - X-raying fine-bore feeding tubes prior to use to exclude inadvertent bronchial intubation.

Tips and problems
- *Patient has problems swallowing.* Ask the patient to swallow sips of water as the tube is passed.
- *Constant coiling in the mouth.* Your tube may be too soft—cool it in the fridge.
- *Resistance to passing.* There may be an anatomical reason for this, e.g., esophageal stricture. The tube may need to be passed under X-ray guidance.

Urethral catheterization

Indications
- Perioperative monitoring of urinary output
- Acute urinary retention
- Chronic urinary retention
- Aid to assess fluid status after surgery
- Incontinence

Male catheterization

Equipment
- Foley catheter (size 12–20G)
- Dressing or catheter pack containing drapes
- Cleansing solution
- Gloves (two pairs)
- lidocaine gel or lubricant jelly
- Gauze
- Drainage bag
- 10 mL syringe

Preparation
- Have patient lie supine.
- Expose the genital area and cover with a sterile drape with a hole in it.

Method
- Clean your hands and put on sterile gloves.
- Pick up the glans penis with your non-dominant "dirty" hand, through the hole in the drape: the other hand will be your "clean" hand.
- Holding a swab soaked in betadine with your clean hand, retract the foreskin and clean the urethral orifice and glans thoroughly, so that your gloved fingers only touch the swab, not the glans penis.
- In an awake patient, lidocaine gel may be used; otherwise, any lubricant jelly will work. Without letting go of the penis, discard the swab and pick up the sterile gel with your clean hand and inject it into the urethra (or coat the tip of the catheter).
- Still holding the penis in a vertical position, introduce the catheter with the clean hand and advance gently for ~10 cm.
- Lower the penis to lie horizontally and advance the catheter fully until there is urine flow through the catheter.
- Inflate the balloon now in the bladder via the smaller catheter channel with the 10 mL sterile water.
- ► *Never* inflate the balloon until there is return of urine, as this risks inflating balloon within the prostatic urethera, causing urethral rupture.
- Attach a catheter bag firmly to the catheter.
- ► Replace the foreskin to avoid paraphimosis.

Tips and problems
- *No urine immediately*
  - The bladder has just been emptied: insert a 2-mL syringe into the end of the catheter and aspirate any residual urine.
  - The catheter tip may be blocked with lubricant jelly—try gently instilling 15–20 mL of sterile water and gently aspirating.
- *Still no urine*. The patient may be anuric or a false passage may have been created—palpate to see if the bladder is empty or if you can feel the catheter balloon (which should not normally be palpable).
  - Treat anuria appropriately.
  - Consult a senior colleague if a false passage may have been created.
- *Inability to insert*. Try a smaller catheter or a silastic (firmer). If unsuccessful, ask a senior colleague for help. In the case of an enlarged prostate, a Coude catheter may be needed.
- *Decompression of grossly distended bladder*. Rapid decompression of a distended bladder (e.g., from chronic retention) may result in mucosal hemorrhage. Empty the bladder by 250–500 mL every 30 min until empty. Then monitor urine output closely, as a brisk diuresis and dehydration may follow.
- *Bypassing catheter*. This is usually due to catheter blockage. Check urine output, flush the catheter, and observe. If urine is flowing down the catheter and bypassing it, the catheter may be too small—try a slightly larger size.
- *Catheter stops draining*. The catheter may be blocked. Flush as above. If unsuccessful, try inserting a new catheter. Is the patient oliguric or anuric? Treat appropriately.

Female catheterization

Equipment As for male catheterization.

Preparation Lay patient on back with knees bent. Ask the patient to place heels together and allow knees to fall apart as far as possible.

Method

A similar technique to male catheterization is used here, but note:
- Separate the labia minora with the non-dominant "dirty" hand and ensure that the whole genital area is adequately cleaned using the dominant "clean" hand.
- Identify the external urethral orifice. If this proves difficult in obese patients, an assistant may help by retracting the dependent fat from the pubic area.
- Lubricate the tip of the catheter with sterile lubricant jelly or lidocaine gel and pass gently into the urethra.

Suprapubic catheterization

Indications
- Urinary retention with failed or contraindicated urethral catheterization

Cautions
- Do not perform suprapubic catheterization on a patient with a known bladder tumor or previous bladder surgery—seek expert advice.
- Ensure by clinical examination (and, if available, ultrasound bladder scanning) that the bladder is full and distended.

Equipment
- Dressing pack
- Gloves
- Cleansing solution
- Two 10 mL syringes
- 25G and 21G needle
- 10 mL 1% lidocaine
- Prepacked suprapubic catheter set (usually containing catheter, trocar, and scalpel)
- 1/0 silk suture
- Catheter bag

Preparation
- Lay patient supine and expose abdomen.
- Confirm clinically an enlarged, tense bladder.
- Identify catheterization site, 3–4 cm (two finger breadths) above the symphysis pubis (see Fig. 3.7).

Method
- Clean the skin thoroughly around the site and apply drapes.
- Inject lidocaine into the skin and subcutaneous tissues, injecting and aspirating in turn *until urine is withdrawn*.

Two systems for introducing a suprapubic catheter are available.

Nottingham introducer (uses trocar)
- Make a 1-cm incision at the identified site.
- Advance the catheter, with the trocar in place, through the incision and subcutaneous tissues. A "give" will be felt as the bladder is entered.
- Withdraw the trocar and ensure that there is free flow of urine from the catheter.
- Inflate the catheter balloon and suture the flange of the catheter to the skin.
- Attach a catheter bag.

Bonano (based on the Seldinger technique)
- Make a 5-mm nick in the skin.
- Take the introducer needle and advance it, aspirating until urine is withdrawn.

- Remove the syringe and pass the guidewire down the needle into the bladder, then remove the needle, holding the guidewire in place.
- Pass the dilator firmly over the wire, into the bladder.
- Remove the dilator and pass the catheter into the bladder, securing it as above.

Tips and problems

- *Bypassing urine*. With some types of catheters and trocars, urine may initially bypass the catheter. This will cease with full advancement of the catheter and decompression of the bladder.
- *No urine, or feculent matter in catheter*. Obtain help—you may have entered the peritoneum or bowel.

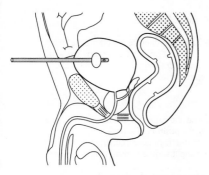

Fig. 3.7 Site of typical suprapubic catheter placement.

Abdominal paracentesis

This is a useful technique in some patients for the diagnosis and management of ascites, often in a patient with malignancy. In many institutions, it is performed by interventional radiologists, under ultrasound guidance.

Indications
- Diagnostic evaluation of ascites
- Therapeutic drainage of ascites

Equipment
- Dressing pack
- Gloves
- Cleansing solution
- 10 mL syringe and 21G and 25G needles
- 10 mL 1% lidocaine
- 60 mL syringe with 16G aspiration needle for diagnostic "tap"
- Bonano catheter or paracentesis catheter, three-way tap, and collecting bag for therapeutic drainage
- Specimen container if appropriate
- Dressing

Preparation
- Position the patient supine and expose the abdomen.
- Percuss out and identify the position of ascites.
- Identify a suitable tap site: the right lower quadrant is the most common one, with the patient turned semilaterally to ensure the ascites fills this area.
- Avoid the suprapubic area and sites of old scars from surgery.

Method
- Prepare the skin at the appropriate site and place sterile drapes.
- Infiltrate local anesthetic into the skin and subcutaneous tissues down to the peritoneum. Aspirate as the needle is advanced, to avoid accidental vessel puncture.

Diagnostic tap
- Introduce the aspiration needle through the skin and subcutaneous tissues while aspirating. A "give" should be felt and fluid freely aspirated as the peritoneal cavity is entered.
- Withdraw 15–20 mL of fluid for diagnostic evaluation. Send for CBC, culture and sensitivity, TB culture, protein, glucose LDH, amylase, and cytology.
- Remove the aspiration needle carefully and apply an occlusive dressing.

Therapeutic drainage
- Introduce catheter into the abdominal wall until "give" is felt. Trial aspirate with a syringe to ensure that ascites returned.
- Slide catheter over the needle into the peritoneal cavity. Stop if resistance is encountered.
- Allow up to 1000 mL of ascites slowly over 1–2 hr.

Tips and problems

- *Unable to aspirate adequate quantity of fluid.* The ascites may be loculated. Drainage under ultrasound guidance may be helpful.
- *Blood or feculent material.* Continual staining of the ascitic fluid with fresh blood or any staining with feculent material may indicate puncture of a vessel or viscus. This is potentially serious and needs evaluation.
- *Peritoneal catheter.* Some patients who require repeated ascitic taps might benefit from placement of a temporary intraperitoneal catheter to allow daily drainage of ascites for symptomatic relief. There is a risk of peritonitis with these devices and usually only a short period of use is recommended, e.g., 2–3 days.

The volume of ascites drained should be closely monitored, along with the patient's serum albumin and overall fluid balance. A maximum drainage of 2 L/day is usually advised.

Rigid sigmoidoscopy

This is a useful skill to learn. It can be performed in the outpatient setting as part of the investigation of lower GI complaints or trauma, but may also be performed on the ward, e.g., in acute admissions with rectal bleeding.

Indications
- Investigation of anorectal symptoms
- Visualization of the rectum

Equipment
- Rigid sigmoidoscope with obturator and light source
- Lubricating jelly
- Gloves
- Gauze

Preparation
- Position the patient in the left lateral position with the hips flexed as fully as possible and knees partially extended.
- Carry out a digital examination of the rectum to identify low-placed lesions or fecal loading, which may prevent safe insertion or obscure a useful view.

Method
- Lubricate the sigmoidoscope with jelly.
- With the obturator in place, introduce the scope gently through the anal sphincter in the direction of the umbilicus for ~5 cm.
- Remove the obturator; attach light source, insufflator, and eyepiece.
- Introduce small amounts of air to open up the lumen.
- Advance the instrument slowly under direct vision, ensuring that a patent lumen is identified prior to advancing the scope further.
- Note the appearance of the mucosa and the presence of any mucosal lesions. The level of any lesion should also be noted using the marked scale on the outer casing of the sigmoidoscope.
- If the patient experiences significant discomfort, do not persist.
- Evacuate any air and withdraw the scope slowly, again under direct vision.
- Clean the area around the patient's anus.

Tips and problems
- *Biopsy.* Unless experienced in the skill, do not attempt biopsy of lesions. Note and document its position and refer to a person skilled in the procedure.
- *Unable to see the upper rectum.* Remember that the rectum has a sacral curvature often pronounced in women. *Gently* use the tip of the scope as a "lever" to push the anterior wall of the rectum forward to open to lumen. If this is not easy and painless, do not persist—it may represent pathology.
- *Rectosigmoid junction.* Negotiation of the rectosigmoid junction can be difficult. The best view that can be hoped for is to see the last sigmoid fold above the junction. Do not attempt to pass the scope into the distal sigmoid—this is the role of flexible sigmoidoscopy.

Clinical pearls—anatomy of the rectum

- The rectum is said to start at the level of S2, but a distance of 15 cm from the anorectal junction is used to the rectum.
- The rectum has two main angles:
  - The first is the acute anorectal angle, which slopes posteriorly and is formed in part by the pull of the sling of levator ani.
  - The second is the sacral curvature, which runs throughout the rectum, sloping progressively anteriorly up to the level of the rectosigmoid junction.
- Three "lateral valves" are commonly described but are only the mucosal folds of the rectum, equivalent to the colonic folds.
- The peritoneal-lined "pouch of Douglas" (or rectovesical pouch in males) extends a variable distance down the anterior wall of the rectum. Its contents (e.g., sigmoid colon) may be easily palpable, particularly in elderly females.
- The upper third is covered by peritoneum anterolaterally and the middle third, just anteriorly. The lower third is entirely extraperitoneal.
- The rectum has a complete outer longitudinal muscle coat (thus diverticular disease does not occur in the rectum).
- The rectum and associated mesorectal fat, blood vessels, and lymph nodes are enclosed and separated from the "true" pelvic organs by a fascial sheet—the mesorectum.

Local anesthesia

Local anesthesia (LA) is used in a variety of settings and is easy to deliver. It is essential to become familiar with the different agents and their relative merits and potential dangers.

Indications
- Minor procedures requiring anesthesia, e.g., insertion of a chest tube, central venous access, suprapubic catheterization, etc.
- Excision of skin or subcutaneous lesions
- Infiltration of surgical wounds postoperatively

Cautions
- **Allergy**. Do not use local anesthesia if there is a history of allergy to local anesthetic.
- **Infection** at site of infiltration. Injection may spread infection. The effect of the local anesthetic will be diminished (due to an acidic environment) and injection may be more painful.
- **Increased risk of toxicity**. Heart block, low cardiac output, epilepsy, myasthenia gravis, hepatic impairment, porphyria, β-blocker, or cimetidine therapy
- **Adrenaline** causes vasoconstriction, reducing bleeding locally and prolonging anesthetic effect. It should not be used for injections into the fingers, toes, ears, or penis (all supplied by end arteries) or where skin flaps are involved, to reduce the chance of flap necrosis.

Anesthetic agents (see Table 3.2)

Equipment
- Syringe
- Needles 21G–25G
- Alcohol swabs

Preparation
- Identify site of infiltration and check for any sign of infection or obvious subcutaneous blood vessels.
- Calculate maximum dose of anesthetic for each individual patient.
- Draw up anesthetic and check details of drug and dose.

Method
- Clean area with alcohol swabs.
- Inject anesthetic slowly with a fine needle to area required, aspirating before each delivery to prevent accidental IV injection.
- Injecting of local anesthetic in a fan-shaped area subcutaneously from a single injection is often more comfortable for the patient.
- Field block. Injecting of anesthetic into the tissues surrounding the area to be anesthetized (e.g., a cutaneous lesion) will often produce a field block, including the area itself.

Table 3.2 Anesthetic agents

Anesthetic	Onset	Duration	Toxic dose	Mg/mL in vial
Bupivacaine (Marcaine)	5–10 min	3–8 hr	2 mg/kg	0.25% = 2.5 mg/mL
				0.50% = 5 mg/mL
Levobupivacaine	5–10 min	3–8 hr	2 mg/kg	0.75% = 7.5 mg/mL
Lidocaine	2–3 min	30–90 min	3 mg/kg	1% = 10 mg/mL
Lidocaine + epi	2–3 min	>90 min	7 mg/kg	2% = 20 mg/mL
Prilocaine	2–3 min	30–90 min	6 mg/kg	4% = 40 mg/mL

Toxicity

This is caused by an overdose of local anesthetic, with systemic absorption, or by accidental IV injection.

Symptoms and signs

- Neurological: mild—slurred speech, light-headedness, tinnitus, and numbness of tongue or mouth, visual disturbance. Severe—confusion, convulsions, and coma
- Cardiovascular: Early tachycardia and hypertension, late bradycardia, hypotension, cardiac arrhythmias, and cardiac arrest may ensue.
- These features usually will occur at a peak of 10–25 min after SC injection, but occur immediately with IV injection.

Treatment

- Stop procedure.
- Maintain the patient's airway and provide oxygen.
- Ensure IV access.
- Perform an ECG.
- Convulsions: give diazepam 5–10 mg IV, slowly.
- Hypotension: raise end of bed and initiate IV fluids.
- Bradycardia usually resolves; atropine is rarely needed.

Tips and problems

- ▶ You are more likely to achieve good anesthetic block with a large volume of less concentrated LA than with a small volume of more concentrated LA: generally use 1% rather than 2%.
- Allow 2–3 min for the LA to take effect: spend this time setting up your instruments and draping the patient.
- *Accidental IV injection.* See Toxicity section above.
- *Inadequate analgesia.* Infiltrate more anesthetic up to the patient's maximum calculated dose. If the patient is still not tolerating the procedure, alternative anesthetic methods may have to be considered, e.g., regional anesthesia (note maximum LA dose), sedation, or general anesthetic.
- The smaller the needle, and the more slowly you inject initially, the less painful it is for the patient.

Intercostal nerve block

This may be a useful skill to learn, although it is usually performed by anesthesiologists.

Indications
- Pain due to fractured ribs
- Post-thoracotomy pain relief

Equipment
- Dressing pack
- Skin antiseptic
- Gloves
- 20 mL syringe and needle
- 20 mL of local anesthetic, e.g., bupivacaine 2.5 mg/mL

Preparation
The patient is positioned sitting forward, resting their arms on a table, and the site of infiltration is identified.
- *Broken ribs*. Medial to the site of fracture on the posterior aspect of the chest wall
- *Post-thoracotomy*. Medial to the posterior edge of the scar on the posterior chest wall

Method
- Ensure that the skin is prepared thoroughly with antiseptic. Place drapes appropriately.
- Insert the needle and syringe containing anesthetic through the skin, first hit the rib and then work inferiorly until just off the edge of the rib (unlike pleural aspiration) associated with the nerve to be blocked.
- Aspirate the syringe to ensure that the needle has not entered a blood vessel or the pleural space. If no blood or air is withdrawn, the site is infiltrated with 4–5 mL of anesthetic.
- This is repeated along the ribs above and below the site.
- Obtain a chest X-ray to ensure that a pneumothorax has not complicated the procedure.

Notes
- *Multiple blocks*. Ensure that the patient does not receive a toxic dose of local anesthetic (📖 p. 567).
- *Air or blood is aspirated*. Withdraw the needle slowly. Get a chest X-ray.

Mechanism of action of local anesthetics

Local anesthetic works by blocking Na channels in the nerve membrane, preventing propagation of the action potential. Small, nonmyelinated pain fibers are blocked first. Large, myelinated fibers that conduct impulses from pressure senses are the last to be blocked.

Head and neck surgery

Michal Mekel, MD
Sareh Parangi, MD

Thyroglossal cyst, sinus, and fistula

Key facts

- Thyroglossal duct cyst is a cystic expansion of a remnant of the thyroglossal duct tract. Thyroglossal duct sinus and fistula represent other classifications of the duct remnant.
- Incidence: <1%
- Male-to-female ratio: 1:1

Anatomy

The thyroid gland arises as a diverticulum at the foramen cecum of the tongue. This diverticulum, with its narrow neck connected to the tongue, descends in the midline of the neck as the thyroglossal tract to reach its normal position at the base of the neck. The path of descent is usually anterior to the hyoid bone. The tract usually atrophies and disappears by the tenth week of gestation. Portions of the tract and remnants of thyroid tissue associated with it may persist at any point between the tongue and the thyroid.

Clinical features

- Usually presents in children or young adults
- Characteristically presents as a painless midline neck mass, may be slightly tender
- In 60% of patients the cyst is at or just below the hyoid bone, although it may occur anywhere along the thyroglossal duct tract.
- Up to 20% of cysts are noted to be slightly off the midline, with a predilection for the left side.
- The cyst is mobile and moves up with swallowing.
- 5% become infected, presenting as a painful, red neck swelling.
- 15% have a fistula to the skin (due to infection or incomplete excision).
- The incidence of thyroglossal duct cyst carcinoma is approximately 1% of all thyroglossal duct cysts, the majority being papillary thyroid carcinoma. Treatment is by excision, with a cure rate of 95%.

Diagnosis and investigations

- Thyroid function should be assessed preoperatively.
- Imaging: Ultrasound should be used to delineate the cystic mass as well as identify a normally located thyroid gland prior to excision. A CT scan is advocated in adult patients presenting with a thyroglossal duct cyst prior to definitive treatment.
- Fine-needle aspiration may reveal a cloudy, infected fluid or a straw-colored fluid (not obligatory).

Treatment

Surgery

- The treatment of choice is surgical excision via a Sistrunk procedure.
- The procedure involves a horizontal incision along a skin crease, elevation of subplatysmal skin flaps, separation of the strap muscles in the midline, and excision of the cyst with a 10–15 mm mid-portion of the hyoid bone together with any proximal tract above it.
- If there is a fistula or sinus in the neck, it should be excised with the cyst.

Infected thyroglossal cyst

- The majority respond to antibiotics.
- Surgical drainage is required if abscess is present or if the patient fails to respond to antibiotics.
- Elective excision of the cyst once acute infection has resolved

Complications

Higher recurrence rates have been attributed to young age of the patient and rupture of the cyst at the time of operation.

Branchial cyst, sinus, and fistula

Key facts

- Comprise up to one-third of congenital neck masses
- May result from the first, second, or third branchial cleft
- Incidence: <1%
- Male-to-female ratio: 1:1
- The first-arch branchial cleft cysts account for less than 1% of all branchial cleft anomalies. The tract of the cyst is intimately associated with the facial nerve.
- Second-cleft branchial cyst is the most common cause of congenital neck lumps.
- A branchial abscess is an infected branchial cyst.

Anatomy

The pharyngeal pouches are lateral out-pouchings of the region of the primitive pharynx. At the extreme lateral wall of each pharyngeal pouch, the endodermal lining contacts the ectodermal epithilium of a branchial cleft. The branchial clefts are named in relation to the pharyngeal pouch with which they are apposed. A developmental alteration of the branchial clefts or pouches can result in the following:

- Cyst: has no communication with the body surface
- Sinus: communicates with a single body surface, either the skin or pharynx
- Fistula: communicate with two body surfaces

A cystic dilation of the tract may be associated with either sinus or fistula.

Clinical features

- Presents as a neck lump, usually painless
- Location:
  - First branchial cleft cysts (rare) present near the angle of the mandible.
  - Second branchial cleft cysts are found high in the neck and deep to the anterior border of the sternocleidomastoid muscle.
  - Third branchial cleft cysts (rare) are seen near the upper pole of the thyroid gland.
- Usually presents in young patients
- In adults, 2/3 occur in men and classically appear in the third decade.
- Two-thirds occur on the left side; 2% are bilateral.
- They may become infected during an upper respiratory infection and present with an acute branchial-cyst abscess causing pain, increased swelling, and, occasionally, pressure symptoms (difficulty swallowing or breathing).

Diagnosis and investigations

- Imaging
  - Ultrasound shows a fluid-filled cyst and can differentiate cystic lesions from solid masses.
  - CT and MRI can delineate the relationship of the cyst to surrounding structures.
- Fine-needle aspiration biopsy
  - Abscesses—purulent fluid is obtained that may culture organisms
  - Cysts—straw-colored fluid containing cholesterol crystals
- Differential diagnosis of cystic masses in the lateral neck of young adults must always include a cystic lymph node metastasis from papillary thyroid cancer.

Treatment

Infected cyst

- Manage with antibiotics. Allow inflammation to resolve before excision is attempted.
- In case of an abscess, drain via a transverse incision in the neck at the point of maximum convexity.

Branchial cyst

- Surgical excision is the treatment of choice.
- Excision is done through a transverse incision over the cyst, preferably in a transverse skin crease.

Branchial fistula

- Surgical excision of the sinus or fistula through a horizontal elliptical incision around the neck opening
- A further transverse incision at a higher level may be required if the upper end of the tract cannot be reached ("stepladder" incisions).

Complications

- A branchial cyst at any site often lies near important nerves. Previous infections causing fibrosis will increase the risk of damaging them. The following nerves are at risk:
  - Hypoglossal nerve (tongue deviates to affected side on protrusion)
  - Mandibular branch of the facial nerve (movement of lower lip)
  - Great auricular nerve (numb ear)
  - Spinal accessory nerve (paralysis of trapezius: weakness of arm abduction, asymmetry, and chronic pain)

Salivary calculi

Key facts

- The three major salivary glands (parotid, submandibular, and sublingual) are subject to the development of stones; 80% occur in the submandibular gland, less than 20% occur in the parotid, and approximately 1% occur in the sublingual gland.
- Composed of calcium phosphate and carbonate
- More common in men, ages 30–60 years

Clinical features

- Pain and swelling of the affected gland upon eating and drinking
- If there is partial obstruction of the duct, the swelling can last minutes or several hours and then disappear.
- May be complicated by sialadenitis (inflammation of a salivary gland)
- Complete obstruction leads to persistent swelling and infection.

Points in examination of the submandibular gland

- Examine the duct orifice from the front. Ask patient to open his mouth wide and point tongue upward. The ducts lie near the midline at the root of the tongue. Is it red? Is there pus? Can you see an impacted stone?
- Examine the gland bimanually from the front. Place the finger of one hand over the gland. The index of the other hand is placed in the mucosal surface of the mandible and the gland palpated between the two.

Diagnosis and investigations

- Plain films are effective in detecting radio-opaque stones. Despite their similar chemical makeup, 90% of submandibular calculi are radio-opaque, whereas 90% of parotid calculi are radiolucent with standard facial X-rays.
- Ultrasound (US): More than 90% of stones 2 mm in diameter or larger can be detected by US. US may also assess periglandular structures.
- Sialography: The duct is cannulated and radio-opaque dye is injected, followed by plain film. This procedure is technically difficult and invasive. It may show a filling defect, and may provide therapeutic benefit due to the flushing effect. It is contraindicated in patients with acute sialadenitis or contrast allergy.
- CT: High-resolution, non-contrast CT scanning is currently the imaging modality of choice for evaluation of salivary stones.
- MR sialography: Standard MRI will not detect calculi. MR sialography does not require intraductal contrast, but it is not yet widely used.

Treatment

- Conservative management: Patients should be instructed to keep well hydrated, massage the gland, and "milk" the duct.
- If infection is suspected, anti-staphylococcal antibiotics should be administered for 7–10 days. Surgical intervention is typically avoided during acute infection.
- Stones less than 2 mm in diameter can typically pass with the assistance of ductal dilation alone.
- Surgical intervention
  - Submandibular stones can be removed via a transoral approach approximately 50% of the time. Stones palpable within the mouth are generally amenable to this procedure.
  - For parotid stones, parotidectomy is performed for stones that are not within approximately 1.5 cm of the orifice of the duct.
- Less invasive approaches
  - Lithotripsy: For patients in whom a simple transoral approach is not possible (stone in the proximal duct or inside the salivary gland) or when it fails
  - Wire basket retrieval: Removal of stones with a wire basket extractor under fluoroscopic guidance
  - Sialoendoscopy: To visualize the ductal anatomy and remove small stones beyond the reach of transoral surgical procedures

Clinical pearls—anatomy and physiology of salivary glands

- Salivary glands produce saliva containing water; electrolytes (especially K^+ and HCO_3); varying amounts of mucus and enzymes.
- Saliva functions to lubricate, aid mastication, aid taste, suppress oral bacteria, and initiate starch digestion.
- The facial nerve trunk lies between the deep and superficial lobes of the parotid gland.

Inflammatory disorders of the salivary glands

Key facts

- Inflammation of the salivary glands can be caused by the following:
  - Bacterial infection: caused by retrograde bacterial contamination of the salivary ducts from the oral cavity (penicillin-resistant *Staphylococcus aureus*—in hospitalized patients, *Streptococcus* species and *Hemophilus influenza*—in community-acquired cases)
  - Salivary calculi (sialolithiasis)
  - Viral infection, e.g., mumps (paramyxovirus), HIV
  - Granulomatous infections, e.g., tuberculosis (TB)
  - Noninfectious inflammatory disorders, e.g., Sjogren's syndrome, sarcoidosis

Clinical features

- May present as a unilateral facial lump, pain, dry mouth, or drooling
- The gland is often tender on palpation.
- Acute suppurative (bacterial) infection of the parotid has a quick onset of signs and symptoms, usually occurring in elderly debilitated patients. The patient may be toxic and pus may exude from the opening of the parotid duct, opposite the crown of the second upper molar tooth.
- Patients who are elderly, debilitated, or dehydrated with poor oral hygiene or who have had anticholinergic drugs occasionally develop parotitis in the postoperative period.
- Chronic sialadenitis is characterized by repeated episodes of pain and swelling. There is often a history of recurrent, intermittent swelling.
- Systemic viral infections can produce localized salivary gland disease in any age group.
- Granulomatous salivary gland infections can occur in children and in elderly patients. They often cause asymptomatic gradual enlargement within the gland.

Diagnosis and investigations

- If pus is present, take a bacteriology swab and send it to the lab.
- Order plain X-rays to determine whether radio-opaque calculi are present in the duct or gland.
- CT scanning may help differentiate between stones, inflammation, and tumor.

Treatment

Acute suppurative infection

- Most patients respond to antibiotics.
  - Give anti-staphylococcal penicillin (naficillin, oxacillin, augmentin) 10–14 days, IV if necessary.
  - Rehydrate dehydrated and debilitated patients.
  - Provide good oral hygiene.
- Examine patients after the infection has subsided to rule out obstruction due to a parotid tumor.

- In case of an abscess, a surgical drainage may be necessary. This involves elevation of an anterior-based facial flap with abscess drainage by radial incisions in the parotid fascia parallel to the facial nerve branches. A drain should be placed and wound edges loosely approximated.

Chronic sialadenitis

- Teach patients with recurrent parotitis to massage the gland in order to express saliva from the duct.
- Chewing a sour candy promotes ductal secretions and is often helpful.
- Dilatation of the duct with lacrimal probes can assist drainage.
- Remove calculi if possible.
- Consider surgical removal of the gland when conservative management has failed to control symptoms.

Other inflammatory processes

- Acute viral parotitis: Supportive measures include bed rest, oral hygiene, hydration, and dietary modifications to minimize glandular secretory activity.
- Tuberculous mycobacterial disease: Triple drug therapy
- Sjogren's syndrome: Symptomatic treatment and prevention of irreversible damage to the teeth and eyes

Salivary gland tumors

Key facts
- Malignant salivary gland tumors are rare, accounting for 0.4% of all malignant tumors.
- They can arise from the major salivary glands (parotid, submandibular, sublingual) or the minor glands; 80% arise in the parotid gland.

Clinical features
- Most patients present with slow-growing, asymptomatic masses.
- Clinical indicators suggestive of malignancy include rapid growth, pain, facial nerve involvement, bleeding from the duct, and cervical lymphadenopathy.
- Pain may indicate neural invasion by the tumor.
- Minor salivary gland tumors usually present as non-ulcerated, painless masses involving the oral cavity.

Benign tumors
Pleomorphic adenoma (benign mixed tumor)
- Accounts for 65% of all salivary gland tumors
- Most often found in the parotid gland
- Histologically is incompletely encapsulated with pseudopod extensions. These features contribute to recurrence after simple enucleation.
- Surgical therapy requires resection with adequate margins.

Warthin tumor (papillary cystadenoma lymphomatosum)
- The second-most common neoplasm of the parotid gland
- The majority occur in the parotid gland.
- Usually affects men >50 years
- Usually presents as a slow-growing mass in the tail of the parotid gland
- Tumors can be multicentric; 10% are bilateral.
- Treatment is complete surgical excision; recurrence is rare.

Malignant tumors
Mucoepidermoid carcinoma
- The most common malignant neoplasm of the parotid gland
- Accounts for 30% of all malignant tumors of the salivary glands
- Low-grade tumors are usually small and partially encapsulated. High-grade tumors are usually larger and locally invasive.

Adenoid cystic carcinoma
- Accounts for 10% of all salivary gland neoplasms
- The most common malignancy of the submandibular and minor glands
- Slow growing with tendency toward neural involvement
- Multiple local recurrences can occur despite adequate surgical intervention.
- Distant metastasis to the lungs, liver, and bones is common; regional lymph node metastases are rare.

Acinic cell carcinoma
- 5%–11% of all salivary gland cancers
- The majority occur in the parotid gland.
- Can be multicentric (2%–5%) or occur bilaterally

Adenocarcinoma
- Most commonly occurs in the minor salivary glands
- Represents 15% of malignant parotid neoplasms
- Aggressive tumor with strong propensity to recur and metastasize

Squamous cell carcinoma
- A rare neoplasm. More common in males, usually in seventh decade
- Occurs more often in the submandibular gland
- Usually presents as a firm indurated mass
- High incidence of regional and distant metastases
- Prognosis is poor.

Undifferentiated carcinoma
- A rare tumor, usually affects the parotid gland
- The tumor is closely related to infection with Epstein–Barr virus.
- Extremely aggressive with marked local invasion and distant metastasis

Diagnosis and investigations
- Complete head and neck examination including tumor characteristics of size, location, mobility, tenderness, and cranial nerve function
- FNA: to obtain a definitive diagnosis; controversial
- CT and MRI provide important diagnostic information about overall dimension, adjacent tissue involvement, and vascular invasion.
- Metastatic workup with emphasis on cervical lymph nodes

Treatment
- The treatment of choice for most salivary gland neoplasms is complete surgical excision with identification and preservation of the facial nerve.
- Facial nerve involvement by tumor requires facial nerve resection.
- Neck dissection is considered depending on tumor type and stage.
- For high-grade mucoepidermoid carcinomas, elective neck dissection should be considered, given the high rate of occult neck metastases.
- Postoperative radiation therapy for high-grade malignant tumors

Complications of parotid surgery
- Facial nerve injury
  - Higher risk with reoperations and operations for malignancy
  - 10%–30% temporary facial nerve paralysis
  - <3% permanent paralysis
- Frey's syndrome
  - Common long-term complication of surgery; up to 25% of patients
  - Facial flushing and sweating of the skin in anticipation of food, due to alternate nerve regeneration after surgery

Prognosis
- Factors affecting survival include tumor stage, location, grade, size, recurrence, and regional and distant metastases. Facial nerve paralysis, skin involvement, pain, and gender also affect the prognosis.
- The 5-year survival rate ranges from 80% to 90% in low-grade tumors to as low as 30%–40% in undifferentiated carcinoma.

Squamous cell carcinoma of the oral cavity

Key facts
- 95% of the malignancies of the oral cavity are SCCs.
- Incidence is 6 per 100,000.
- SCC accounts for 0.6%–5% of all cancers in the United States, and up to 45% of cancers in India.
- Male-to-female ratio: 2.2:1; usually occurs in seventh decade of life
- Predisposing factors include alcohol, tobacco use, and betel nut chewing (in India). Human papillomavirus (HPV) may also play a role in the etiology.
- The most important prognostic factor is status of the cervical lymph nodes.
- 6% of patients have a synchronous SCC present in the aerodigestive tract (mouth, larynx, lungs, esophagus).

Clinical features
- The presentation is usually of an exophytic lesion or a nonhealing ulcer. Ulcers may easily bleed on touching and produce pain.
- Symptoms depend on the site of the tumor.
  - Cancer of the tongue may cause referred pain to the ears, slurring of speech, and difficulty eating.
  - Cancer of the floor of the mouth may invade the mandible, causing loosening of the lower anterior teeth.
- Other symptoms may include odynophagia, bleeding, dysphagia, oral discomfort, reduced movement of oral structures, and trismus.

Diagnosis and investigations
- Physical examination of the mouth and teeth. Removal of prosthetics is important for full examination.
- Examination of the neck is mandatory and should include all levels of lymph nodes
- A biopsy may be performed under local anesthesia.
- CT or MRI
  - Show the extent of disease and bone involvement
  - Used for staging of cervical disease
- Endoscopy (nose, pharynx, hypopharynx, larynx, and esophagus)
  - Evaluates the primary lesion
  - Identifies synchronous tumors
- Evaluation of distant metastases (lung, liver, or bone)
  - Chest radiograph, laboratory studies (liver function tests, alkaline phosphates, serum calcium)
  - With abnormal findings proceed with chest CT, abdominal US or CT, or bone scan.

Table 4.1 Clinical classification of SCC of the oral cavity (AJCC)

T (primary tumor)	N (nodes)	M (metastasis)
T1, <2 cm	N0, no lymph nodes	M0, no metastases
T2, 2–4 cm	N1, single ipsilateral <3 cm	M1, distant metastases
T3, >4 cm	N2a, single ipsilateral 3–6 cm	
	N2b, multiple ipsilateral <6 cm	
	N2c, bilateral/contralateral <6 cm	
T4, involvement of other structures	N3, any nodes >6 cm	

Stage grouping

- Stage 1, T1, N0, M0
- Stage 2, T2, N0, M0
- Stage 3, T3, N0, M0 or T1–T3, N1
- Stage 4, T4, any N; any T, N2/N3; any T, any N, M1

Treatment

T1 and T2 lesions

- The common treatment for early-stage cancer is surgical excision.
- Equal survival with surgical excision vs. radiation therapy
- Because of occult neck metastasis in 20%–30% of patients, treatment of the neck is required for some tumors with N0, either with lymphadenectomy or with radiation; supraomohyoid neck dissection (levels I, II, and III) is appropriate.

T3 and T4 lesions

- Combination therapy: surgical resection with either pre- or postoperative radiation therapy
- Radical neck dissection or modified radical neck dissection (preservation of the spinal accessory nerve, sternocleidomastoid muscle, and jugular vein) should be done for all cases; decision is based on number of nodes, extracapsular spread, and fixation to adjacent structures.

Reconstruction

- Split-thickness skin grafts are used for resurfacing small superficial defects of the oral cavity that cannot be primarily closed.
- Optional myocutaneous flaps for large floor-of-mouth and tongue resections include the following:
  - Regional flaps:
    Pectoralis major myocutaneous flaps
    Delto-pectoral flaps—for large skin-surface coverage
  - Free flaps:
    A radial forearm free flap—osteomyocutaneous flap
    For mandibular reconstruction—fibula, iliac crest, or scapula

Prognosis

- Early stage: 75% 5-year survival
- Advanced stage: 35% 5-year survival

Endocrine surgery

Michal Mekel, MD
Sareh Parangi, MD

Nontoxic goiter

Key facts

- *Goiter* refers to an enlarged thyroid gland.
- Sporadic nontoxic goiter is associated with normal thyroid function and develops in subjects living in iodine-sufficient area.
- Endemic goiter develops in iodine-deficient areas, occurs in more than 10% of the population, and shows biochemical evidence of hypothyroidism.

Clinical features

- Patients present with a thyroid mass.
- Endemic goiters are usually noted during childhood and continue to grow with age.
- Symptoms may be caused by compression of structures in the neck and superior mediastinum, including dyspnea, dysphagia, and hoarseness (due to stretching of the recurrent laryngeal nerve).
- Obstructive symptoms are more likely in patients with substernal goiter.

Diagnosis and investigation

- Thyroid-stimulating hormone (TSH) measurement: the degree of thyroid dysfunction is often mild or subclinical.
- Ultrasound often reveals a heterogeneous thyroid gland or confluent nodules.
- Fine needle aspiration (FNA) is for selected patients with a discrete nodule within the thyroid gland.
- Chest X-rays, CT, and MRI are used for evaluation of mediastinal goiters, to reveal extent of goiter and possible tracheal deviation.

Treatment

- Surgery
  - Treatment of choice
  - Extent of surgery: lobectomy and isthmusectomy for unilateral goiter, total thyroidectomy for bilateral disease
  - Complications of surgery include injury to recurrent laryngeal nerve (1%–2%), hypoparathyroidism (2%–4%), and bleeding (<1%).
- Thyroxine therapy is rarely helpful for small goiters; TSH suppression may slow further goiter development.
- Radioablation therapy is an alternative to surgery in poor surgical candidates.

Graves' disease

Key facts
- Graves' disease is the most common cause of hyperthyroidism.
- It is the most prevalent autoimmune disorder in the United States.
- It is more common in women.

Pathogenesis

Graves' disease is caused by thyroid-stimulating antibodies that bind to and activate the thyrotropin receptor on thyroid follicular cells, stimulating the synthesis of thyroid hormones. Antibodies are also produced against thyroid peroxidase and thyroglobulin. This leads to abnormalities in most organ systems, including the cardiovascular and central nervous system.

Clinical features
- A firm, diffuse goiter
- Thyrotoxicosis symptoms, including nervousness, fatigue, irritability, palpitations, heat intolerance, weight loss, and tremor
- Ophthalmopathy, due to infiltration of T cells in the extraocular muscles and orbital connective tissue. These changes displace the eyeball forward. It is clinically evident in 50% of patients.
- Infiltrative dermopathy occurs in 1%–2% of patients.

Diagnosis and investigations
- Thyroid function tests reveal low serum TSH, high serum-free T3, high or normal serum-free T4, and high serum thyroid-stimulating antibodies.
- Radionuclide scan shows high radioactive iodine uptake.

Treatment
Antithyroid medications
- Methimazole, propylthiouracil (PTU)
  - Interfere with biosynthesis and secretion of thyroid hormone
  - Patients usually become euthyroid within 6 to 12 weeks.
  - Side effects include hepatotoxicity and agranulocytosis (PTU).
  - If hyperthyroidism during pregnancy is severe enough to warrant treatment, PTU is used and thyroid function tests are checked monthly.
- Propranolol is used to control catecholamine response of hyperthyroidism.
- Used for 12–24 months. Remission can be seen in 60% of patients with a recurrence rate of 60%.

Radioactive iodine (131-I)
- Euthyroidism may take 4–6 months, requiring multiple doses.
- May cause transient worsening of ophthalmopathy
- Contraindicated in pregnancy, which should be avoided for 1 year after taking radioactive iodine

Surgery
- Indicated for pregnant women not controlled with anti-thyroid medication, patients with local compressive symptoms or recurrence after medical treatment, many children, and those who fear the administration of radioactive iodine or wish to become pregnant rapidly after treatment.
- Sub-total or near-total thyroidectomy

Thyroid nodules

Key facts

- The prevalence of palpable thyroid nodules in adult Americans is 4%–7%.
- The prevalence of thyroid nodules in autopsy studies is 50%.
- Thyroid nodules are more frequent in women.
- Most thyroid nodules are benign (but see Box 5.1).

Clinical features

- Most thyroid nodules are asymptomatic, discovered as a chance finding by the patient or during physical examination.
- A sudden presentation of painful swelling in the thyroid is probably hemorrhage into a colloid nodule; spontaneous resolution will occur.

Box 5.1 Clinical risk factors for malignancy in a thyroid nodule

- Age <20 years
- Previous neck irradiation
- Male gender
- Family history of thyroid cancer
- A hard, fixed, >4 cm nodule
- Presence of lymph nodes
- Recurrent laryngeal nerve palsy
- Pressure symptoms

Diagnosis and investigations

- Thyroid function tests (TSH, free T4, free T3); most patients are euthyroid
- Calcitonin (optional)
- Thyroid scintigraphy (123-I), done for patients with low TSH (hyperfunctioning gland) for the identification of autonomously functioning thyroid nodule
- Ultrasonography defines nodule characteristics, including size, borders, echogenicity, vascular flow, and microcalcifications.
- FNA
  - Procedure of choice in differentiating benign from malignant nodules
  - Usually done with ultrasound guidance.
  - False-negative rate, 5%; false-positive rate, 3%
  - In general, nodules that are larger then 1 cm should be investigated.
- Results of FNA include the following:
  - Benign (macrofollicular)
  - Malignant (papillary, anaplastic, or medullary cancer)
  - Suspicious
  - Indeterminate (atypical or microfollicular)
  - Other—lymphoma, metastatic disease
  - Hurthle cell neoplasm
  - Nondiagnostic

- FNA cannot differentiate between benign and malignant follicular neoplasm, since capsular or vascular invasion is used to differentiate between the two.

Treatment

- Benign FNA, nodule ≤4 cm with no pressure symptoms: observe, follow up with ultrasound in 6–12 months
- Nondiagnostic FNA: repeat FNA, consider surgery if repeat FNA is nondiagnostic.
- Toxic nodule <3 cm: radioiodine treatment (^{131}I)
- Indications for surgery
  - FNA results: malignant, suspicious, indeterminate
  - Pressure symptoms, increasing size
  - Nodule size >4 cm
  - Toxic nodule >3 cm
  - Significant substernal extension

Surgery

- Thyroid lobectomy (including isthmus and pyramidal lobe) is performed for nonmalignant nodules or indeterminate cytology.
- Total thyroidectomy is performed for a malignant nodule, presence of contralateral nodules, or with history of neck radiation.
- Consider total thyroidectomy for a suspicious nodule or nodules >4 cm.

Important structures that need to be preserved during thyroid surgery (see Fig. 5.1):
- Recurrent laryngeal nerve
- Parathyroid glands
- Superior laryngeal nerve—external branch

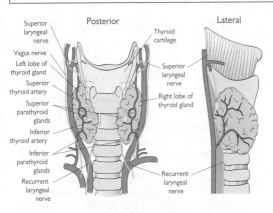

Fig. 5.1 Anatomy of the region of the thyroid gland. Taken from Longmore M, et al. (2007). *Oxford Handbook of Clinical Medicine*, 7th ed. Oxford: Oxford University Press.

Thyroid cancer

Key facts
- Makes up <1% of all malignancies in the United States
- Thyroid cancer classification:
  - Well-differentiated tumors: arising from follicular cell origin, 90%–95% of all thyroid cancers. These include papillary, follicular, and Hurthle cell carcinomas.
  - Medullary thyroid cancer: 4% of all thyroid cancers
  - Anaplastic carcinoma: <1% of thyroid carcinomas

Clinical features
- Usually presents as a painless thyroid mass
- Hoarseness and firm fixation of the mass suggest advanced disease and a poor prognosis.
- Papillary carcinoma may be found incidentally in a thyroid sample resected for a benign process.

Differentiated thyroid cancer
Papillary carcinoma
- Most common thyroid cancer; 70%–80% of all thyroid malignancies
- Associated with an excellent prognosis
- A papillary thyroid cancer <1 cm is defined as a *microcarcinoma*.
- Associated with history of radiation exposure
- Typical histologic characteristics include intranuclear inclusion bodies (orphan Annie nuclei) and psammoma bodies.
- Multicentricity can be found in up to 70% of patients.
- Lymph node metastases can be found in 30%–50% of patients. Central neck nodes are usually involved first. This does not affect long-term survival.
- More aggressive subtypes include insular, columnar, and tall-cell carcinomas.

Follicular carcinoma
- Age is usually >50 years.
- A subtype of follicular carcinoma, which consists of oxyphilic cells, is termed *Hurthle cell* carcinoma and occurs usually in older patients.
- The histologic diagnosis of follicular cancer depends on capsular or vascular invasion (which can be determined only on final pathology).

Medullary thyroid carcinoma (MTC)
- MTC originates from the parafollicular cells (C cells).
- It is associated with secretion of calcitonin, which is used as a marker.
- 70%–80% of MTCs are sporadic; 20%–30% of MTCs are associated with multiple endocrine neoplasia (MEN) 2A or 2B;. Familial MTC carries a genetic risk for MTC without the other associated endocrine dysfunction associated with MEN. The inherited disorders share a *RET* oncogene mutation that predisposes to MTC. Sporadic MTC may also have a somatic RET mutation.

- MTC is multicentric in 90% of patients with hereditary forms and in 20% of patients with the sporadic form.
- Nodal metastases are present in >70% of patients with palpable disease.

Anaplastic thyroid cancer

- This is the most aggressive form of thyroid cancer.
- It occurs usually in older patients and those with previously existing goiter disease.
- Patients typically present with dysphagia, cervical tenderness, and a painful mass.
- There is rapid deterioration with local invasion of surrounding structures with tracheal obstruction.

Diagnosis and investigations

- Thyroid function tests should be obtained: most patients are euthyroid.
- Ultrasonography, for characterization of the nodule, visualization of the contralateral lobe, and evaluation of cervical lymph nodes
- FNA should be done for any suspicious nodule and any enlarged suspicious cervical lymph node.
- CT scan of the neck and chest and laryngoscopy, for evaluation of vocal cords, should be done for large tumors with compressive symptoms before surgery, and for those with voice changes.
- For medullary thyroid cancer diagnosed by FNA, investigation should include the following:
  - Calcitonin level
  - A detailed family history for MEN characteristics and screening for pheochromocytoma (24-hr urinary catecholamines) and hyper-parathyroidism (serum calcium levels and parathyroid hormone)
  - Staging—imaging of neck and chest

Table 5.1 TNM Classification for differentiated thyroid cancer

Stage	Patient age < 45 years	Patient age > 45 years
I	Any T, any N, M0	T1, N0, M0
II	Any T, any N, M1	T2, N0, M0
III		T3, N0, M0; T1–T3, N1a, M0
IV		T4, any N, any M; N1b, any T, any M; any T, any N, M1

T1: Tumor <2 cm	N0: No metastatic nodes	M0: No metastases
T2: Tumor 2–4 cm	N1a: Metastases to level VI	M1: Distant metastases
T3: Tumor >4 cm	N1b: Metastases to cervical or mediastinal nodes (see Fig. 5.1)	
T4: tumor invades adjacent structures		

Treatment
Differentiated thyroid cancer
- Papillary thyroid cancer: total thyroidectomy with removal of suspicious central lymph nodes or with central neck dissection (level VI)
- Papillary thyroid cancers smaller than 1 cm (microcarcinoma): lobectomy plus isthmusectomy is appropriate (usually discovered after lobectomy for a benign lesion).
- Follicular thyroid carcinoma: the diagnosis is made after lobectomy and isthmusectomy are done for a follicular neoplasm. A completion total thyroidectomy should be done in that case.
- Modified radical neck dissection should be done in patients with clinically and cytologically evident lymph node metastases in lateral neck.
- Radioiodine ablative treatment is used postoperatively to destroy any residual thyroid tissue or metastatic disease to lymph nodes or distant sites in select patients.

Medullary thyroid cancer
- Total thyroidectomy with central node dissection is the appropriate treatment.
- An ipsilateral neck dissection is recommended for patients with palpable cervical nodes, patients with central neck nodes, and patients with primary tumors >2 cm.
- For patients with MEN 2A, subtotal parathyroidectomy should be carried out at the same time.
- Radioactive iodine therapy is ineffective.

Anaplastic thyroid cancer
- Complete resection is often not possible.
- The most effective therapy for local control of the disease is a multimodality therapy consisting of a combination of radiotherapy and chemotherapy, followed by surgical resection of as much tumor as safely possible, followed by combined chemoradiotherapy.
- Tracheostomy for airway management may be necessary.

Surgical complications
- Hypocalcemia (2%–4%). Every effort should be made during surgery to evaluate parathyroid tissue intraoperatively and autotransplant glands that appear to be devascularized.
- Recurrent laryngeal nerve injury (1%–2%). Be careful during dissection in the nerve pathway, including the tracheoesophageal groove and ligament of Berry. Do not use electrocautery close to the nerve.
- Bleeding (<1%). Wound hematoma may require immediate re-exploration. In case of airway compromise, the wound should be opened at the bedside.

Prognosis
- 10-year survival rate: stage I, 95%; stage II, 50%–95%; stage III, 15%–50%; stage IV, <15%
- Prognosis of papillary cancer is better than for follicular cancer.
- Medullary carcinoma: cure rate is 40%–50%.
- Anaplastic carcinoma: expected life span is <6 months after diagnosis.

Hyperparathyroidism

Key facts
Primary hyperparathyroidism (pHPT)
- The most common cause of hypercalcemia in outpatients
- Usually caused by a single adenoma. More than one abnormal gland is present in 20% of patients.
- The incidence of double adenomas increases with age.
- Can occur with MEN 1 and less frequently with MEN 2A; patients have hyperplasia of four glands.
- Parathyroid carcinoma is present in 0.5% of patients with pHPT.

Secondary hyperparathyroidism (sHPT)
- Caused by chronic extrinsic overstimulation of normal parathyroid glands
- Most commonly caused by chronic renal failure
- Pathogenesis consists of decreased 1,25-$(OH)_2D_3$, hyperphosphatemia, and altered parathyroid hormone (PTH) metabolism.
- Long-term treatment with lithium is also associated with parathyroid hyperplasia.

Clinical features
- The pentad of symptoms: "painful bones, kidney stones, abdominal groans, psychic moans, and fatigue overtones."
- Other complications include memory impairment and higher risk for cardiovascular diseases.
- Manifestations of sHPT include bone pain, bone deformities, fractures, metastatic calcifications, and skin manifestations (pruritus, calciphylaxis).

Diagnosis and investigations
- pHPT: hypercalcemia, increased blood level of intact PTH, and normal or increased urinary calcium concentration. Patients will often have low blood phosphorus level.
- Rule out familial hypocalciuric hypercalcemia (FHH) by measurement of 24-hr urine calcium. FHH patients will have urinary calcium levels <100 mg/24 hr.
- Preoperative localization studies
  - Ultrasound: sensitivity 22%–82%; specificity 80%–90%
  - Sestamibi scan: sensitivity 39%–92%; specificity 90%–95%
- A thorough clinical history should be taken to rule out other endocrinopathies (MEN syndrome).

Treatment
Primary HPT
- Surgery is the only definitive treatment for pHPT.
- Surgery is recommended for patients with overt complications and symptoms such as nephrolithiasis, fractures, and neuromuscular syndrome.

- Consider a targeted exploration (minimally invasive surgery) for a localized hyperfunctioning gland with intraoperative monitoring of PTH.
- For HPT associated with MEN syndrome, a subtotal parathyroidectomy or total parathyroidectomy with parathyroid autotransplantation should be done.

Indications for surgery in asymptomatic pHPT
- Serum calcium >1 mg/dL above upper limit of normal
- 24-hr urine calcium >400 mg
- Creatinine clearance reduced by >30%
- Bone density >2.5 SD below peak bone mass
- Age under 50 years

Secondary HPT
- Parathyroidectomy is indicated when medical treatment fails to control progressive disease.
- All four glands should be explored during the operation.
- A subtotal parathyroidectomy or a total parathyroidectomy with parathyroid autotransplantation should be done.

Complications of surgery
- Recurrent laryngeal nerve injury
- Bleeding
- Postoperative hypocalcemia
- Failure to cure
- Recurrence

Adrenal masses

Key facts

- Adrenal masses are classified as functional (hormone secreting) and nonfunctional tumors.
- Functional tumors include
  - Cortisol-producing adenomas
  - Aldosterone-producing adenomas (aldosteronomas)
  - Pheochromocytoma
  - Adrenal cortical carcinoma
- Nonfunctional tumors include ganglioneuromas, myelolipomas, benign cysts, or metastases.
- Adrenal incidentalomas are adrenal lesions discovered incidentally on imaging; they are seen with increased frequency over the age of 40.
- 80% of patients with incidentalomas have nonfunctional tumors.

Clinicopathological features

Cortisol-secreting adrenal tumor

- Originates from the adrenal cortex
- Accounts for 10%–20% of cases of Cushing's syndrome
- Symptoms include fatigue, depression, weight gain, menstrual irregularities, glucose intolerance, and easy bruising.
- Signs include central obesity, cervical fat pad, thinned skin, purple striae, acne, hirsutism, and proximal muscle wasting.

Aldosterone-secreting adrenal tumor

- Originates from the adrenal cortex
- Should be differentiated from adrenal hyperplasia as a cause of primary hyperaldosteronism
- Results in primary hyperaldosteronism (Conn's sundrome)
- Characterized by refractory hypertension and hypokalemia
- Occurs at ages 30–60 years

Pheochromocytoma

- Originates from the adrenal medulla
- Symptoms include severe hypertension, tachycardia, palpitations, arrythmias, anxiety attacks, and sweating.
- Can be part of a familial syndrome—MEN2
- The 10% tumor: 10% malignant, 10% bilateral, 10% familial, 10% children, 10% extra-adrenal
- Malignancy is determined with tumor invasion to adjacent structures or with metastatic disease.

Adrenal cortical carcinoma

- A rare malignancy with poor prognosis
- Comprises 5% of all adrenal incidentalomas
- Risk for malignancy is correlated with tumor size—25% risk for lesions larger than 6 cm.
- Two-thirds of tumors are functional, and present with rapidly progressive symptoms, usually hypercortisolism or virilization.
- Nonfunctional tumors can present with flank or abdominal pain.

Diagnosis and investigations
Biochemical evaluation
- Cushing's syndrome
  - High blood or salivary cortisol levels; low ACTH levels
  - 1 mg overnight dexamethasone suppression test; serum cortisol >1.8 μg/dL is suggestive of Cushing's syndrome
  - Confirmed by 24-hr urinary free cortisol and high-dose dexamethasone test.
- Aldosteronoma: ratio of serum aldosterone/renin >20 is suggestive of hyperaldosteronism
- Pheochromocytoma: measurement of blood or 24-hr urinary catecholamines, metanephrines, normetanephrines, and vanillylmandelic acid (VMA)

Imaging
- CT scan
  - Delineates tumor size, location, enhancement characteristics, invasion to adjacent structures, contralateral adrenal, and metastases.
  - Benign lesions are suggested by size smaller than 4 cm, homogeneous mass, smooth borders, and attenuation value of <10 HU on unenhanced CT scan.
- MRI: characteristic brightness of pheochromocytoma on T2 images
- MIBG scan (^{131}I-metaiodobenzylguanidine): useful in patients with biochemical evidence of pheochromocytoma whose tumors cannot be localized by CT or MRI
- FNA
  - May be useful in patients with history of cancer (particularly lung, breast, and kidney) when metastasis is suspected
  - Pheochromocytoma should be excluded before FNA.
- Bilateral adrenal venous sampling with measurements of aldosterone and cortisol may be necessary to localize the secreting tumor.

Treatment
- Resection of the involved adrenal gland is the treatment of choice for hormonally functioning and malignant (or suspected malignant) adrenal tumors.
- Adrenalectomy may be performed via open (transabdominal, thoracoabdominal or retroperitoneal approach) or laparoscopic approach.
- For adrenal carcinoma, tumor >6–7 cm, or those with evidence of local invasion, open adrenalectomy is the procedure of choice.
- Preparation for surgery for pheochromocytoma includes α-blockade (usually phenoxybenzamine) for 1–3 weeks before surgery. β-Blockers may be given for tachycardia or arrhythmias only after complete α-blockade. Adequate hydration is also required.
- After adrenal surgery for Cushing's syndrome, patients should be treated with glucocorticoids until the hypothalamic–pituitary–adrenal axis recovers (12–24 months).

- Tumors smaller than 4 cm with no laboratory evidence of hypersecretion or suspicious imaging may be treated conservatively with annual hormonal and imaging study. Tumors larger than 4 cm should be surgically excised.
- Adrenalectomy for adrenal metastasis should be considered with solitary metastasis.

Breast surgery

Michelle Specht, MD

Breast cancer

Key facts

- 1 in 8–9 lifetime risk for women
- Most common in Western Europe; least common in Japan and Africa
- Incidence increases with age.
- <1% occurs in men
- 5%–10% is related to identifiable genetic abnormality (*BRCA1*, *BRCA2*, *p53*, *PTEN*, etc.)
- 60% present as symptomatic disease; 40% during screening

Pathological features

Of all breast cancer cases, 80% are ductal adenocarcinoma and 20% are lobular, mucinous tubular, or medullary adenocarcinoma. Most carcinomas are believed to originate as in situ carcinoma before becoming invasive, and 70% express estrogen or progesterone receptors.

Clinical features

Breast lump

- Most common presenting symptom
- Usually painless (unless inflammatory carcinoma)
- Firm; ill defined; irregular with poorly defined edges
- May be immobile (held within breast tissue), tethered (attached to surrounding breast tissue or skin), or fixed (attached to chest wall)
- Disease progression may lead to skin retraction, nipple inversion, skin changes (peau d'orange), bleeding, and ulceration.

Nipple abnormalities

- The nipple may be the prime site of disease (Paget's disease), presenting as an eczema-like change.
- The nipple may be affected by an underlying cancer:
  - Inverted
  - Deviated
  - Associated bloody discharge

Skin changes

- Carcinoma beneath the skin causes dimpling, puckering, or color changes.
- Late presentation may be with skin ulceration or fungating.
- Lymphedema of the skin (peau d'orange) suggests local lymphatic involvement.

Systemic features

- Systemic features include weight loss, anorexia, bone pain, jaundice, malignant pleural and pericardial effusions, and anemia.

Diagnosis and investigations

Diagnostic tests
- Clinical examination (as above)
- Radiological assessment. All patients with a clinically suspicious lesion should undergo diagnostic workup with bilateral mammography (if age >30) and targeted ultrasound.
- Cytological assessment with fine needle aspiration cytology (FNAC), core biopsy, or excisional biopsy. Core or excisional biopsy is preferred in most cases because tissue invasion is able to be assessed, which distinguishes invasive cancer from DCIS.

Staging investigations
Systemic staging is usually reserved for patients after surgical treatment with a tumor who are at risk of systemic disease or have symptoms suggestive of systemic disease.
- Chest CT
- Abdomen and pelvic CT
- Bone scan
- CT of the head if symptoms are present

Treatment
Therapy of nonmetastatic breast cancer includes surgery, radiation therapy, and chemotherapy.

Surgical treatment of breast cancer

Surgical options for local treatment include excision, mastectomy, and surgical management of affected lymph nodes and metastatic disease.

Wide local excision (lumpectomy)

- Excision of the tumor with clear margins
- Surgical excision maybe guided by palpation or preoperative needle localization by ultrasound, mammography, or breast MRI.
- Contraindications to lumpectomy include previous radiation therapy, multicentric breast cancer, and large tumor relative to breast size.
- Excision is usually followed by radiation therapy to reduce risk of local recurrence.

Simple mastectomy

- For large tumors (especially in small breast), central location, and late presentation with complications such as ulceration and inflammatory breast cancer
- Also used for multicentric tumors or where there is evidence of widespread in situ changes
- Adjuvant breast radiotherapy is used when there is a high risk of recurrence, multiple lymph node involvement, or close margins.
- Performed with reconstruction at the same time or at a later stage:
  - Latissimus dorsi flap
  - TRAM flap
  - Implant reconstruction (📖 p. 456)

Studies show no difference in overall or disease-free survival when comparing lumpectomy with radiation to simple mastectomy.

Surgical management of regional lymph nodes

Sentinel lymph node biopsy

- Isosulfan blue dye or methylene blue dye or sulfur technicium colloid is injected into the breast to identify the first draining lymph node(s).
- Sentinel lymph node(s) are excised and undergo enhanced pathologic assessment.
- If there is no evidence of metastases, no further treatment is necessary.
- If positive for metastatic disease, patients undergo axillary lymph node dissection.
- Contraindications to sentinel lymph node biopsy include a clinically positive axillary lymph node with FNA biopsy positive for metastatic disease, pregnancy, and preoperative chemotherapy.

Axillary lymph node dissection

- Optimizes staging and prognostication and helps direct adjuvant treatment
- Decreases local recurrence in the setting of lymph node–positive disease
- Increases risk of lymphedema

Surgery for metastatic disease

Surgery in metastatic disease is limited to procedures for symptomatic control of local disease (pain, bleeding, and fungating cancer).

Radiation therapy

- Used to decrease local recurrence, particularly after wide local excision
- May be omitted in elderly women with small hormone-positive tumors
- Contraindicated during pregnancy and in women with a history of ipsilateral breast radiation therapy

Chemotherapy

In nonmetastatic disease, medical therapy is used to reduce the risk of systemic recurrence and is usually given after primary surgery.

- *Endocrine therapy*: anti-estrogens, e.g., tamoxifen, aromatase inhibitors LHRH antagonists. This is most effective in ER-positive tumors.
- *Chemotherapy* (e.g., anthracyclines, cyclophosphamides, and taxanes): offered to patients with a high risk of systemic recurrence (positive lymph nodes, large tumors, and/or high grade). May decrease systemic recurrence by 30%–40%. Trastuzumab is a monoclonal antibody to HER2 that may be used with HER2/*neu*+ breast cancer patients.

In metastatic disease, medical therapy is palliative to increase survival time and includes

- Endocrine therapy—as above
- Chemotherapy (e.g., anthracyclines, taxanes)
- Radiotherapy—to reduce pain of bony metastases or symptoms from cerebral or liver disease

Breast cancer screening

Aims

- To identify asymptomatic breast cancer at an early stage
- Mammography is recommended annually for asymptomatic women >40 years of age.
- Two-view (lateral and oblique) mammography of both breasts
- Suspicious- or malignant-looking lesions are called back for clinical assessment by standard triple assessment.

High-risk screening

- Women with a first-degree relative diagnosed with breast cancer should begin screening mammography 10 years prior to the year the incident cancer was detected but not prior to age 25.
- Women at high risk (greater than 20% lifetime risk) should get an MRI and a mammogram annually. (Lifetime risk is estimated using various models: BRCAPRO, Claus, or Gail risk model.) This includes patients who have tested positive for a *BRCA* mutation.
- Women at moderately increased risk (15%–20% lifetime risk) should talk with their doctors about the benefits and limitations of adding MRI screening to their yearly mammogram.
- Yearly MRI screening is not recommended for women whose lifetime risk of breast cancer is less than 15%.
- Patients with a history of mantle radiation therapy are eligible for such screening.

Results

- Absolute reductions in cancer deaths due to screening over 10 years are as follows:
  - 0.5 per 1000 at age 40
  - 2 per 1000 at age 50
  - 3 per 1000 at age 60
  - 2 per 1000 at age 70
- Studies suggest up to a 30% reduction in mortality from screening-detected early-stage breast cancer.

Benign breast disease

Fibroadenoma

Fibroadenoma is benign overgrowth of one lobule of the breast. Usually isolated, it may be multiple or giant. It is most common under age 30 but may occur at any age up to menopause.

- *Features*: painless, mobile, discrete lump
- *Diagnosis*: ultrasound followed by FNA, core or excisional biopsy
- *Treatment*: excision if there is concern over diagnosis, cosmesis, or symptoms.

Cysts

Cycsts are almost always benign. They are often associated with fibrocystic disease (see below).

- *Features*: round, symmetrical lump(s). They may be discrete or multiple and are occasionally painful.
- *Diagnosis*: ultrasound. If the cyst is simple there is no need for aspiration or biopsy; if complicated or complex, aspiration or excision should be considered.
- *Treatment*: aspiration of simple cyst if symptomatic. It often recurs.

Fibrocystic disease

This disease is a combination of localized fibrosis, inflammation, cyst formation, and hormone-driven breast pain. It occurs almost exclusively between menarche and menopause (15–55 years of age).

- *Features*: Cyclical pain and swelling, "lumpy" breasts, multiple breast cysts
- *Diagnosis*: Lumps usually require intensive assessment (once a diagnosis of fibrocystic disease is made, any woman *may* develop a carcinoma).
- *Treatment*: Reassurance, anti-inflammatories, supportive bra, and/or hormonal manipulation (e.g., primrose oil).

Breast infections

Lactational mastitis

This condition is due to acute staphylococcal infection of mammary ducts. It may degenerate into an acute lactational abscess. Treat with oral antibiotics and (repeated) aspiration if abscess occurs. There is no need to stop lactating. Incision and drainage of an abscess may put the patient at risk for a milk fistula.

Recurrent mastitis/mammary duct ectasia

This condition is due to dilated, scarred, chronically inflamed subareolar mammary ducts and is associated with smoking. Patients present with recurrent yellow-green nipple discharge or recurrent breast abscesses. Infection is usually mixed anaerobic. Surgery is rarely necessary. Treatment is smoking cessation.

Traumatic fat necrosis

This posttraumatic disorder of breast tissue is caused by the organization of acute traumatic injury by

- fibrosis;
- organized local hematoma; and
- occasionally calcification.

It presents with a new, painless, or painful breast lump, often poorly defined. It may occur after reduction mammoplasty.

Diagnosis may be difficult. Failure to resolve the necrosis or doubt about the diagnosis after assessment is an indication for excisional biopsy.

Phyllodes tumor

- Most common nonepithelial breast tumor
- Associated with large, painless, mobile, and rapidly growing lesion that pathologically has a leaf-like appearance
- Classified as benign or malignant (cystosarcoma phyllodes)
- Wide local excision is indicated with a minimum of 1-cm margins.
- In large or recurrent tumors, perform mastectomy.
- Axillary lymph node dissection is not indicated, as metastatic spread is usually hematologic.

Syndromes of the breast

Mondor's syndrome

Sclerosing thrombophlebitis of the anterior chest wall follows breast surgery and presents as a cord-like mass. Treat with NSAIDs.

Poland's syndrome

This syndrome consists of hypoplasia or absence of pectoralis major with lack of breast development and an ipsilateral hand development anomaly.

Acute breast pain

Causes and features

Breast origin

- *Breast abscess.* Acute, severe, localized pain in the breast, associated with swelling, redness, and sometimes purulent nipple discharge. Abscess is most common in breast-feeding women and may be due to chronic mastitis/mammary duct ectasia (see 🔲 p. 256). It is occasionally recurrent.
- *Mastitis.* Recurrent, intermittent breast pain with swelling, tenderness, seropurulent nipple discharge. Mastitis is most common in smokers and is associated with mammary duct ectasia (see 🔲 p. 256).
- *Fibrocystic disease* (see 🔲 p. 256). Usually recurrent or chronic breast pain, but may be an acute, isolated episode. Often multifocal, this disease is associated with tender, vague swelling or "lumpiness."

Non-breast origin

- *Musculoskeletal.* Often onset after exercise, coughing, or straining but not always. There are no associated breast symptoms. Pain is usually sharp and precipitated by movement or breathing. Patients are often tender deep to breast tissue and over other chest wall areas (e.g., costochondral junctions in costochondritis).
- *Visceral.* May be due to atypical angina or acute coronary syndrome
- *Skin pathology.* Such as infected sebaceous cysts, cellulitis, skin abscess

Chapter 7

Upper gastrointestinal surgery

Denise Gee, MD

Upper gastrointestinal endoscopy

There are three types of endoscopy looking at the upper GI and pancreaticobiliary tracts.

Gastroscopy

Correctly termed esophago-gastro-duodenoscopy (EGD), gastroscopy allows direct visualization of pathology and small-channel biopsies to be taken.

Indications

- Investigation of dysphagia
- Investigation of dyspepsia, reflux disease, upper abdominal pain
- Investigation of acute or chronic upper GI bleeding
- Investigation of iron deficiency anemia (with colonoscopy)
- Therapeutic interventions for upper GI pathology
  - Balloon dilatation of benign strictures
  - Endoluminal stenting of malignant strictures
  - Injection, coagulation, or banding of bleeding sources, including ulcers, varices, tumors, and vascular malformations

Preparation and procedure

- The patient should be npo for 4 hr (except in emergency indications).
- IV access is required.
- Often performed with local anesthetic throat spray (topical benzocaine)
- Often performed with IV sedation (e.g., midazolam 5 mg)

Risks and complications

- Perforation (usually of the esophagus)—median risk is approximately 1/3000; highest in elderly, with esophageal pathology, during therapeutic interventions
- Bleeding—most common after biopsies or therapeutic procedures
- Respiratory depression and arrest—related to overmedication with sedative; most common in frail, low–body weight, elderly patients

Endoscopic retrograde cholangiopancreatography (ERCP)

Indications

- Investigation of possible biliary disease (common bile duct stones, biliary strictures, biliary tumors, biliary injuries, intrahepatic biliary disease)
- Investigation of pancreatic disease (pancreatic duct strictures, pancreatic duct abnormalities)
- Therapeutic interventions for pancreaticobiliary disease
  - Stenting for common bile duct stones, strictures, tumors
  - Sphincterotomy for extraction of biliary stones

Preparation and procedure

- The patient should be npo for 4 hr (except in emergency indications).
- IV access is required.
- Often performed with local anesthetic throat spray (topical lidocaine)

- Always performed with IV sedation (e.g., midazolam 5 mg) and occasionally analgesia (e.g., fentanyl 50 μg)
- Performed under fluoroscopic guidance
- May be performed under general anesthesia (GA).

Risks and complications
- Perforation (of the esophagus or of the duodenum)—median risk is approximately 1/1000; highest in elderly, with pathology, during therapeutic interventions, especially sphincterotomy
- Bleeding: after biopsies or therapeutic procedures, especially sphincterotomy. Usually controlled by balloon pressure; may require open surgery
- Respiratory depression and arrest: related to overmedication with sedative. Seen in frail, low–body weight, elderly patients.

Ileoscopy
Often termed *push endoscopy*, ileoscopy is performed with a long-length, thin-caliber endoscope aiming to intubate past the duodenojejunal junction and visualize the first loops of the upper small bowel.

Indications
- Investigation of undiagnosed upper GI bleeding (possibly due to proximal small bowel pathology)
- Investigation of abdominal pain
- Investigation of upper small-bowel Crohn's disease

Preparation and procedure
These are as for gastroscopy.

Risks and complications
These are as for gastroscopy.

Esophageal motility disorders

Key facts

These disorders comprise a spectrum of diseases involving failure of coordination or contraction of the esophagus and its related muscular structures.

Pathological features

In some cases, degeneration of the inner and outer myenteric plexuses can be demonstrated but often no structural abnormality is seen.

Clinical features

Achalasia

- Peak ages of incidence are in young adulthood (idiopathic) and old age (mostly degenerational).
- Slowly progressive dysphagia, initially worse for fluids than for solids.
- Frequent regurgitation of undigested food is common late in the disease course.
- Secondary recurrent respiratory infections are due to aspiration.

Diffuse esophageal spasm

- Most commonly seen in young adults; males > females
- Characterized by acute pain along the length of the esophagus, induced by ingestion, especially of hot or cold substances (odynophagia)

Diagnosis and investigations

Achalasia

- *Barium swallow.* A characteristic failure of relaxation of the lower esophagus tapering to a "bird's beak."
- *Esophageal manometry.* Hypertonic lower esophageal high-pressure zone with failure of relaxation normally induced by swallowing. In chronic cases the proximal esophagus may be aperistaltic.
- *Esophagoscopy* is used to exclude benign and malignant strictures.

Diffuse esophageal spasm

- *Barium swallow.* A "corkscrew" appearance of the esophagus is caused by discoordinated diffuse contractions.
- *Esophageal manometry.* Diffuse hypertonicity and failure of relaxation. There is little or no evidence of coordinated progressive peristalsis during episodes, but normal peristalsis occurs when asymptomatic.
- *Esophagoscopy.* Required to exclude underlying associated malignancy

Treatment

Achalasia

- Endoscopically guided controlled balloon dilatation (fixed pressure) is successful in up to 80% of patients, with a low complication rate (perforation). Results are often short term; multiple procedures may be needed over time.
- Botulinum toxin injections have success in some patients failing dilatation.

- Surgical myotomy (**Heller myotomy**) is an open or laparoscopically performed division of the lower esophageal muscle fibers. It is highly successful, especially in resistant cases.
  - Specific complications include reflux, obstruction of the gastroesophageal junction, and esophageal perforation.
  - Often performed with partial fundoplication

Diffuse esophageal spasm

- Oral calcium channel blockers, or relaxants, e.g., benzodiazepines
- Long-acting nitric oxide donors (smooth-muscle relaxant)
- Widespread esophageal pneumatic dilatations (often repeated)
- Long surgical myotomy is rarely undertaken.

Clinical pearls—anatomy and physiology of the esophagus

- Upper two-thirds. Stratified squamous epithelial-lined (develops squamous carcinoma), striated skeletal muscle, lymphatic drainage to neck and mediastinal nodes, somatic innervation of sensation (e.g., moderately accurate location of level of pathology)
- Lower third. Transition to columnar epithelium (develops adenocarcinoma), transition to smooth muscle, lymphatic drainage to gastric and para-aortic nodes, visceral innervation (poor localization of pathology)
- The gastroesophageal junction, the site of portosystemic anastomosis (between left gastric and (hemi)azygous veins), may develop gastric or esophageal varices.
- Upper esophageal sphincter (UES) = cricopharyngeus
- Lower esophageal sphincter (LES) = functional zone of high pressure above the gastroesophageal junction. Relaxants include alcohol and caffeine.
- Swallowing requires intact and coordinated innervation from vagus (UES, esophagus, LES) and intramural myenteric plexus.

Zenker's diverticulum (pharyngeal pouch)

Key facts

- An acquired "pulsion" diverticulum arising in the relatively fibrous tissue between the inferior constrictor and cricopharyngeus muscle: Killian's triangle
- Arises primarily as a result of failure of appropriate coordinated relaxation of the cricopharyngeus, causing increased pressure on the tissues directly above during swallowing
- Typically occurs in the elderly
- Associated with lower cranial nerve dysfunction (e.g., motor neuron disease, previous CVA)

Pathological features

- Acquired diverticulum: fibrous tissue and serosa without muscle fibers in most of the wall
- Tends to lie to one side of the midline (usually to the left) because the cervical spine is directly behind it.

Clinical features

- Halitosis
- Upper cervical dysphagia
- Intermittent "lump" appearing to the side of the neck on swallowing
- Regurgitation of food—undigested

Diagnosis and investigations

- Diagnosis may be made on observed swallowing with a transient neck swelling appearing.
- Barium swallow will show filling of the pouch.

▶ Gastroscopy should be avoided unless there is a question of associated pathology, since the pouch can be easily missed and easily damaged or perforated by inadvertent intubation.

Treatment

Cricopharyngeal myotomy must be performed. Zenker's diverticulum can be resected or suspended. More recently, endoscopic stapled pharyngoplasty has also been introduced, involving side-to-side stapling of the pouch to the upper esophagus, which also divides the cricopharyngeus muscle.

Hiatus hernia

Key facts

Hiatus hernia entails presence of part or all of the stomach within the thoracic cavity, usually by protrusion through the esophageal hiatus in the diaphragm (see Fig. 7.1).

- Very common; women > men; most are asymptomatic
- May or may not be associated with gastroesophageal reflux disease (GERD)
- Predisposing factors: obesity, previous surgery

Clinicopathological features

Sliding hernia

- Results from axial displacement of upper stomach through the esophageal hiatus, usually with stretching of the phrenoesophageal membrane.
- The gastroesophageal junction is above the diaphragm.
- It is by far the most common form and may result in GERD.

Rolling (paraesophageal) hernia

Rolling hernia results from displacement of part or all of the fundus and body of the stomach through a defect in the phrenoesophageal membrane such that it comes to lie alongside the normal esophagus.

- Much less common type
- The gastroesophageal junction is below the diaphragm.
- Symptoms include hiccups, "pressure" in the chest, odynophagia, and early satiety.
- May result in volvulus or become incarcerated and cause obstruction

Diagnosis and investigations

- Barium swallow usually identifies the type and extent.
- CT scanning of the thorax may be helpful in acute presentations.

Treatment

Medical (mainly for GERD symptoms)

- Reduce acid production. Patient should stop smoking, lose weight, and reduce alcohol consumption.
- Counteract acid secretion with proton pump inhibitors (PPI) and provide symptomatic relief with antacids.

Surgical

Surgery is indicated for the following:

- Persistent symptoms despite maximal medical therapy
- Established complications of rolling (paraesophageal) hernia, such as volvulus or obstruction

The elective procedure of choice is open or laparoscopic reduction of the hernia with crural repair and often a complete or partial fundoplication, depending on whether GERD symptoms predominate. Acute presentations may require a partial gastrectomy.

Sliding hernia   **Rolling hernia**

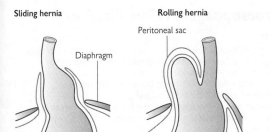

Fig. 7.1 Hiatus hernia—sliding and rolling. Taken from Longmore M., et al. (2007). *Oxford Handbook of Clinical Medicine*, 7th ed. Oxford: Oxford University Press.

Gastroesophageal reflux disease

Key facts

- Pathologically excessive entry of gastric contents into the esophagus
- Reflux occurs in "normal" patients up to 5% of the time.
- Highest prevalence is in middle-aged adults.
- GERD is usually due to gastric acid but also to bile reflux.
- Contributory factors include the following:
  - **Reduced tone in the lower esophageal sphincter**: idiopathic, alcohol, drugs, previous surgery, secondary to existing peptic stricture
  - **Increased intragastric pressure**: coughing, obesity, delayed gastric emptying, large meal

Pathological features

Esophagitis

- Results in inflammatory changes in the squamous-lined esophagus.
- Varies in severity from minor mucosal erythema and erosions to extensive circumferential ulceration and stricturing

Stricture

- Chronic fibrosis and epithelial destruction may result in stricturing.
- GERD may eventually lead to shortening and narrowing of the lower esophagus.
- It may lead to fixation and leave patient susceptibile to further reflux.

Esophageal metaplasia—Barrett's esophagus

- May develop as a result of gastroesophageal reflux; possibly more common in biliary reflux.
- Normal **squamous epithelium** is replaced by **columnar epithelium**.
- **Dysplasia** and premalignant change (**metaplasia**) may occur in the columnar epithelium.

Clinical features

- Dyspepsia may be the only feature and may radiate to the back and left neck.
- True reflux may occur with acid and regurgitation in the pharynx.
- GERD is commonly worse at night, after large meals, and when recumbent.
- Dysphagia may occur if there is associated ulceration or a stricture.

Diagnosis and investigations

Empiric treatment is with acid suppressive medications such as H_2 blockers and proton pump inhibitors for up to 12 weeks. If symptoms fail to respond to treatment, GERD can be confirmed by 24-hr continuous pH monitoring. EGD should be performed to exclude esophageal malignancy. Esophageal manometry will help exclude a motility disorder that may present with similar symptoms.

Treatment

Medical

- **Reduce acid production**: ↓ smoking, ↓ weight, ↓ alcohol consumption
- **Counteract acid secretion**: H_2 blockers, proton pump inhibitors, symptomatic relief with antacids

Surgical

The procedure of choice is laparoscopic fundoplication, **Nissen fundoplication** (wrapping fundus of the stomach around the intra-abdominal esophagus to augment high-pressure zone).

It is indicated for
- Persistent symptoms despite maximal medical therapy
- Large-volume reflux with a risk of aspiration pneumonia
- Complications of reflux, including stricture and severe ulceration

There is an uncertain role in the prevention of progressive dysplasia in Barrett's esophageal metaplasia in the absence of symptoms. The procedure of choice in patients with high-grade dysplasia is esophagectomy.

Esophageal tumors

Key facts and pathological features

There are several types of esophageal tumors.

Adenocarcinoma

- Rapidly increasing incidence in Western world; men to women, 5:1
- Most common in Japan, northern China, and South Africa
- Associated with dietary nitrosamines, GERD, and Barrett's metaplasia
- Typically occurs in the lower half of the esophagus

Squamous carcinoma

- Incidence is slightly reducing in Western world; men to women, 3:1
- Associated with smoking, alcohol intake, diet lacking in fresh fruit and vegetables, chronic achalasia, and chronic caustic strictures
- May occur anywhere in the esophagus

Rhabdomyo(sarco)ma is a malignant tumor of skeletal muscle wall of the esophagus. It is very rare.

Lipoma and gastrointestinal stromal tumors (GIST; 📖 p. 278) are rare.

Clinical features

- **Dysphagia**. Any new symptoms of dysphagia, especially over the age of 45, should be assumed to be due to tumor until proven otherwise.
- **Hematemesis** is rarely the presenting symptom.
- **Incidental/screening**. Occasionally these tumors are identified as a result of follow-up or screening for **Barrett's metaplasia**, achalasia, or reflux disease. Presence of high-grade dysplasia in Barrett's is associated with the presence of an occult adenocarcinoma in 30%.
- **Symptoms of disseminated disease** include cervical lymphadenopathy, hepatomegaly due to metastases, and epigastric mass due to para-aortic lymphadenopathy.
- **Symptoms of local invasion** include dysphonia in recurrent laryngeal nerve palsy, cough and hemoptysis in tracheal invasion, neck swelling in SVC obstruction, and Horner's syndrome in sympathetic chain invasion.

Diagnosis and investigations

- Diagnosis is usually by flexible esophagoscopy and biopsy.
- Barium swallow is indicated for failed intubation or suspected post-cricoid carcinoma (which is often missed by endoscopy).

Staging investigations

- **Local staging**: endoluminal ultrasound scan to assess depth of invasion
- **Regional staging**: CT scanning to evaluate local invasion, locoregional lymphadenopathy, and liver disease
- **Disseminated disease**. PET scanning may be used to exclude occult disseminated disease in patients otherwise considered for potentially curative surgery.

Treatment

Palliative

Most patients present with incurable disease and require palliation.

- Dysphagia can be treated by endoluminal self-expanding metal stenting (SEMS) and external beam radiotherapy. Surgery is very rarely indicated for palliation.
- Metastases require systemic chemotherapy if symptomatic.

Potentially curative

- Squamous carcinoma is treated with radical external beam radiotherapy followed by surgery (radical resection).
- Adenocarcinoma (large) is treated with neoadjuvant chemoradiotherapy followed by surgery (radical resection).
- Adenocarcinoma (small) or high-grade dysplasia in Barrett's requires surgical resection.

Peptic ulcer disease

Key facts

- Peptic ulceration develops when a breakdown in the mucosal defense of the stomach or duodenum leads to a mucosal breach.
- It may be acute and transient (e.g., stress ulceration after surgery, in acutely unwell ICU patients).
- If the repair system fails to deal with the breakdown of the mucosa, it may become chronic.
- The term *peptic* refers to ulcers in columnar mucosa in the lower esophagus, stomach, duodenum, or small bowel—usually due to the action of acid.

Classification

Peptic ulcers can be broadly classified into the following types:
- Type I: located on lesser curve
- Type II: two ulcers—lesser curve and duodenal (due to high acid secretion)
- Type III: prepyloric (due to high acid secretion)
- Type IV: high near gastric cardia
- Type V: associated with NSAIDs

Type I and IV

- Men to women, 3:1. Peak age of incidence is 50 years.
- Associated with *Helicobacter pylori* in 45% of cases, and with high alcohol intake, smoking, and normal or low acid secretion

Type II and III

- Men to women, 5:1. Peak age of incidence is 25–30 years.
- Associated with *H. pylori* in 85% of cases, and with high acid secretion and smoking

Atypical ulceration

- Usually due to either atypical sites of gastric acid secretion (e.g., ectopic gastric mucosa in a Meckel's diverticulum) or abnormally high levels of acid secretion (e.g., **Zollinger–Ellison syndrome**; see next page)
- Associated with ulceration that fails to respond to maximal medical therapy, multiple ulcers, or ulcers in abnormal locations (e.g., distal duodenum or small bowel)

Clinical features

- Nausea and epigastric pain
- Duodenal ulceration is typified by hunger pains with central back pain **relieved by food**. Pain is often cyclical and occurs in the early hours of the morning.
- Gastric ulceration is typified by **pain precipitated by food**, with associated weight loss and anorexia. Pain is less cyclical.
- Vomiting and upper abdominal distension suggest gastric outlet obstruction.

Diagnosis and investigations
- **Gastroscopy**
- **Barium swallow** may be obtained if gastroscopy is contraindicated.
- **Urease testing** to assess for presence of *H. pylori* can be performed on antral biopsies from gastroscopy or as a CO_2 breath test.
- **Fasting serum gastrin levels** should be checked if hypergastrinemia is suspected.

Complications
- Acute upper GI bleeding (see 📖 p. 280)
- Iron deficiency anemia due to chronic low level bleeding
- Perforation (see 📖 p. 282)
- Gastric outlet obstruction due to chronic scarring at or around the pylorus

Treatment
Medical
- Advise patient to reduce alcohol intake, stop smoking, and avoid NSAIDS.
- H_2 blockers or PPIs are most effective at acute symptom control.
- Give topical antacids, especially for acute ulceration postoperatively or in ICU patients.
- *H. pylori* eradication therapy (usually triple therapy of metronidazole, PPI, and clarithromycin)

Surgical
Surgery is rarely necessary with very highly effective acid-reducing drugs and eradication therapy. Indications for surgery include the following:
- Gastric outlet obstruction not responsive or suitable for endoscopic dilatation
- Failure to respond to maximal medical treatment with severe symptoms or habitual recidivism
- The usual procedure is truncal vagotomy and pyloroplasty or partial gastrectomy ± highly selective vagotomy.
- Emergency indications include
  - Perforation (see 📖 p. 282).
  - Bleeding (see 📖 p. 280).

Zollinger–Ellison syndrome
- Due to hypergastrinemia, causing extensive, persistent, or typical ulceration
- Suspect benign secretory gastrinoma (usually intrapancreatic). Occasionally the cause is malignant gastrinoma (associated with MEN syndromes).
- This syndrome is diagnosed by elevated serum gastrin level, tumor located by CT scanning, angiography, and selective pancreatic venous cannulation at surgery.
- Treatment is resection of pancreatic tissue containing tumor.

Gastric tumors

These tumors may arise from tissues of the mucosa (adenocarcinoma), connective tissue of the stomach wall (previously known as leiomyoma or leiomyosarcoma but part of the spectrum of disease called *gastrointestinal stromal tumors* [GISTs]; see 📖 p. 278), neurendocrine tissue (carcinoid tumors; see 📖 p. 278), or lymphoid tissue (lymphomas).

Key facts

Adenocarcinoma's average age of incidence is >50 years; men to women: 3:1. Predisposing factors include the following:

- Diet rich in nitrosamines (smoked or fresh fish, pickled fruit)
- Chronic atrophic gastritis
- Blood group A
- Chronic gastric ulceration related to *H. pylori*

Clinical features

Symptoms

- Dyspepsia (any new onset of dyspepsia over the age of 45 should raise suspicion of adenocarcinoma until proven otherwise)
- Weight loss, anorexia, and lethargy
- Anemia (iron deficiency due to chronic blood loss)
- Occasionally gastric tumors present as acute upper GI bleeding (see 📖 p. 280).
- Dysphagia is uncommon unless involving the proximal fundus and gastroesophageal junction.

Signs

- Weight loss
- Palpable epigastric mass
- A palpable supraclavicular lymph node (Virchow's node) suggests disseminated disease.

Diagnosis and investigation

- Diagnosis is usually by gastroscopy (barium swallow may be required if gastroscopy is contraindicated).
- Staging (see Table 7.1) tests include the following:
  - Thoracoabdominal CT scan to assess for distant metastases and local lymphadenopathy
  - Endoluminal ultrasound to assess for local disease
  - Laparoscopy (for patients considered for potential resection) to exclude small-volume peritoneal metastases

Treatment

Surgery is the only curative treatment for gastric cancer. This involves partial to total gastrectomy, depending on the size of tumor. Margins of 5 cm are required. Lymph node dissection is also performed; the extent is controversial. Unless the patient has T1/N0/M0 tumor, chemoradiation is recommended in addition to surgical resection.

Table 7.1 TNM staging of gastric cancers

T (tumor)	N (nodes)	M (metastases)
Tis, in situ within mucosa	N0, no lymph nodes	**M0, no metastases**
T1, confined to submucosa	N1, tumor spread to 1–6 lymph nodes	M1, metastases
T2, confined to muscle wall	N2, tumor spread to 7–15 lymph nodes	
T3, involvement of serosal surface	N3, tumor spread to >15 lymph nodes	
T4, involvement of other organs		

Clinical pearls—anatomy and physiology of the stomach

- The fundus is predominantly a storage zone with few active cells.
- The body contains mostly chief cells (which secrete pepsinogen and are stimulated by gastrin and local ACh release), and oxyntic cells (which secrete H^+, are stimulated by gastrin, histamine, and Ach, and are inhibited by H^+, secretin, and gastric inhibitory protein [GIP]).
- The antrum contains G cells (which secrete gastrin, are stimulated by ACh from vagus, stretch, and are inhibited by vasoactive inhibitory protein [VIP], secretin, and H^+).
- The pyloric sphincter is a functional sphincter of circular muscle.
- Arterial supply is profuse (gastric ischemia is rare) via the celiac axis—left gastric, splenic, and common hepatic arteries.
- Lymphatic drainage follows arteries and is profuse.

Chronic intestinal ischemia

This condition is caused by a chronic reduction in blood supply to the intestine without acute threat to the viability of the bowel.

Key facts

Chronic intestinal ischemia is uncommon. It usually presents with vague symptoms and diagnosis is often prolonged. Causes include the following:

- Progressive atherosclerosis affecting the visceral vessels, usually requiring more than one vessel to be affected (e.g., superior mesenteric artery occlusion and celiac artery stenosis)
- Obliterative small-vessel disease (e.g., thrombangiitis obliterans, systemic sclerosis, severe diabetic vasculopathy)

Clinical features

Symptoms

- **Mesenteric angina**: chronic central abdominal pain is brought on by eating; associated with nausea and vomiting
- May present with weight loss, general anorexia, and malnutrition
- Often associated with other features of extensive vascular disease, such as renal impairment, coronary disease, and claudication

Signs

- Weight loss, central abdominal tenderness

Diagnosis and investigations

- Intestinal ischemia is usually diagnosed by imaging of the visceral arteries in combination with clinical symptoms. Methods of imaging visceral vessels include
  - CT angiogram
  - MR angiogram
  - Transfemoral digital subtraction angiogram or aortogram
- Other tests should include
  - Assessment of renal function
  - Assessment of coronary circulation
  - Exclusion of aneurysmal disease
- Small-vessel disease may require autoimmune screening.

Complications

- Acute intestinal ischemia is less common because of the development of collaterals; although, if undiagnosed, loss of all visceral vessels results in eventual pan-intestinal infarction.
- Chronic ischemic strictures are due to focally severe ischemia.

Treatment

Medical

- Stop smoking
- Control of hypertension; treatment of hyperlipidemia
- Aspirin 81 mg qd to prevent thrombembolic events
- Control diabetes if present
- Treatment of autoimmune disease if present

Interventional

Treatment for large-vessel stenosis is radiologically guided stenting. There is a risk of converting stenosis to acute occlusion with the risk of precipitating emergency surgery. Stenting is not possible if the stenosis is at the aortic ostium of the vessel affected.

Surgical

- Surgery is infrequently done with the advent of stenting. Either supraceliac-to-mesenteric bypass or iliac-to-mesenteric bypass is done.
- Overall prognosis is poor, as the underlying disease process is often widespread and progressive.

Clinical pearls—anatomy and physiology of the small intestine

- The duodenum is a secretory and digestive organ. It is described in four parts (the second part admits the common bile and pancreatic ducts via the ampulla of Vater on the medial wall).
- The jejunum is a secretory and digestive organ. Typical features include a thick, red-purple wall, prominent plicae circulares, and single arterial arcades with long mesenteric vessels.
- The ileum is predominantly an absorptive organ. Typical features include a thin blue-purple wall, prominent lymphoid aggregates, and multilayered mesenteric arterial arcades.
- The terminal ileum is a specialized area of ileum particularly concerned with absorption of bile salts and the vitamin B_{12}–IF (intrinsic factor) complex.

Small-bowel tumors

Key facts
The small bowel is a rare location for tumors. Tumors may arise from
- **Mucosa**—adenocarcinoma (<5% of all GI malignancies)
- **Neuroendocrine** tissue, e.g., carcinoid tumors
- **Connective tissue** of the bowel wall, e.g., GIST, lipoma
- **Lymphoid tissue** (lymphoma)

Adenocarcinoma of small bowel
- 40% of all small-bowel tumors
- Most frequent in the duodenojejunal junction and proximal jejunum; least common in the middle and distal ileum
- Associations:
  - Familial adenomatous polyposis (third most common location of adenocarcinoma after colorectal and duodenum)
  - Peutz–Jegher's syndrome
  - Crohn's disease
  - Untreated long-standing celiac disease

Carcinoid tumors
- 25% of all small-bowel tumors
- Tumors are most frequent in the distal small bowel; they may arise in the appendix or Meckel's diverticulum.
- Most are benign (nonmetastatic).
- They may produce enteric hormones (e.g., 5-HT, kallikrein, substance P). Hormone effects only occur when the primary tumor is able to secrete hormones into the systemic circulation, or when hepatitic metastases secrete into the caval circulation (carcinoid syndrome; see next page).

GIST (gastrointestinal stromal tumors)
- 10% of small-bowel tumors
- These arise from mesenchymal tissues of the bowel wall and mesentery (smooth muscle cells, fibroblasts, lipocytes).
- Previously they were called leiomyo(sarc)oma or lipo(sarco)ma.
- Tumors of myenteric plexus tissues are a variant called *GANT* (gastrointestinal autonomic nerve tumors).

Primary lymphoma
- 20% of small-bowel tumors
- Arise from the lymphoid tissue of the small-bowel wall
- This type is almost always non-Hodgkin's. Most often, B-cell lymphomas arise from the mucosa-associated lymphoid tissue (MALT).

Clinical features
- **Adenocarcinoma of small bowel** often presents late with metastases. It may present with small bowel obstruction, recurrent abdominal pain, or recurrent or occult GI bleeding.
- **Carcinoid tumors** are usually found incidentally after appendectomy or Meckel's diverticulectomy.

- **Carcinoid syndrome** is rare (typified by flushing, tachycardia, colicky abdominal pain, diarrhea, and wheezing).
- **GISTs** often present with a slow-growing abdominal mass and vague abdominal pain; they may present with occult GI bleeding from tumor ulceration.
- **Primary lymphoma** presents with malaise, abdominal pain, and diarrhea. It may present with acute perforation or small-bowel obstruction.

Diagnosis and investigations

Common diagnostic tests:

- CT of chest and abdomen identifies primary tumor, assesses extent of involvement of other tissues, and assesses possible metastatic disease.
- Small-bowel contrast study is rarely required for the identification of primary tumors.
- Ileoscopy may demonstrate proximal lesions presenting with occult, recurrent upper GI bleeding.

Complications

- Bleeding is common with adenocarcinoma and some GISTs.
- Obstruction is seen, especially in adenocarcinoma, GISTs, GANTs, and lymphoma.
- Perforation is seen in lymphoma, especially shortly after starting chemotherapy (due to bowel wall replacement by tumor, which then melts away with chemotherapy); it also occurs with adenocarcinoma.
- Malabsorption occurs often with lymphoma if it is widespread.

Treatment

Surgery

- Primary surgical resection with macroscopic clearance of tumor is required for adenocarcinoma, carcinoid, GISTs, and GANTs.
  - Potentially curative for nonmetastatic disease
  - Palliative to prevent complications if disease is metastatic
- Surgical resection may be indicated for primary lymphoma prior to chemotherapy if there is a high risk of perforation of primary tumor.
- Surgical resection of metastases is uncommon.

Medical

- Chemotherapy is used for lymphoma and metastatic adencarcinoma.
- Hepatic abalation and embolization is used to treat carcinoid metastases to treat symptoms of carcinoid syndrome.
- Imatinib (Gleevac®) (anti-CD113) is used as treatment for GISTs that are positive for cKIT.

Acute hematemesis

Key facts

- *Hematemesis* is vomiting of blood, usually due to bleeding proximal to the duodenojejunal junction.
- *Melena* is the passage of altered blood (dark purple, pitch black, or "tarry," usually due to bleeding below the gastroesophageal junction).
- 20% of cases require intervention because of ongoing bleeding or re-bleeding.

Causes and features

- Peptic (gastric or duodenal) ulceration (benign; 50%)
  - Fresh red blood with clots, occasionally mixed with food
- Esophageal varices
  - Copious dark red venous blood with little mixing with food; features of portal hypertension (e.g., caput medusa)
- Esophageal ulceration
  - Small volumes of bright red blood or streaks are typical.
- Esophageal trauma (Mallory–Weiss tear)
  - Small volumes of fresh bright blood preceded by violent or prolonged vomiting or retching
- Vascular malformations and lesions (e.g., Dieulafoy lesions)
- Gastric carcinoma, leiomyoma
- Aortenteric fistula
  - Copious bright red blood (often rapidly fatal)

Associated or predisposing conditions

- Agents affecting mucosal health include NSAIDs, steroids, alcohol, major trauma, or massive burns.
- Agents worsening risk of bleeding are anticoagulants.

Emergency management

Resuscitation

- Establish large-caliber IV access—give 1–2 L of crystalloid if patient is tachycardic or hypotensive. Only use uncross-matched blood if the patient is in extremis; otherwise wait for cross-matched blood if transfusion is needed.
- Catheterize and monitor strict in's and out's if patient is hypotensive.
- Send blood for CBC, chemistry, LFTs, coagulation panel, type and cross-match (at least 4 units).
- Consider alerting the ICU if patient is unstable.
- Monitor pulse rate, BP, and urine output (with urinary catheter).
- Insertion of a Sengstaken–Blakemore gastroesophageal tube may be a life-saving maneuver but is rarely used.

Establish a diagnosis

- Urgent EGD is the test of choice (at least within 24 hr).
  - This may require ongoing resuscitation with an anesthetist present.
  - EGD allows diagnosis and biopsy if appropriate.
  - EGD may enable therapeutic interventions, including epinephrine injection, heater probe coagulation, and banding of varices.

- Angiography
  - Rarely suitable for active bleeding. It may allow selective embolization in some patients with recurrent bleeding.

Early treatment
- Give IV PPI (e.g., omeprazole 40 mg IV); stop all NSAIDs.
- Blood transfusion if large-volume hematemesis or a drop in Hb
- Ensure that the appropriate surgical team knows of the patient in case surgical intervention is required.
- For known or suspected liver disease consider FFP or vitamin K to correct clotting.
- Surgery may be required if there is
  - Massive hemorrhage requiring ongoing resuscitation
  - Failed initial endoscopic treatment with ongoing bleeding
  - Re-bleeding not suitable for repeated endoscopic treatment
  - A >6-unit bleed

Definitive management
Varices (see 📖 p. 280)
- Endoscopy coagulation or banding, interventional radiology, or surgery
- IV vasopressin or analogues

Gastric or duodenal ulcer
- Endoscopic coagulation or injection. This may be repeated.
- Surgery for failed primary management or re-bleeding that is unsuitable for attempted repeat endoscopic treatment.
- Surgical options include local excision of gastric ulcer or vagotomy and antrectomy; vagotomy and pyloroplasty with oversewing of the duodenal ulcer.
- *Helicobacter pylori* eradication (triple therapy)

Gastric carcinoma
- Endoscopic treatment is often not effective.
- Partial or subtotal gastrectomy (often palliative, rarely curative)

Esophageal trauma
- Oral antacids

Aortoenteric fistula
- Surgery if the patient survives beyond diagnosis

Acute upper GI perforation

Causes and features

- Duodenal ulceration
- Gastric ulceration (usually anterior prepyloric; less commonly anterior body)
- Gastric carcinoma
- Traumatic, e.g., fishbone perforation
- Ischemic (usually secondary to gastric volvulus)

Symptoms

- Acute-onset upper abdominal pain is severe, constant, and worse with breathing and moving; it may radiate to the back or shoulders.
- Prodrome of upper abdominal pain (in benign or malignant ulceration)
- Copious vomiting and upper abdominal distension suggest volvulus.
- Prodrome of weight loss, dyspepsia, and anorexia suggests carcinoma.

Signs

- Generalized peritonitis is common ("board-like" generalized rigidity with marked guarding and tenderness).
- Localized upper abdominal peritonitis may occur, especially with previous surgery where adhesions may act to contain the contamination.
- Mild fever, pallor, tachycardia, and hypotension (often profound due to autonomic reaction). Typically these symptoms respond quickly to modest fluid resuscitation.

Emergency management

Resuscitation

- Establish large-caliber IV access. Give 1–2 L crystalloid if patient is tachycardic or hypotensive.
- Catheterize and monitor strict in's and out's if patient is hypotensive.
- Send blood for CBC, chemistries, coagulation panel, type and screen.

Establish a diagnosis

- Obtain upright chest X-ray (looking for free air). If the chest X-ray is nondiagnostic, a lateral decubitus abdominal film can be performed, although a CT is more common.
- Obtain CT scan if the diagnosis is unclear on chest X-ray, as it may demonstrate presence of gastric carcinoma.

Early treatment

- Once the diagnosis of perforation is confirmed on clinical or radiological grounds, the treatment is surgical, unless
  - the patient declines; or
  - the patient is considered unlikely to survive and supportive care is deemed more appropriate.
- Conservative management—IV PPI, npo, IV antibiotics—has a very limited role in management. It offers an outcome similar to that of surgery only in cases where the perforation has sealed at the time of presentation, there is no hemodynamic instability, and there are no signs of peritonitis.

Definitive management

Duodenal ulcer

- Sutured closure with omental patch (Graham patch)
- Empirical oral triple therapy for *H. pylori*
- Definitive surgery vagotomy and antrectomy should only be performed for recurrent perforation, failed fully compliant medical therapy, or in a recidivist noncompliant patient. However, some would perform a vagotomy and pyloroplasty if the perforation can be included in the pyloroplasty

Gastric ulcer

- Sutured closure with omental patch if prepyloric
- Local excision with concern for gastric cancer if located in the gastric body

Gastric carcinoma

- Partial gastrectomy (usually palliative)

Traumatic

- Sutured closure

Volvulus with ischemia

- Usually subtotal gastrectomy

Acute appendicitis

Causes and features

▶ Acute appendicitis can affect any age but is uncommon under the age of 4 and over the age of 80. The peak age of incidence is early teens to early twenties. There are three types:

- **Mucosal**: mildest form, usually diagnosed by pathology reporting
- **Phlegmonous**: typified by slow onset and relatively slow progression
- **Necrotic**: often due to acute bacterial infection with ischemic necrosis. This type leads to perforation unless treated by surgery.

Differential diagnosis

- Children:
  - Nonspecific abdominal pain, including mesenteric adenitis
  - Meckel's diverticulitis
  - Ovarian cyst or menstrual symptoms (perimenarchal girls)
- Adults:
  - Terminal ileal pathology: Crohn's disease, Meckel's diverticulitis, gastroenteritis
  - Retroperitoneal pathology: pancreatitis, renal colic
  - Ovarian pathology: ectopic pregnancy, cyst, infection, menstrual pain
- Older adults:
  - Ileocecal pathology: cecal diverticulitis, cecal tumors
  - Colonic pathology: sigmoid diverticulitis
  - Ovarian pathology: cysts, infection, tumors

Clinical features

Symptoms include the following:

- Malaise, anorexia, and fever
- Diarrhea is common and may be mistaken for acute (gastro)enteritis.
- Abdominal pain starts periumbilically and localizes to the right lower quadrant.
- Abdominal pain caused by coughing and moving

Signs include the following:

- Fever, right lower quadrant pain
- Peritonitis may suggest perforation (local or generalized). Often it is maximal over **McBurney's point** but only if the appendix is in the conventional anatomical position.
- Palpation and release of left lower quadrant cause pain in the right lower quadrant (**Rovsing's sign**).

Investigations may be normal and none are diagnostic or exclusive.

Complications include the following:

- Perforation (localized or generalized)
- Right lower quadrant phlegmon (usually appendicitis with densely adherent cecum and omentum forming a "mass")
- Right lower quadrant abscess (usually secondary to perforated retrocecal appendicitis)
- Pelvic abscess (usually secondary to perforated pelvic appendicitis)

Emergency management
Resuscitation
- Establish IV access.
- Catheterize and monitor strict in's and out's if patient is hypotensive.
- Draw CBC, chemistries, and urinalysis.

Establish a diagnosis
- The diagnosis is a clinical one in all but exceptional cases and tests can often be unnecessary.
- CT is appropriate in menstruating females to differentiate menstrual-related cause from pelvic etiologies or in older adults to differentiate from diverticulitis and cancer.
- CT is the best test in suspected appendiceal phlegmon or abscess.
- An ultrasound scan (pelvic) is indicated in young women of childbearing age if ovarian pathology is suspected.
- In some circumstances, laparoscopy may be a useful surgical diagnostic maneuver allowing diagnosis of pelvic pathology.

Definitive management
Acute appendicitis
- Open or laparoscopic appendectomy
- Preoperative antibiotics should be given.

Appendiceal phlegmon or abscess
- IV antibiotics (e.g., levofloxacin and flagyl)
- If symptoms settle: delayed (interval) appendectomy after 6 weeks
- If symptoms fail to settle: patient may need an operation
- Appendiceal abscess should be amenable to CT-guided drainage followed by interval appendectomy.

Clinical pearls—anatomy of appendectomy

- Commonly **retrocecal** but may be pelvic or retrocolic
- **Tenia coli of cecum converge at base of appendix** and aid localization, especially in difficult locations
- Small mesentery with sole blood supply from **appendicular artery** (a terminal branch of the ileocolic), which may thrombose, causing gangrene
- Principles of **appendectomy** are as follows:
  - **Muscle-splitting incision** is centered at **McBurney's point**.
  - The **laparoscopic approach** is increasingly popular.
  - The mesentery of the appendix is divided and ligated.
  - The appendix is clamped and tied at the base, and excised or divided at its base with a stapler if done laparoscopically.
  - Some surgeons invaginate the stump using a purse-string in the wall of the cecum around the base of the appendix in an open operation.

Acute peritonitis

Acute peritonitis is defined as acute inflammation in the peritoneal cavity.

Causes
Causes of this condition may be primary (rare) or secondary (common).
- Primary peritonitis is typically streptococcal with probable portal of entry via the bloodstream rather than the intra-abdominal organs.
- The most common causes of secondary peritonitis are as follows:
  - **Acute perforated appendicitis** (📖 p. 284), especially in patients under age 45
  - **Acute perforated diverticular disease** (📖 p. 347) is most frequently in patients over 45.
  - **Upper GI perforation** (see 📖 p. 282)
  - Perforated tumors (colonic or gastric)
  - Perforated ischemic bowel
  - Acute pancreatitis (usually inflammatory rather than infective)
  - Peritoneal dialysis related: often atypical or cutaneous organisms gain entry via contaminated dialysate bags or catheter
  - Postsurgical intervention, e.g., anastomotic leak, enteric injury

Clinical features
There are features common to all causes. Additional features suggestive of an underlying cause should also be sought, particularly in the history.

Symptoms
- Anorexia and fever
- Severe generalized abdominal pain radiating to the shoulders and back
- Abdominal pain that is worse with movement, coughing, or sneezing

Signs
- Fever, tachycardia
- Generalized abdominal tenderness with guarding and rigidity
- Differential maximal tenderness *may* indicate the possible underlying cause.
- Gentle palpation may allow identification of an underlying mass.

Emergency management
Resuscitation
- Establish large-caliber IV access.
- Catheterize and monitor strict in's and out's if patient is hypotensive.
- Send blood for CBC, chemistries, amylase and lipase, LFTs, and type and screen.

Establish a diagnosis
Most causes of acute peritonitis require surgery to correct them, with the exception of acute pancreatitis.

Diagnostic tests are indicated if the patient would otherwise be a candidate for surgical intervention.
- Blood tests usually reveal an elevated WBC.
- It is always necessary to send and check an amylase level to rule out pancreatitis.

- Abdominal CT scanning is the test of choice for diagnosis. It should reliably exclude acute pancreatitis and may locate the source of the pathology.
- Laparoscopy is occasionally useful in patients in whom a formal laparotomy should be avoided if possible.

Early treatment
- IV antibiotics may be appropriate without a clear diagnosis.

Definitive management

Acute appendicitis See 📖 p. 284.

Upper GI perforation See 📖 p. 282.

Perforated diverticular disease
- IV antibiotics (e.g., levofloxacin and flagyl)
- Surgical treatment involves resection of the affected segment. Often acute repair of perforation requires sigmoid resection with a Hartmann's turn-in and end colostomy.

Perforated tumor
Surgical resection is required even if palliative. The ends of the bowel may be reanastomosed or exteriorized as stomas, depending on the circumstances (degree of contamination, underlying pathology).

Primary peritonitis or CAPD-related peritonitis
- A diligent and systematic search is necessary to ensure there is no occult source of perforation as a cause.
- Primary treatment is extensive lavage of all quadrants and treatment with appropriate antibiotics (guided by culture results from peritoneal fluid).

Acute abdominal pain

This type of pain is often a daunting challenge to the admitting team because of the huge differential diagnosis possible and the wide range of tests available to try and establish a diagnosis. Be methodical and remember some simple rules:

- Perform a proper history and physical—do not work to the diagnosis given to you by the referring doctor,
- Resuscitate the patient properly and give adequate analgesia—this often helps to clarify the diagnosis. There is *no* reason to withhold analgesia prior to senior clinical examination.
- Try to clarify if you think the patient has signs of peritonitis (localized or generalized)—this will narrow the differential and may require surgery as part of the diagnostic workup.

Etiology

A differential diagnosis is best formulated on the basis of area of discomfort (see Box 7.1). Although a good guide, it is wise to remember that viscera are often mobile and pain often radiates to adjacent sections of the abdomen.

Clinical features

Although each condition has its own clinical features, there are some general rules to follow.

Symptoms and signs

- Constant pain, gradual in onset but progressively worsening, suggests an underlying inflammatory cause.
- Intermittent pain that is poorly localized suggests colic arising from visceral distension.
- Central and lower abdominal pain in children (under the age of 12) is self-limiting (nonspecific) in 70% of cases, from benign gynecological causes in 25% (girls), and only pathological in 10%–20%.
- Severe pain out of proportion to the clinical signs suggests ischemic bowel until proven otherwise.
- Pain in the flank or back arises from (at least partially) retroperitoneal structures—consider the pancreas, renal tract, and abdominal aorta.

Emergency management

Resuscitation

- Establish IV access.
- Catheterize and monitor strict in's and out's if patient is hypotensive.
- Give adequate analgesia. If intra-abdominal pathology is suspected, 5–10 mg morphine IV is reasonable. IV morphine *never* hides established clinical signs—it often helps to clarify the diagnosis through its anxiolytic effect on patients.
- Send blood for CBC, chemistries, LFTs, amylase, and type and screen.

Box 7.1 Causes of acute abdominal pain arranged according to abdominal region

Right upper quadrant	*Epigastric*	*Left upper quadrant*
• Right lower lobe pneumonia/embolism	• Pancreatitis	• Left lower lobe pneumonia/embolism
• Cholecystitis	• Gastritis	• Large-bowel obstruction
• Biliary colic	• Peptic colic	
• Hepatitis	• Myocardial infarction	
Right lumbar	*Umbilical*	*Left lumbar*
• Renal colic	• Small-bowel obstruction	• Renal colic
• Appendicitis	• Intestinal ischemia	• Large-bowel obstruction
	• Aortic aneurysm	
	• Gastroenteritis	
	• Crohn's disease	
Right lower quadrant	*Hypogastric*	*Left lower quadrant*
• Appendicitis	• Cystitis	• Sigmoid diverticulitis
• Crohn's disease	• Urinary retention	• Left tubo-ovarian pathology
• Right tubo-ovarian pathology	• Dysmenorrhea	
	• Endometriosis	

Establish a diagnosis

The time frame for diagnosis of acute abdominal pain varies according to presentation. It is not uncommon for 12–24 hr of "masterful inactivity" to be used to allow the diagnosis to be clarified. Some causes of acute abdominal pain require diagnosis and management immediately upon admission or within 6–8 hr or less. Try to be thoughtful in ordering diagnostic tests—many may be requested but usually only one or two are really useful.

- Blood tests are very rarely diagnostic. Serum amylase more than 3× the normal maximum is highly suggestive of acute pancreatitis.
- Always request a plain upright chest radiograph—it is the first-line test of choice for free abdominal air.
- An upper-abdominal ultrasound is an excellent test for suspected hepatobiliary pathology.
- Pelvic ultrasound (transabdominal or transvaginal) is a good test for suspected tubo-ovarian disease.
- CT scanning is indicated in many situations.

Early treatment

- IV antibiotics are inappropriate without a clear diagnosis—they will suppress but may not adequately treat developing infection.
- Until a definitive management plan is established, concentrate on fluid balance, analgesia, and monitoring vital signs.

Gynecological causes of lower abdominal pain

Gynecological pathologies are a common cause of lower abdominal pain in not only women of childbearing age but also postmenopausal women.

Causes

- Complications of menstruation—retrograde menstruation, mid-cycle ovulation pain ("Mittelschmerz")
- Ovarian cyst—acute swelling, rupture, torsion
- Tubo-ovarian infection, including PID, abscess
- Ectopic pregnancy including rupture

Clinicopathological features

Complications of menstruation

- May have marked tenderness bordering on peritonitis
- Typically cyclical pains with sharp and sudden onset
- Normal blood tests; self-limiting

Ovarian cyst complications

- May have severe pain with few clinical signs
- Normal blood tests

Tubo-ovarian infection

- Commonly caused by *Escherichia coli*, *Bacteroides fragilis*, or *Streptococcus* spp.
- Associated with cervical disease or instrumentation
- Sexually transmitted infections can cause tubo-ovarian sepsis, which may be more chronic and recurrent: *Neisseria gonorrheae*, *Chlamydia trachomatis*
- Associated with multiple sexual partners and unprotected intercourse
- Pyrexia, mild tachycardia, occasional purulent vaginal discharge
- Often affects both sides, causing bilateral pain and tenderness

Ectopic pregnancy

- May occur at any age
- The most common site is the Fallopian tube (ampulla, tube, or isthmus).
- Associated with previous tubal disease or surgery
- Menstrual irregularity or a late period is common but not uniform.
- May give rise to symptoms while enlarging with unilateral pelvic pain
- Symptoms increase with complications (bleeding into site of pregnancy, free rupture with bleeding into pelvis and peritoneal cavity).
- Typified by lower abdominal pain without fever
- Hypotension with tachycardia suggests active intra-abdominal bleeding but is fortunately rare at presentation.

Emergency management

Resuscitation

- Establish large-caliber IV access if an ectopic pregnancy is suspected.
- Catheterize and monitor strict in's and out's if patient is hypotensive.
- Give adequate analgesia (5–10 mg morphine IV is reasonable).
- Send blood for CBC, chemistries, and type and screen.

Establish a diagnosis

- Obtain urine β-hCG (and serum β-hCG when urine test is positive, since this is more reliable). All women of childbearing age should be assumed to be pregnant until proven otherwise. Pregnancy testing may be negative in ectopic pregnancy if the fetus has already expired by the time of presentation.
- High vaginal swabs should be taken if tubo-ovarian sepsis is suspected.
- Pelvic ultrasound (transabdominal or transvaginal) is the diagnostic test of choice unless the patient is acutely unstable. It has a high sensitivity and good specificity.
- Laparoscopy is a very common diagnostic test. It allows a firm diagnosis of most gynecological pathology and may be therapeutic (e.g., pelvic lavage, cyst treatment).

Early treatment

- IV antibiotics for a clear diagnosis of pelvic infection
- If ruptured or bleeding ectopic pregnancy is seriously considered, make sure the surgical and gynecological teams are aware. Direct transfer to operating room may be necessary.

Definitive management

- **Complications of menstruation**. Conservative management—pelvic lavage if laparoscopy is performed
- **Ovarian cyst complications**. Ovarian preservation if below the age of menopause. Cystectomy or drainage where possible
- **Tubo-ovarian infection**. Levofloxacin po and metronidazole po for non-sexually transmitted infections. Metronidazole po for chlamydia; IV penicillin for neisserial infections
- **Ectopic pregnancy**. Conservation or reconstruction of the affected tube or ovary wherever possible. If it is not salvageable, perform unilateral salpingo-oophrectomy.

Intra-abdominal abscess

Key facts

Intra-abdominal sepsis can present as an intra-abdominal abscess if the sepsis is contained by tissues or anatomy. Common locations are as follows:

- Usually alongside the organ of origin (e.g., paracolic in diverticulitis, parapancreatic after infected pancreatitis)
- Pelvic (especially after pelvic sepsis such as appendicitis or after generalized peritoneal infection)
- Subphrenic (e.g., after upper GI perforation)

Causes

- Sigmoid diverticulitis (see 📖 p. 347)
- Acute appendicitis (see 📖 p. 284)
- Severe acute cholecystitis (see 📖 p. 300)
- Upper GI perforation (see 📖 p. 282)
- Infected acute pancreatitis (see 📖 p. 306)
- Post-trauma

Clinical features

Depending on the source, the preceding pathology may have specific clinical features but the development of an abscess gives rise to certain common features independent of the origin.

Symptoms

- Malaise, anorexia
- Localized abdominal pain is constant.

Signs

- High fever typically peaks in excess of 38.5°C, occurring twice a day.
- Tachycardia tends to follow the temperature.
- Localized abdominal tenderness with a possible mass if abscess in an accessible position (e.g., paracolic)

Emergency management

Resuscitation

- Establish large-caliber IV access if the patient is unwell.
- Catheterize and monitor strict in's and out's if patient is hypotensive.
- Give adequate analgesia (e.g., 5–10 mg morphine IV).
- Send blood for CBC, chemistries, and type and screen.

Establish a diagnosis

- Helical CT scanning is the diagnostic test of choice.
- Pelvic ultrasound (transabdominal or transvaginal) is occasionally useful if a pelvic abscess is suspected and CT scanning is to be avoided because of age.

Early treatment

IV antibiotics are appropriate if the patient is septic and should be given according to the most likely underlying diagnosis and organisms.

Definitive management

- Radiologically guided drainage by ultrasound or CT scanning wherever possible. Limitations include abscesses with dangerous access or complex multiloculated abscesses.
- Open surgical drainage is usually only indicated if
  - Radiological drainage not possible or safe
  - Radiological drainage fails to deal with the clinical symptoms or abscess recurs
  - Surgical treatment is required for the primary underlying pathology.

Liver, pancreatic, and biliary surgery

Cristina Ferrone, MD

Jaundice—causes and diagnosis

Key facts

Physiology

- Unconjugated bilirubin is formed mainly in the spleen by the breakdown of hemoglobin.
- It is insoluble and is transported in the plasma bound to albumin.
- Taken up by the liver by active transport, it is converted in the hepatocytes into conjugated bilirubin (water-soluble).
- It is excreted into the bile canaliculi and via the main bile ducts into the duodenum.
- 10% of the unconjugated bilirubin is reduced to urobilinogen by small-intestinal bacteria and is reabsorbed in the terminal ileum and then excreted in the urine (enterohepatic circulation).
- 90% is converted by colonic bacteria to stercobilinogen, which is excreted in feces.

Jaundice is clinically apparent at serum bilirubin levels above 2 mg/dL (34 µmol/L).

Causes and features

Prehepatic jaundice (hemolytic)

- Congenital abnormalities of red cell structure or content (e.g., hereditary spherocytosis, sickle cell disease)
- Autoimmune hemolytic anemia
- Transfusion reactions
- Drug toxicity

Hepatic jaundice (hepatocellular)

- *Hepatic unconjugated hyperbilirubinemia*
  - Gilbert's syndrome: deficiency or abnormalities of unconjugated bilirubin uptake system
  - Crigler–Najjar syndrome: abnormality of conjugation process enzymes
- *Hepatic conjugated hyperbilirubinemia*
  - Infection: viral (e.g., hepatitis A, B, and C, Epstien–Barr virus [EBV], CMV); bacterial (e.g., liver abscess, leptospirosis); parasitic (e.g., amebic)
  - Drugs, e.g., acetaminophen overdose, antipsychotics, antibiotics
  - Noninfective hepatitis, e.g., alcohol-related chronic hepatitis

Posthepatic jaundice (obstructive)

- *Intraluminal abnormalities of bile ducts*
  - Gallstones
  - Blood clot
  - Parasites (e.g., flukes)
- *Mural abnormalities of bile ducts*
  - Cholangiocarcinoma
  - Congenital atresia
  - Sclerosing cholangitis

- Biliary cirrhosis (primary [autoimmune] or secondary [sepsis])
- Choledochal cysts (Caroli's disease)
- Traumatic or postsurgical stricture
• *Extrinsic compression of bile ducts*
  - Pancreatitis
  - Tumors, e.g., head of pancreas, ampulla of Vater
  - Lymphadenopathy of porta hepatis nodes

Diagnosis and investigations

History

Common aspects overlooked in the clinical history of jaundiced patients:
- Family history of blood disorders and pancreaticobiliary cancers
- Recent travel to foreign countries; chemical exposure in work place
- Recent drugs or changes in medications
- Recent surgery or anesthesia
- History of gallstones
- Alcohol intake, cholangitis (pain, fever, rigors), and carcinoma

Basic tests

- Reticulocytosis, abnormal blood smear (hemolysis)
- ↑ Prothrombin time
- Hepatitis screen (viral titers for hepatitis A, B, and C, CMV, EBV)
- Immunology (anti-smooth muscle antibodies [chronic active hepatitis] and anti-mitochondrial antibodies [primary biliary cirrhosis])
- LFTs (see Table 8.1)

Advanced tests

- Ultrasound scan (liver, gallbladder, bile ducts, and pancreas)
  - Excludes the presence of extrahepatic obstruction (dilated common bile duct)
  - May locate cause of obstruction
  - Examines hepatic parenchyma in possible hepatitis
- Magnetic resonance cholangiopancreatography (MRCP) or CT if no cause is identified on ultrasound
- ERCP to further evaluate the bile ducts and pancreatic duct
- Liver biopsy (ultrasound-guided) for suspected hepatitis
- Pancreatic-protocol CT scan to evaluate the pancreatic head if pancreatic cancer is suspected
- Abdominal or pelvic CT scan with oral and IV contrast to evaluate extent of intrahepatic and extrahepatic biliary dilatation

Table 8.1 Liver function tests in jaundice

	Hemolytic	Hepatocellular	Obstructive
Unconjugated bilirubin	Increased	Increased	Normal
Alkaline phosphatase	Normal	Normal	Much increased
γ-glutamyl transferase	Normal	Increased	Much increased
Transaminases	Normal	Increased	Normal
Lactate dehydrogenase	Normal	Increased	Normal

Jaundice—management

Complications of jaundice

- Biliary infection (cholangitis) is most often seen in obstructive jaundice or with a previously damaged or manipulated biliary tree (after ERCP). It is commonly due to gram-negative bacteria (e.g., *Escherichia coli*, *Pseudomonas*).
- Disordered coagulation is due to decreased synthesis of vitamin K–dependent clotting factors (II, VII, IX, X) because the absorption of vitamin K is bile-dependent, and to impaired platelet function.
- Renal failure (hepatorenal syndrome) is caused by a combination of infection, dehydration, and a direct effect of high levels of bilirubin and other toxic products of metabolism on the kidney. Mortality is highest when the patient is over 65 with an elevated blood urea.
- Relative immunosuppression predisposes to systemic infections (e.g., chest infection) and reduces wound healing through combinations of jaundice, infection, and reduced proteosynthesis.

Acute presentation—general treatment

Fluid balance

- Correct dehydration. Give up to 1000 mL IV crystalloid if there is no preexisting liver disease. Sodium input should be carefully monitored in preexisiting liver disease. Monitor hourly urine output, use urethral catheter.
- Treat the obstruction through gallstone extraction or stenting via ERCP or intraoperative common bile duct exploration, etc.
- Treat infection. Obtain blood cultures if the patient has a temperature over 101. Give IV antibiotics according to local protocol. Treatment of bile duct obstruction may be required urgently (e.g., radiologically guided drainage, ERCP, surgery). Consider prophylactic antibiotics.
- Check clotting times (APTT, PT). Give vitamin K 10 mg IV stat if PT is prolonged or begin infusion of fresh frozen plasma.
- Ensure adequate nutrition. Enteral feeding is optimum but may require a fine-bore nasogastric tube (NGT) or a surgical gastrostomy, jejunostomy, or percutaneous endoscopic gastrostomy (PEG) tube.

Acute presentation—specific treatments

- Endoscopic procedures (ERCP)
  - Sphincterotomy is used for common bile duct stone extraction and treatment of ampullary strictures due to tumors or inflammation.
  - Stent insertion (plastic or expanding metal) is used for benign or malignant strictures and external compression of bile duct.
- Percutaneous transhepatic cholangiogram (PTC) is used for stent insertion (often in combination with ERCP) and temporary external drainage of obstructed biliary system.
- Surgical drainage (e.g., choledochoduodenostomy) is very rarely used.

Elective presentation—specific treatments
Hemolytic jaundice
- Steroids for an autoimmune disease;
- Splenectomy (laparoscopic), rarely used for hereditary causes and failed medical treatment

Obstructive jaundice
- ERCP and PTC may be used as above for stones, strictures, and compression.
- Surgical drainage (e.g., choledochoduodenostomy or cholecystojejunostomy) is used for failed interventional treatments.
- Surgical resection, e.g., pancreaticoduodenectomy (Whipple procedure), is used for cases of pancreatic or distal bile duct tumors that are benign or malignant but considered resectable on staging. Staging of potentially suitable patients may include endoscopic ultrasound, CT scan, ERCP or MRCP, visceral arteriography, or laparoscopy.

Hepatocellular jaundice
- Remove causative agent and support liver function.
- Consider transplantation in specific circumstances.

Selective arteriography
Selective arteriography of the hepatic, celiac, and superior mesenteric arteries gives information about anatomical variants, vessel invasion, and tumor resectability.

Prognosis in acute jaundice
Adverse risk factors include the following:
- Older patients
- Uncontrolled sepsis and multiple-organ dysfunction (typically acute tubular necrosis)
- Underlying malignant disease
- Underlying comorbidities

Gallbladder stones

Key facts

Gallstones present in roughly 10% of people >50 years of age.

Pathological features

Bile has three major constituents:

- Bile salts (primary: cholic and chenodeoxycholic acids; secondary: deoxycholic and lithocholic acids)
- Phospholipids (90% lecithin)
- Cholesterol

Bile containing excess cholesterol relative to bile salts and lecithin is predisposed to gallstone formation.

Types of gallstones

- Pure cholesterol (10%). Often solitary, large (>2.5 cm), round
- Pure pigment (bile salts; 10%). Pigment stones are of two types:
  - Black (associated with hemolytic disease)
  - Brown (associated with chronic cholangitis and biliary parasites)
- Mixed (80%). Most common; usually multiple

Predisposing conditions

- Increasing age
- Female (pregnancy and use of the oral contraceptive)
- Obesity
- Multiparity
- Chronic hemolytic disorders (only for pigment stones)
- Long-term parenteral nutrition (alteration of bile composition)
- Previous surgery (e.g., vagotomy or resection of the terminal ileum), short-gut syndrome or disease involving the distal small bowel (e.g., Crohn's disease)—alteration of bile composition

Clinical features (common presentations)

Biliary colic

Intermittent, severe epigastric and right upper quadrant pain is usually associated with nausea and vomiting. Pain resolves after a few hours; there is tenderness over the gallbladder during acute episodes.

Acute cholecystitis

Severe, continuous right upper quadrant pain often radiates to the right flank and back; it is associated with anorexia and pyrexia. Tenderness the over gallbladder occurs during inspiration (Murphy's sign).

Complications of acute cholecystitis include the following:

- Formation of an empyema or abscess of the gallbladder, indicated by fever and severe localized pain
- Jaundice due to compression of the adjacent common bile duct by edema and direct compression by a gallbladder stone (Mirizzi syndrome)
- Perforation with biliary peritonitis
- Cholecystoenteric fistula formation (may lead to a gallstone entering and obstructing the distal ileum (gallstone ileus)

Chronic cholecystitis

This chronic, inflammatory cell infiltration of the gallbladder is due mainly to mechanical irritation of gallstones or recurrent attacks of cholecystitis.

Diagnosis and investigations

- CBC, electrolytes, LFTs, blood culture, lipase, serum amylase—in acute presentations
- Ultrasound is the procedure of choice, as it identifies stones, determines wall thickness, and assesses ductal dilatation.
- Abdominal X-ray. Only 10% of calculi are radio-opaque.
- HIDA scan is useful when ultrasound findings are equivocal, as it evaluates gallbladder emptying.
- Oral cholecystogram (Graham–Cole test) is rarely used.

Surgical treatment

Cholecystectomy

The vast majority are done laparoscopically, often as outpatient surgery. Cholecystectomy is indicated for

- Patients with symptoms deemed to be due to gallbladder stones.
- Asymptomatic patients with gallbladder stones who are at risk of complications involving porcelain (flecks of calcium in gallbladder wall), gallbladder (7-fold increase in risk of developing gallbladder carcinoma), gallbladder mass, gallbladder polyp, history of pancreatitis, or long-term immunosuppression

Risks of laparoscopic cholecystectomy

- Conversion to open operation
- Common bile duct injury
- Bleeding
- Bile leak from the cystic duct stump or from hepatic parenchyma

Nonsurgical treatments

Percutaneous drainage of gallbladder (cholecystostomy tube)

- Done under ultrasound or CT guidance
- Used for empyema or acute cholecystitis in patients too ill to undergo surgery
- If the patient has gallstones and is fit for an operation, the patient should undergo cholecystectomy ~6 weeks after percutaneous drainage.

Dissolution therapy

- Rarely used. Requires a functioning gallbladder, small stones
- Problems: requires prolonged treatment; less than 70% response; high rate of recurrence of stones; toxicity of medication

Extracorporeal shock wave lithotripsy

This procedure is hardly ever used, as there is risk of visceral injury and a high risk of stone recurrence.

Common bile duct stones

Key facts

- Types of stones as per gallbladder stones (see 🕮 p. 300).
- Common bile duct (CBD) stones are involved in 10% of patients with gallstones.
- Most pass from the gallbladder into the CBD (secondary duct stones).
- These stones rarely form within the CBD (primary duct stones); they are almost always associated with partial duct obstruction.

Clinicopathological features

Asymptomatic

CBD stones are usually found incidentally on ultrasound for gallbladder stones.

Obstructive jaundice

- Usually due to CBD stone causing obstruction; rarely due to stone-induced CBD stricture
- Anorexia, nausea, itching
- Dark urine and pale stools
- Epigastric pain and fever is due to associated low-grade bile infection.
- A palpable, distended gallbladder is rare with CBD stones.

Courvoisier's law

"If in the presence of jaundice the gallbladder is palpable, then it [the jaundice] is unlikely to be due to stone."

The reason for this is that CBD stones originate in the gallbladder, which is usually scarred and fibrotic, preventing distension.

Ascending cholangitis

- Constant, severe right upper quadrant pain, obstructive jaundice, and high fevers (Charcot's triad)

Acute pancreatitis

Alcohol ingestion and gallstones are the top two causes of acute pancreatitis in adults (see 🕮 p. 306).

Diagnosis and investigations

Basic tests

- CBC (↑ WBC in cholangitis and pancreatitis), creatinine, LFTs (↑ conjugated bilirubin and alkaline phosphatase), serum amylase and lipase (↑ in pancreatitis), clotting studies

Advanced tests
Ultrasound (transabdominal)
- Best first-line investigation
- Findings suggestive of cholecystitis include gallbladder wall thickening, stones, and pericholecystic fluid.
- Accuracy is lowest for distal CBD stones and acute presentation, in cases of obesity, and when there is extensive overlying bowel gas.

Abdominal CT scan
- Visualizes the CBD well and also demonstrates the pancreatic head
- Significantly better than ultrasound at imaging the CBD and documenting CBD stones

Magnetic resonance cholangiopancreatography (MRCP)
- Noninvasive, avoids radiation exposure, highly accurate
- Helps evaluate for a common bile duct mass, pancreatic head mass, or ampullary mass
- Gives a more detailed evaluation of the biliary tree and liver than abdominal CT

Endoscopic retrograde cholangiopancreatography (ERCP)
- Used diagnostically and for therapeutic interventions
  - Endoscopic sphincterotomy (ES) and stone extraction or destruction (lithotrypsy)
  - Stent insertion for unextractable stones or after fracturing large stones
  - Patients unable to tolerate MRCP (claustrophobia)
- Risks of ERCP (↑ with ES)
  - Hemorrhage
  - Acute pancreatitis
  - Ascending infection
  - Perforation (usually retroduodenal, may involve peritonitis)

Percutaneous transhepatic cholangiography (PTC)
- Used for failure of ERCP as therapeutic procedure (often in combination with ERCP)
- Involves cannulation of either the left or right hepatic duct through the top of the liver, used primarily for drainage of stagnant bile due to distal obstruction
- Risks: sepsis, tube movement, leakage around the tube, patient discomfort and dehydration

Treatment
Principles of treatment of CBD stones are as follows.

Emergency treatment of CBD stones
- ERCP with extraction
- Occasionally PTC is required.
- Laparoscopic or open cholecystectomy and common bile duct stone extractions

Elective treatment of CBD stones
- Indicated for all patients having had complications (pancreatitis, cholangitis, obstructive jaundice)
- Usually by ERCP or combined ERCP/PTC
- Rarely, a CBD exploration is required at the time of surgery (laparoscopic or open), only if ERCP fails.
  - Open CBD exploration requires a T-tube to be left in the CBD.

Treatment of persistent CBD stones after cholecystectomy
- Rarely necessary with more accurate preoperative diagnosis and more effective preoperative treatments
- Postoperative ERCP
- Stones can be extracted via a T-tube track, if present (6 weeks after surgery with radiologically guided basket extraction).

Acute pancreatitis

Causes and features

This disorder is caused by an inflammatory process in which cascade of a release of inflammatory cytokines (TNF-α, IL-2, IL-6) and pancreatic enzymes (trypsin, lipases, co-lipases) is initiated by pancreatic injury; it may develop into full-blown MODS or SIRS (see 📖 p. 136).

Causes

- Gallstones
- Alcohol
- Hyperlipidemia
- Direct damage (trauma, ERCP, post-surgery, cardiopulmonary bypass)
- Toxic
  - Drugs, e.g., azathioprine, estrogens, thiazides, isoniazid, steroids, NSAIDs
  - Infection, e.g., viral (mumps, CMV, hepatitis B), mycoplasma
  - Venom (scorpion, snake bites).
- Idiopathic.

Classification and complications

- Edema (70%). May be simple or associated with phlegmon formation of the pancreas. Transient fluid collections common.
- Pancreatic pseudocyst
- Severe/necrotizing (25%). Necrosis may be sterile or infected.
- Hemorrhagic (5%)

Clinical features

- Severe epigastric pain radiating to the back
- Epigastric tenderness associated with guarding and, in severe cases, rigidity, which may be generalized
- Severe nausea and vomiting
- Fever, dehydration, hypotension, and tachycardia
- Left flank ecchymosis (Grey–Turner's sign) and periumbilical ecchymosis (Cullen's sign), 1%–3% of cases are secondary to hemorrhagic pancreatitis

Emergency management

Resuscitation

- Establish large-caliber IV access. Give crystalloid fluid up to 1000 mL if patient is tachycardic or hypotensive. The patient may require ongoing fluids IV.
- Catheterize and moniter in's and out's if patient is hypotensive.
- Send blood for CBC (Hb, WBC), electrolytes (Na, K), LFTs (albumin), amylase, lipase, PT, and PTT.
- Monitor pulse rate, BP, and urine output (urinary catheter).
- Consider insertion of a central line and manage patient in an ICU if patient is hemodynamically unstable or fails to respond to early resuscitation.
- Assess severity of the attack with Ranson's criteria (see Box 8.1).

Box 8.1 Ranson's criteria

Three or more positive criteria within 48 hr of admission = severe attack
- Age >55 years
- WBC >16,000/mm^3
- Glucose >200 mg/dL
- LDH >350 IU/L
- BUN >5 mg/dL
- AST >250 IU/dL
- Serum Ca <8 mg/dL
- Hct ↓ 10%
- Base defect >4 mEq/L
- PaO$_2$ <60 mmHg
- Fluid sequestration >6 L

Establish a diagnosis
- Serum amylase >1000 U is diagnostic but may be normal even in severe cases. Elevated amylase may occur in a wide range of other acute abdominal events (intestinal ischemia, leaking aneurysm, perforated ulcer, cholecystitis).
- Serum lipase remains elevated longer than serum amylase: this test is more specific but less sensitive.
- Abdominal X-ray (nonspecific findings): absent psoas shadows; sentinel loop sign (dilated proximal jejunal loop adjacent to pancreas because of local ileus); colon cutoff sign (distended colon to mid-transverse colon with no air distally); may show gallstone, pancreatic calcification
- CT may be required if the diagnosis is uncertain (shows pancreatic edema, swelling, loss of fat planes; may show hemorrhagic complications).
- An ultrasound scan should be done upon admission to identify gallstones in the bile duct.

Early treatment
ERCP and stone extraction are only indicated for proven bile duct stones with cholangitis or severe obstruction.

Definitive management
Treatment of early complications
- Fluid restriction with close monitoring of fluid status
- Urgent ERCP with stone extraction
- Respiratory, renal, and cardiovascular support
- CT-guided FNA if suspected pancreatic necrosis
- Debridement of infected necrosis
- An acute pseudocyst rarely needs drainage unless it is very large.

Overall outcome
Mortality is associated with pancreatic necrosis and the presence of sepsis, including MODS.

Chronic pancreatitis

Key facts

- Chronic pancreatitis is characterized by recurrent or persistent abdominal pain arising from the pancreas.
- It is often associated with exocrine and/or endocrine pancreatic insufficiency.
- It is characterized by irreversible destruction and fibrosis of pancreatic parenchyma.
- It may arise following one or more episodes of acute pancreatitis or may be a chronic progressive process de novo.

Pathological features

- The process may affect all or part of the gland (focal).
- The head tends to be the most severely involved in chronic alcohol disease.
- Features of acute pancreatitis may occur: edema, acute inflammatory infiltrate, focal necrosis, intraparenchymal hemorrhage.
- Chronic inflammatory changes cause progressive disorganization of the pancreas:
  - Glandular atrophy and duct ectasia
  - Microcalcification and intraductal stone formation with cystic change secondary to duct occlusion
  - Pancreatic duct strictures from chronic inflammation

Causes and clinical features

Causes

- Recurrent acute pancreatitis of any cause, especially alcohol
- Secondary to pancreatic ductal obstruction
  - Pancreatic head cysts, tumors
  - Pancreatic duct strictures—post-surgery, ERCP, parasitic infestation
  - Congenital pancreatic abnormalities (pancreas divisum, annular pancreas)
  - Cystic fibrosis
- Associated with autoimmune diseases (primary biliary cirrhosis, primary sclerosing cholangitis)
- Congenital idiopathic chronic pancreatitis

Features of chronic inflammation

- Recurrent or chronic abdominal pain
  - Typically epigastric, radiating to the back and requiring opiates
  - Worse with food, alcohol.

Features of exocrine failure

- Anorexia and weight loss (due to protein malabsorption)
- Steatorrhea (due to fat malabsorption); soft, greasy, foul-smelling stools that typically float on water.

Features of endocrine failure

- Insulin-dependent diabetes mellitus (due to loss of β-islet cells)

Diagnosis and investigations

Basic tests
- Plain abdominal X-ray may show pancreatic calcification.
- Transabdominal ultrasound may show cystic change and duct dilatation within the pancreas.

Advanced tests
- Pancreatic CT scan
  - May identify a cause, e.g., anatomical variants, tumors, cysts
  - May show extent of disease—pancreatic atrophy, disorganization of pancreatic ducts, altered acinar pattern with fibrosis, calcification, and cystic change
- MRCP scan may show the same changes as those on CT.
- ERCP demonstrates irregularity of the pancreatic duct strictures, calculi, dilated segments ("chain of lakes"), and changes in first- and second-order branches and cyst formation. A secondary effect from involvement of the head is stricture of the common bile duct, leading to an obstructive pattern of liver function tests.

Treatment

Prevention of cause and progressive damage
- Patient should stop alcohol use. Treat gallstones, autoimmune disease.
- Encourage a diet rich in antioxidants (vitamins A, C, E, selenium).

Control symptoms and complications
- Dietary modifications: adequate carbohydrates and protein; reduced fat
- Pancreatic exocrine enzyme supplements (e.g., Creon®)
- Analgesia—may require opiates or celiac plexus block
- Control of diabetes mellitus often requires insulin. Control is often difficult because of variable pancreatic function.

Surgical treatment
Indications include the following:
- Treatment of reversible cause (anatomical abnormalities, tumors, cysts, ductal strictures, or stones). Operations used include those to remove causes and those to drain an obstructed pancreatic duct:
  - Pancreaticoduodenectomy (Whipple procedure)
  - Middle pancreatectomy; distal pancreatectomy
  - Pancreaticojejunostomy (Peustow, Beger, or Frey procedure)
- Treatment of severe intractable pain or multiple relapses. Operations are done usually to resect the affected portion:
  - Transverse pancreaticojeunectomy(Peustow)
  - Duodenal preserving pancreatic head resection (Beger)
  - Transverse pancreaticojeunectomy and pancreatic head resection (Frey procedure)
  - Whipple procedure
  - Complications (pseudocyst, obstruction, fistula, infections, portal hypertension)

All surgery is associated with a risk of symptom recurrence due to recurrent or progressive disease.

Portal hypertension

Key facts

Normal portal vein pressure is 5–10 mmHg. Portal hypertension (PH) develops when the mean portal pressure is greater than 12 mmHg.

Causes and pathological features

Causes

- Prehepatic: congenital portal vein atresia, or portal vein thrombosis, trauma, or a thrombosed portocaval shunt
- Hepatic: cirrhosis (e.g., being an alcoholic most frequently the cause), chronic active hepatitis, and parasitic diseases (e.g., schistosomiasis)
- Posthepatic: Budd–Chiari syndrome (hepatic venous thrombosis), constrictive pericarditis, or tricuspid valve incompetence (rare)

Features and complications

- Decreased or reversed portal blood flow to the liver promotes the development of portosystemic collaterals between the portal system and systemic circulation:
  - Left gastric vein into the esophageal veins at the gastroesophageal junction—esophageal and gastric varices
  - Superior rectal into inferior rectal veins at the lower rectum—rectal varices
  - Obliterated umblical vein into the epigastric veins—caput medusa
- Esophageal or gastric varices may bleed torrentially.
- Liver cell dysfunction or liver failure occurs in hepatic and posthepatic causes.
- Ascites is due in part to portal hypertension but may also be due to associated liver dysfunction.
- Splenomegaly (hypersplenism may result)
- The Child–Pugh classification is used to assess the severity of liver dysfunction (see Table 8.2).

Diagnosis and investigations

- Electrolytes, LFTs, albumin, coagulation factors
- Screening tests for causes of cirrhosis (see 🕮 p. 312)
- MRI and ultrasound scan to assess liver morphology, diagnose PH, and assess cause
- Transabdominal Doppler ultrasound to assess blood flow in the portal vein and hepatic artery
- Gastroscopy in acute variceal bleeding (see 🕮 p. 280)

Treatment

Cause

- Cessation of alcohol use
- Anticoagulation for Budd–Chiari syndrome
- Antiviral treatment for hepatitis

Chronic complications
- Ascites: oral spironolactone. In cases of tense ascites, paracentesis may be required, with IV albumin replacement.
- Esophagogastric varices
  - Beta-blockers (e.g., propranolol or esmolol) reduce portal venous pressure
  - Repeated injection sclerotherapy or variceal ligation
  - Elective portal–systemic shunts (e.g., splenorenal anastomosis and transjugular intraparenchymal portosystemic shunt/stent [TIPS])
  - Liver transplant may be considered for treatment if condition associated with severe liver disease.
- Rectal varices: injection sclerotherapy
- Symptomatic splenomegaly or hypersplenism: splenectomy (laparoscopic or open)

Acute complications
These include bleeding esophagogastric varices.

Table 8.2 Child–Pugh classification of liver disease

	1 point	2 points	3 points
Bilirubin (mg/dL)	<2	2–3	>3
Albumin (g/L)	>3.5	2.8–3.5	<2.8
PT (seconds over control)/INR	<4/<1.7	4–6/1.7–2.3	>6/>2.3
Ascites	Absent	Slight	Moderate
Encephalopathy	None	Grade 1–2	Grade 3–4

Clinical pearls—anatomy of portal circulation

- The hepatic portal circulation carries blood from the GI tract (from the distal esophagus to the anorectal junction) to the liver.
- Portosystemic anastomoses occur in "junctional" areas of venous drainage:
  - Left gastric veins (portal) and esophageal veins (hemi/azygous veins) at the gastroesophageal junction
  - Superior rectal veins (portal) and inferior rectal veins (pudendal veins) in the lower rectum
  - Pancreatic and duodenal veins (portal) and retroperitoneal (hemi/azygous) veins in the upper retroperitoneum
  - Umbilical vein (portal) into the epigastric veins at the umbilicus
- Portal venous blood drains into liver venous sinusoids and subsequently into the hepatic veins.

Cirrhosis of the liver

Key facts
- The most common cause is alcohol related.

Causes
Acquired
- Alcohol intake
- Chronic hepatitis (autoimmune, infective types B, C, and D, drug-induced)
- Primary biliary cirrhosis
- Secondary biliary cirrhosis (gallstones, strictures, cholangitis)
- Venous obstruction, e.g., Budd–Chiari syndrome
- Idiopathic

Congenital
- Hemochromatosis
- Wilson's disease
- Other metabolic disorders (e.g., $\alpha 1$ anti-trypsin def)

Pathological features
Cirrhosis is characterized by fibrosis of the liver parenchyma, nodular regeneration, and hepatocellular necrosis.
- Micronodular form: small and uniform nodules (<4 mm in diameter) separated by thin fibrous septa uniformly throughout the liver
- Macronodular form: larger nodules separated by wider scars and irregularly distributed throughout the liver
- Mixed

Clinical features
- One-third of cirrhosis patients are compensated, i.e., do not produce any clinical symptoms, and their condition is incidentally discovered during a medical examination, at operation, or at autopsy.
- Two-thirds are decompensated, i.e., have features of liver cell dysfunction or complications.

Features fall into three broad groups.

Portal hypertension

See 📖 p. 310.

Hepatocellular failure
- Ascites
- Hypoalbuminemia
- Clotting disorders
- Gynecomastia and testicular atrophy
- Spider nevi
- Jaundice
- Encephalopathy
- Hepatorenal syndrome (renal failure in the setting of hepatic failure, due to renal vasoconstriction of unknown etiology)

Malignant change
- Hepatocellular carcinoma

Diagnosis and investigation

Diagnosis of cause
- Hepatitis screen (A, B, C, D, E; EBV, CMV)
- Metabolic screen (e.g., serum Cu)
- Autoimmune screen (anti-mitochondrial antibodies, anti-smooth muscle antibodies)
- MRI and ultrasound may show the type of cirrhosis, intra- or extra-hepatic biliary dilatation, and extrahepatic obstructive causes.
- Liver biopsy is used to confirm the diagnosis and establish type, activity, evolution, and cause.
- AFP

Investigation of severity or complications
- LFTs (transaminases, γGT, albumin, bilirubin)
- Clotting studies (PT)
- Transabdominal ultrasound or CT scan for splenomegaly and ascites

Treatment

Removal of the cause and prevention of progression
- Abstinence from alcohol
- Combination therapy for hepatitis (interferon-α and ribavirin for 6 months)—moderate to severe hepatitis C
- Immunosuppression for autoimmune causes

Treatment of complications
- Portal hypertension (see 📖 p. 310)
- Encephalopathy treatment aims to lower the amount of nitrogen absorbed from the gut:
  - Administration of oral lactulose
  - Oral, nonabsorbable antibiotics
  - Careful IV fluid replacement to prevent sodium overload
  - Diet high in carbohydrates, low in salt, moderate in protein
- Ascites: oral spironolactone. In cases of tense ascites, paracentesis may be required, with IV albumin replacement.
- Decompensated hepatocellular failure: consider liver transplant

Pancreatic cancer

Key facts

- There are ~37,000 new cases in the United States per year.
- 80% of cases occur between the sixth and seventh decades.
- Risk factors include cigarette smoking, increasing age, high-fat diet, diabetes mellitus, alcoholism, chronic pancreatitis, race, and family history.
- Occupational hazards, e.g., exposure to naphthylene and benzene
- Hereditary factors, including a family history of pancreatic cancer, *BRCA* mutations, and Peutz–Jehger syndrome

Pathological features

- 90% ductal adenocarcinoma
- 7% cystic neoplasms (intraductal papillary mucinous tumors, serous cystadenomas, mucinous cystadenoma or cystadenocarcinoma, papillary cystic tumors)
- 3% islet cell tumors

Clinical features

Carcinoma of the head of pancreas (65%)

- Obstructive jaundice due to compression or invasion of the common bile duct. The gallbladder is typically palpable.
- Pain is epigastric or in the left upper quadrant, often vague, and radiates to the back.
- Anorexia, nausea and vomiting, fatigue, malaise, dyspepsia, and pruritus
- Acute pancreatitis is rarely the first presenting feature.
- Thrombophlebitis migrans (10%) presents as emboli. Splenic vein thrombosis may lead to splenomegaly in 10% of patients.
- Diabetes mellitus

Carcinoma of the body (25%) and tail (10%)

- Usually asymptomatic in the early stages
- Weight loss and back pain
- Epigastric mass
- Jaundice suggests spread to hepatic hilar lymph nodes or metastases.
- Thrombophlebitis migrans
- Diabetes mellitus

Diagnosis and investigations

- CBC, LFTs, blood sugar level
- Elevated serum CA 19–9
- Pancreatic-protocol CT scan of pancreas with triple-phase IV contrast to assess size of the primary lesion, vascular invasion, and distant metastasis
- Fine-needle aspiration cytology (FNAC; usually CT- or ultrasound-guided) is not necessary.
- Endoscopic ultrasound (EUS) to evaluate involved lymph nodes and assess respectability

- ERCP is 85% accurate; it can provide cytology as well as achieve biliary drainage via insertion of a stent.
- Laparoscopy with cytology is used to rule out peritoneal disease and liver metastasis smaller than 1 cm prior to offering surgical resection.

Treatment
Palliative treatment
The majority of tumors (80%) are not suitable for surgical resection because of presence of metastases, local invasion, age, or comorbidities.

Relief of jaundice
Obstructive jaundice is associated with pruritus, coagulopathy, immunological and nutritional derangement, deterioration in liver function, risk of acute renal failure (hepatorenal syndrome), and increased susceptibility to infection. Relief of jaundice is achieved by the following:
- Endoscopic biliary stenting via ERCP
- Percutaneous biliary drainage: percutaneous transhepatic cholangiography (PTC) and internal stenting, or insertion of an internal–external drainage catheter
- Surgical biliary drainage by cholecystojejunostomy or choledochojejunostomy.

Relief of duodenal obstruction
- Surgical gastrojejunostomy or endoscopic duodenal stent

Relief of pain
- Oral narcotics
- Chemical ablation of the celiac ganglia (percutaneous celiac nerve block and thoracoscopic division of the splanchnic nerves are alternatives)

Curative treatment
Radical surgical resection is the only hope of cure if patient is suitable.
- Proximal pancreatoduodenectomy for periampullary tumors and cancer of the pancreas confined to the head
- Distal pancreatectomy for tumors in the tail
- Rarely is a total pancreatectomy indicated.

Adjuvant therapy
Gemcitabine has been shown to improve survival after resection of the pancreatic cancer. It is unclear if radiation improves survival.

Prognosis
In patients with resectable disease, the 5-year survival is 12%–19%.

Cancer of the liver, gallbladder, and biliary tree

Key facts
- Metastatic disease represents the majority of liver tumors (pancreas, colon, stomach, esophagus).
- 35% of patients who die of malignant disease have hepatic metastases.

Clinicopathological features

Hepatocellular carcinoma (HCC)
- 90% of primary liver tumors
- Common in Africa and Asia; occurs in men more than in women
- Risk factors:
  - Cirrhosis, especially due to chronic viral hepatitis (HBV/HCV) or alcohol consumption
  - Aflatoxin exposure, contraceptives, and androgens
- HCC arises from liver parenchymal cells, spreads via local invasion, via portal vein invasion to other sites in the liver, or via hepatic vein invasion and distant metastases (e.g., lung).
- The most common presentation is rapid deterioration in background cirrhosis.

Cholangiocarcinoma
- Usually arises in the extrahepatic biliary tree but may be intrahepatic
- Typical sites are distal common bile duct, common bile duct, confluence of bile ducts (Klatskin tumor), and peripheral bile ducts.

Adenocarcinoma of the gallbladder
- Gallstones are found in 70% of cases.
- Associated with ulcerative colitis and primary sclerosing cholangitis
- Often diagnosed incidentally as an unexpected finding during or after cholecystectomy for "benign" disease causing right upper quadrant pain and nausea
- May present as a gallbladder mass or obstructive jaundice due to local invasion of the common hepatic duct
- Spread is direct into liver tissue (possibly resectable) or to hilar lymph nodes or is blood-borne (incurable).

Ampullary carcinoma
- Typically this carcinoma is small and presents relatively early because of the early onset of painless, obstructive jaundice.
- It has the best prognosis of all upper hepatobiliary cancers because of its early presentation, before local or lymphatic spread.

Other primary liver cancers
- Fibrolamellar carcinoma (FLC)
  - Usually affects younger patients (third and fourth decades)
  - Does not occur on a background of liver disease
  - Presents as a large vascular mass

- Angiosarcoma.
  - <1% of liver tumors (most common sarcoma of the liver)
  - Associated with exposure to arsenic, vinyl chloride, anabolic steroids, and contraceptives

Diagnosis and investigations

- AFP >200 ng/mL is diagnostic of HCC in the setting of cirrhosis and appropriate imaging characteristics.
- An ultrasound scan often identifies the site and cause of biliary obstruction; it is a good assessment of liver parenchyma.
- Needle biopsy is used to confirm diagnosis of HCC if the diagnosis is unclear.
- ERCP is used for diagnosis of ampullary and bile duct carcinoma; it allows biopsy or brush cytology of distal tumors, and enables therapeutic stenting.
- MRCP is used to diagnose proximal tumors or when ERCP is not possible.
- PTC is used for diagnosis of intrahepatic biliary tumors, therapeutic stenting, or external drainage of proximal biliary tumors.
- CT scanning is used for assessment of local spread (including blood vessels), lymph nodes, and distant metastases.

Treatment

Curative

Surgery offers the only cure for primary liver or biliary cancers. Patients suitable for resection must

- Be fit for major surgery
- Have no evidence of metastases or involved lymph nodes (rare)
- Have tumors technically suitable for complete resection

Surgical options for resection include the following:

- Partial hepatectomy
- Liver transplantation (HCC associated with chronic hepatitis)
- Radical cholecystectomy and portal lymph node dissection (adenocarcinoma of gallbladder)
- Radical excision of bile duct with reconstruction (cholangiocarcinoma)
- Pancreaticoduodenectomy (Whipple procedure)—distal cholangiocarcinoma or ampullary carcinoma

Palliative

- Endoscopic or percutaneous stenting for unresectable cholangiocarcinoma or ampullary carcinoma
- Chemotherapy is of minimal benefit in treating any primary liver or biliary cancers.
- Radiofrequency ablation (HCC and colorectal cancer metastases)

Prognosis

- About 20% of these tumors are resectable at the time of diagnosis.
- Prognosis depends on whether the patient is resectable and on the stage of disease.

Acute variceal hemorrhage

Key facts

The mortality rate of first variceal bleed with established portal hypertension is 30%.

Features

See 📖 p. 280 for differential diagnosis.

Typical variceal bleeding

- Is rapid-onset, copious, dark red venous blood with little mixing with food
- Has features of established portal hypertension, e.g., caput medusa
- May result in hepatic encephalopathy (ingested blood provides an extremely protein-rich "meal")

Emergency management

Resuscitation

- Establish large-caliber IV access. Give crystalloid fluid up to 1000 mL if patient is tachycardic or hypotensive. Only use uncross-matched blood if the patient is in extremis; otherwise, wait for cross-matched blood if transfusion is needed.
- Monitor pulse rate, BP, and urine output (urinary catheter).
- Send blood for CBC, electrolytes, LFTs (albumin), cross-match (at least 4 units if hematemesis is large), and clotting factors.
- Always consider alerting the ICU. Variceal bleeds can deteriorate extremely rapidly.
- Insertion of a Sengstaken–Blakemore gastroesophageal tube may be life saving but is only used as a last resort.
  - If the patient needs a Sengstaken tube, they need to be in the ICU.
  - Most patients need sedation or GA for the tube to be inserted.
  - The tube is inserted and the gastric balloon blown up first and traction applied gently until the tube becomes fixed. This alone may stop the bleeding if the varices are gastric.
  - If bleeding continues, the esophageal balloon is blown up to a pressure of ~20–30 mmHg.
  - The esophageal balloon must be deflated regularly to prevent esophageal necrosis.

Establish a diagnosis

- Urgent EGD is the investigation of choice and usually requires anesthesia and intubation to protect the airway (at least within 24 hr).
  - The patient may require ongoing resuscitation.
  - Never biopsy suspected varices.
  - Therapeutic interventions include sclerotherapy and banding, and these are up to 90% successful at controlling acute bleeds.
- Give IV PPI (e.g., omeprazole 40 mg); stop all NSAIDS.
- Give IV vasopression, somatostatin, or octreotide to lower esophageal variceal pressure.
- Give patient a blood transfusion if there is a large volume of hematemesis or a drop in Hb.

- Ensure that the appropriate surgical team knows of the patient in case surgical intervention is required.
- Consider giving FFP to correct clotting abnormalities.

Definitive management

The following procedures are considered for failed endoscopic treatment and ongoing bleeding.

- A transjugular intraparenchymal portosystemic shunt (TIPS) (intrahepatic shunt) may be placed to rapidly reduce the portal pressure, but this has the risk of inducing portal encephalopathy. A connection is made between the hepatic venous system and the portal venous system with stent placement.
- Extrahepatic shunt: encephalopathy occurs in 50% of survivors and the procedure is now seldom performed. Occasionally, a distal spleno-renal shunt will be performed in a Childs A cirrhotic who has variceal bleeding.
- Esophageal transection
  - Left gastric vein devascularization
  - Extremely high mortality
  - Low incidence of encephalopathy but high incidence of recurrent bleeding

Abdominal wall

Matthew Hutter, MD

Inguinal hernia

A **hernia** is the abnormal protrusion of a viscus or body-cavity content through its normal anatomical boundaries.

Key facts
- Inguinal hernias are the most common type of abdominal hernia.
- They occur through the tissues of the inguinal canal.
- They are classified according to their (surgically determined) relationship to the inferior epigastric artery, and subclassified by behavior and form:
  - **Indirect**. Arises lateral to the inferior epigastric artery and often protrudes through the deep inguinal ring. When due to persistence of a patent processus vaginalis it is congenital in origin. Inguinal hernias in childhood are always indirect and due to a patent processus.
  - **Direct**. Arises medial to the inferior epigastric artery and protrudes through the posterior wall of the inguinal canal. It is commonly due to chronic straining or coughing, causing weakening of the posterior canal tissues.

Behavior
- Reducible: contents can be fully restored to the abdominal cavity.
- Incarcerated: part or all of the contents cannot be reduced.
- Strangulated: incarcerated with compromise of the blood supply of the contents, which may or may not lead to infarction. Not all strangulated hernias are accompanied by bowel obstruction, but it is common.

Form
- Scrotal. Descends via the inguinal canal into the scrotum. This is often the end stage of an indirect hernia.
- Sliding (en-glissade). The sac is formed partly by retroperitoneal tissue from the iliac fossa.
- Pantaloon. Direct and indirect hernias coexist, descending either side of the epigastric artery.

Clinical features
- **Direct**. Typically wide-necked; often not well controlled by pressure over the deep inguinal ring. The hernia tends to protrude directly anteriorly and make the inguinal skin crease more apparent.
- **Indirect**. Typically relatively narrow-necked; when small they may be controlled by pressure over the site of origin (the deep inguinal ring). The hernia tends to descend via the inguinal canal toward the top of the scrotum.

Diagnosis
- CT scanning may show a hernia but may not rule out the possibility of a hernia.

Treatment

- Patients with hernias that are narrow-necked, difficult to reduce, or highly symptomatic or who have had episodes of irreducibility or bowel obstruction should be encouraged to undergo repair.
- Patients with hernias that are moderately symptomatic, cosmetic, or interfering with work or leisure activities should be offered repair.
- For asymptomatic hernias, watchful waiting may be considered.
- A groin truss is of limited symptomatic benefit for nonsurgical patients.

Technical aspects

- Repair in children only involves excision of the sac and plication of the deep inguinal ring, since the inguinal canal is almost never unduly weak.
- Adult repairs may be performed by open surgery or via laparoscopic approach (either transperitoneal or in the pre-peritoneal space).
- General or local anesthesia is needed if done via the open approach.
- The 2-year recurrence rate for mesh repairs is approximately 1%–5%.

Clinical pearls—anatomy and repair of inguinal hernia

Anatomy of the inguinal canal

- The inguinal canal is an oblique passage through the lower abdominal wall.
- Contents of the spermatic cord are (in males):
  - 3 vessels (testicular artery, cremasteric artery, artery to the vas)
  - 3 nerves (genital branch of genitofemoral, autonomic supply to the testicle, ilioinguinal nerve)
  - 3 structures (vas, pampiniform venous plexus, testicular lymphatics)
  - 3 coverings (external spermatic fascia, cremasteric fascia, internal spermatic fascia)
- The **deep ring** is formed through the transversalis fascia and has internal oblique fibers anterolaterally and inferior epigastric vessels medially.
- The **superficial ring** is a V-shaped defect in the aponeurosis of external oblique, above and medial to the pubic tubercle.

Adult inguinal hernia repair

Principles of inguinal hernia repair are as follows.

- Exposure of the defect and reduction of the sac and contents
- Tension-free reinforcement of the transversalis fascia (TVF) layer (usually with nonabsorbable mesh). In open repairs this lies in front of the TVF and/or sometimes behind it; in laparoscopic repair it lies behind the TVF.
- Mesh may be fixed in place by sutures (open) or "tacking" devices (laparoscopic approach).

Femoral hernia

Key facts
- Femoral hernias are more common in women than in men.
- They occur through tissues of the femoral canal.
- They have a high risk of strangulation because the neck of the sac has bony and ligamentous structures limiting it on three sides.
- Approximately 30% of femoral hernias present as emergencies: 50% of these require bowel resection for strangulation and ischemia.

Clinical features
- Appears inferior and lateral to pubic tubercle, medial to femoral pulse
- May be mistaken for an upper medial thigh swelling

Diagnosis
- Differential diagnosis includes the following:
  - Low presentation of inguinal hernia
  - Femoral canal lipoma
  - Femoral lymph node
  - Saphena varix (disappears on lying and has a pronounced thrill on percussion of the saphenous vein)
  - Femoral artery aneurysm (pulsatile)
- Ultrasound scanning may help with the differential diagnosis. If there is significant doubt, exploration is usually indicated because of the high risk of complications in untreated femoral hernia.

Treatment
Once the hernia is reduced, the femoral canal can be narrowed by interrupted sutures or a mesh plug may be used to prevent recurrence. Care must be taken not to narrow the adjacent femoral vein. There are two main approaches.

Infrainguinal approach
- Incision is below the inguinal ligament, approaching the femoral canal from below.
- This approach has the advantage of not interfering with the inguinal structures but provides little or no scope for resecting any compromised small bowel and so is best reserved for elective surgery.

Inguinal approach
- Incision is above the inguinal ligament, approaching the femoral canal from above by dissecting through the posterior wall of the inguinal canal.
- This approach requires repair of the inguinal canal on closure but offers some access to the peritoneal cavity should small-bowel surgery be required, and is the usual approach in emergency presentations.

Clinical pearls—anatomy of the femoral canal

- Lies medial to femoral vein within femoral sheath
- The femoral ring is the abdominal opening of the femoral canal.
- Boundaries to the femoral ring are
  - Anteriorly: inguinal ligament
  - Medially: lacunar ligament
  - Posteriorly: pectineal ligament
  - Laterally: femoral vein
- An aberrant obturator artery branch of the inferior epigastric may cross the lacunar ligament and can cause hemorrhage during surgical repair.
- Femoral hernia repair (open) involves suture-plication of the inguinal and pectineal ligaments or placement of a mesh plug.

Umbilical and epigastric hernias

Key facts

These hernias are sometimes referred to collectively as ventral hernias.

- Umbilical hernias can be divided into the following types:
  - True umbilical hernias occur through the umbilical stalk and are almost always congenital in origin. Those present at birth may close spontaneously before the age of 3 years.
  - Periumbilical hernias occur through the periumbilical tissues and are always acquired.
- Epigastric hernias are defects in the midline tissues of the linea alba. They may be small or extensive.

Clinical features

Umbilical hernia

- Small, centrally placed within the umbilicus
- Often contains pre-peritoneal fat and rarely contains bowel or omentum
- May be painful but rarely strangulates

Periumbilical hernia

- Variable in size: up to moderate
- Placed eccentrically and distorts the shape of the umbilicus
- May contain bowel or omentum
- Often painful and occasionally strangulates

Epigastric hernia

- Varies: up to large defects
- Always placed in the midline, although when large it may lie to one side
- Moderate risk of strangulation

Diagnosis

The diagnosis is rarely in doubt. If there is concern that a palpable lump may be a lipoma or subcutaneous tissue growth, a CT scan can usually confirm the diagnosis.

Treatment

- Congenital umbilical hernias should only be repaired if they persist beyond the age of 2–3 years.
- Surgical repair is offered for symptomatic hernias or those with a high risk of complications.

Principles of repair

- Identify edges of hernia sac and reduce hernia.
- Small defects are usually repaired by an overlapping sutured repair using nonabsorbable suture, e.g., 0 Prolene, without reinforcements.
- Larger defects or recurrent hernias may be repaired with mesh.

Incisional hernias

Key facts

- Incisional hernias are very uncommon outside the abdomen.
- Up to 10% of mid-line laparotomy wounds suffer herniation to some degree. Factors that predispose to incisional herniation include the following:
  - Wound infection
  - Steroid use or malnutrition at the time of original surgery
  - Incisional hernias are probably slightly less common after muscle splitting or transverse incisions, compared to midline laparotomies.
- The peak time of presentation is up to 5 years after surgery.

Pathological features

The hernia occurs through the tissues in which the incision is made. Typically, the sac is made up of peritoneum, eventrated scar tissue, and subcutaneous scar tissue.

Clinical features

- The hernia may vary from a few centimeters to a near complete defect in the anterior abdominal wall through which all the mobile viscera regularly protrude.
- The risk of strangulation is maximal in small to medium-size defects.

In large and very large defects, the viscera are often permanently herniated, and if this has been the case for a long period, they "lose the right of domain" within the true abdominal cavity. This means that the remaining lateral abdominal wall tissues chronically retract, and there may be insufficient room for all the viscera within the revised abdominal cavity when the tissues are reapproximated.

Diagnosis

When assessing incisional hernias, assess the following.

- What is the risk of complications and strangulation?
- Is it likely that the contents of the hernia can be reduced fully?
- Is the patient able to undergo the anesthesia necessary for the surgery required?
- Is there a risk of compromise to respiratory function if a very large incisional hernia is reduced and repaired?

Treatment

- Small defects: simple sutured repair
- Medium-sized defects: overlapping (Mayo) sutured repair with or without reinforcing "on-lay" mesh
- Large defects: interposition mesh (prosthetic or porcine collagen), possibly with lateral relaxing incisions
- Laparoscopic repairs involve placement of intraperitoneal mesh that is tacked and sutured circumferentially with adequate overlap around the edge of the hernia.
- In unfit patients or patients unwilling to have surgery a custom-made support corset or binder may be useful.

Other types of hernia

Spigelian

- Occurs under the lower edge of the linea semilunaris and protrudes along the lateral border of the rectus sheath
- Typically difficult to diagnose in the supine position
- Has a high risk of complications
- Repair can be by direct suture-repair of the rectus sheath or by placement of mesh.

Obturator

- Occurs through the obturator canal from the lateral wall of the pelvis with the sac protruding into the medial upper thigh
- Symptoms include pain or abnormal sensations in the distribution of the obturator nerve in the skin of the inner medial thigh.
- Diagnosis is often very difficult, and is usually made by CT scan. A high proportion present with complications of small-bowel obstruction, as the sac is hidden within the muscles of the adductor compartment.
- The neck is narrow and prone to strangulation.
- Repair can be via exposure of the sac in the medial thigh or, more commonly, at laparotomy for complications.

Lumbar

- Occurs through either the inferior or superior lumbar triangles (bounded by the lumbar muscles, lumbosacral fascia, and bony features of the posterior abdominal wall) or, rarely, through lumbar incisions.
- Usually contains retroperitoneal fat and rarely bowel.
- This type may be repaired by direct suture or mesh repair for larger defects.

Perineal

- Spontaneous perineal hernias occur through the greater or lesser sciatic foramina and are exceptionally rare. They present with acute complications and are diagnosed only at surgery.
- Postoperative perineal hernias occur through the pelvic floor muscles and do so usually as a result of surgical procedures (particularly after abdominoperineal resection of the rectum).
- Repair may be via sutured closure of the defect or, more commonly, filling of the defect with prosthetic material (mesh) or biological tissue (muscle flap).

Acute groin swelling

Causes and features

- **Incarcerated groin hernia** (inguinal or femoral). May or may not be associated with intestinal obstruction. Strangulated hernias can be painful and tender.
- **Acute epididymo-orchitis** (in males). Tenderness is particularly over the spermatic cord and the epididymis.
- **Torsion of the testis**. May present with pain in the groin, but unless the testicle is undescended, the tenderness is primarily over the scrotum (and testis).
- **Iliopsoas abscess**. Tenderness is primarily below the inguinal ligament. It may be fluctuant, with associated tenderness in the right iliac fossa due to underlying pathology.
- **Acute iliofemoral lymphadenopathy** (e.g., from infected toenail). Tender diffuse swelling; often multiple palpable lumps (nodes). Lymphoma tends to be less acute.
- **Acute saphena varix**. Compressible, cough thrill
- Acute complications of femoral artery pseudoaneurysm.

Emergency management

Resuscitation

- Establish IV access. Consider giving crystalloid fluid if there is suspicion of a complicated hernia or an iliopsoas abscess.
- Catheterize and monitor fluid status closely if patient is hypotensive.

Establish a diagnosis

- ▶ Torsion of the testis is a true surgical emergency and should not wait for a diagnosis short of exploration.
  - Color-flow Doppler assessment may be able to confirm the presence of a hyperemic testis but, unless it is immediately available, it should not delay operation.
- ▶ If there is a strong clinical history in a young male, immediate operation remains the diagnostic investigation of choice.
- If an iliopsoas abscess is suspected, abdominopelvic CT scanning is the investigation of choice.

Definitive management

Incarcerated groin hernia

- Repair is indicated for all patients except those considered unfit for any surgical procedure or those declining treatment.
- It may not be possible to establish if the hernia is inguinal or femoral preoperatively. If so, it is safest to approach as if for an inguinal hernia.

- Femoral hernias may be approached via an infrainguinal or transinguinal dissection.
  - Infrainguinal approaches may be limited in exposure if there is necrotic bowel within the hernia requiring resection.
  - A transinguinal approach will involve repair of the inguinal canal as well, but offers an almost unlimited exposure of the femoral canal from above and allows plenty of exposure for bowel resection.
- Inguinal hernias should be approached through a conventional incision.
  - Repair may require a mesh, although there is an increased risk of infection if there is an associated bowel resection.
- Anesthesia may be general or local with sedation.

Psoas abscess

The underlying cause should be identified as a matter or priority. Incision and drainage of the groin collection may be indicated, but only as part of the overall treatment.

Torsion of the testis

- Once identified, the affected testis should be assessed. If nonviable, a simple orchiectomy is performed; if viable, an orchiopexy.
- If the diagnosis is confirmed, the contralateral testicle should be fixed by orchidopexy to prevent subsequent torsion.

Epididymo-orchitis

- Antibiotics, oral (e.g., ciprofloxacin 500 mg qd) for 14 days or IV if case is severe

Colorectal surgery

Liliana Bordeianou, MD

Ulcerative colitis

Key facts
- Ulcerative colitis is an acute, chronic inflammatory disease originating in the colonic columnar mucosa.
- The precise etiology is unknown but may include a genetic predisposition (family history).
- Peak age of diagnosis is the late teens and twenties. However, the disease may also present in late adulthood.
- It is most common in Caucasians of Anglo-Saxon descent.

Pathological features
- Granular, hypervascular, and mildly edematous mucosa with loss of vascular pattern is seen at endoscopy.
- There is acute neutrophil infiltration of the colonic mucosa and submucosa. Mucosal crypt abscesses with goblet cell mucin depletion are also present.
- With more severe inflammation there are multiple aphthous ulcers, which may become confluent with only islands of inflamed mucosa and granulation tissue remaining (pseudopolyposis).
- Transmural inflammation may occur in severe disease secondary to the widespread loss of mucosa and subsequent severe inflammation.
- Chronic "burnt-out" disease leads to a pale, featureless, ahaustral pattern to the colon.
- Disease tends to be present in the distal colon and rectum and spread proximally as the extent of the disease increases.

Clinical features
- *Proctitis.* Most common presentation. The rectum is always involved unless the patient is already on topical treatment. Symptoms include urgent, frequent defecation due to rectal irritability, and bloody mucus mixed with loose stools (frank bloody diarrhea is rare).
- *Left-sided colitis.* Disease up to the splenic flexure. Symptoms of rectal irritation plus extensive bloody mucus in stools often lead to bloody diarrhea. There are mild associated systemic features.
- *Pancolitis.* Disease involving the entire colon. It may be associated with mild secondary inflammation of the terminal ileum (backwash ileitis). Diarrhea is the predominant feature; other common systemic features include fever, malaise, anorexia, and tachycardia. It may be associated with anemia (due to blood loss), hypoalbuminemia, and hypokalemia (due to mucus loss).

Diagnosis and investigations
Basic tests
Raised WBC and ESR; low Hct and albumin, especially during episodes of inflammation. KUB may show edematous colonic mucosa ("thumbprinting") but is unreliable for diagnosis or extent of disease. Sigmoidoscopy usually shows erythematous, granular, or frankly ulcerated rectal mucosa with mucus and blood. Biopsies should be taken before starting treatment.

Advanced tests

The extent of disease is best assessed with colonoscopy and biopsies. (In most cases this will also exclude colonic Crohn's disease.)

Treatment

See 📖 p. 360 for management of acute severe colitis.

Medical treatment

Principles are to reduce inflammation and prevent complications. Acute electrolyte derangements should be corrected.

Proctitis
- Steroid suppositories
- Topical 5-aminosalicyclic acid (5-ASA) suppositories

Left-sided colitis
- Steroid foam enemas (penetrate up as far as the splenic flexure)
- Topical 5-ASA foam enemas
- May require systemic steroid treatment (prednisone)

Pancolitis
- Topical steroids or 5-ASA treatments for local symptoms
- Usually needs systemic treatment, e.g., oral steroids (prednisone), 5-ASA treatment
- Oral immunosuppressive agents, e.g., azathioprine, 6-mercaptopurine.
- Anti-TNF-α antibodies, such as Infliximab

Surgical treatment

Surgery is indicated for acute colitis that fails to respond to treatment and for chronic colitis in the following cases:
- The patient is chronically symptomatic despite maximal medical therapy.
- Medical therapy is associated with unacceptable side effects.
- Recurrent exacerbations are affecting growth or development in children and adolescents.
- Confirmed diagnosis reveals dysplasia with or without a dysplasia-associated lesion or mass (DALM), or carcinoma of colon.

Surgical treatment may be as follows:
- Proctocolectomy (removal of colon and rectum) with ileoanal pouch formation
- Proctocolectomy with an abdominoperineal resection (removal of colon, rectum, and anus) with end ileostomy formation (permanent)
- Total abdominal colectomy (removal of colon) with ileostomy (used when the patient is too unwell for major pelvic surgery, e.g., for acute severe colitis)

Crohn's disease

Key facts

- This chronic inflammatory, noncaseating, granulomatous disease affects any part of the GI tract.
- It is associated with several extraintestinal symptoms.
- Its precise etiology is unknown, but may include a genetic predisposition (family history).
- Peak age of onset of symptoms is the teens and early twenties. However, diagnosis is often several years later.
- It is most common in Caucasians of Anglo-Saxon descent.

Pathological features

- Disease is commonly focused in the terminal ileum, but may affect perineum, colon, or the entire small bowel.
- Perineal Crohn's disease is common and may be the first manifestation of disease.
- Colonic Crohn's disease is a long-term risk factor for colorectal cancer formation.
- Affected bowel looks blue-gray, thickened, with spiral surface vessels and encroachment of the mesenteric fat around the bowel ("fat wrapping").
- Transmural inflammation may be in the form of lymphoid aggregates, particularly in the subserosal tissues ("Crohn's rosary"), mucosal crypt ulceration, and fissuring ulceration.
- Mucosal thickening and serpiginous longitudinal ulceration combine to give the appearance of "cobblestoning."
- Perforation, fistulation, and abscess formation are occasional "fistulizing" sequelae of transmural inflammation.
- Extensive fibrosis and smooth muscle hyperplasia may occur, giving rise to stenosis.

Clinical features

- *Inflammatory features.* Fever, malaise, abdominal pain (often right iliac fossa), change in bowel habit (usually diarrhea without blood), and weight loss. Children and adolescents may have failure to thrive or have retarded growth. Rectal bleeding is rare except in Crohn's colitis.
- *Fistulizing features.* Para-enteric abscess formation often with a tender abdominal mass, fistula formation (ileocolic, ileoileal, ileocutaneous). Rarely there is free perforation with features of peritonitis.
- *Stenosing features.* Colicky abdominal pain, weight loss due to poor food intake ("food fear"), palpable or visible distended small-bowel loops
- *Perineal disease.* Atypical severe anal fissures, fistula in ano, anal abscess, anal mucosal thickening, and discoloration

Diagnosis and investigations

Basic tests

Raised CBC and ESR; low Hct and albumin, especially during episodes of inflammation

Advanced tests

- In acute presentations, an abdominal CT may show an inflammatory mass, abscess formation, or localized or free perforation.
- In subacute or chronic presentations, small-bowel disease may be shown by a small-bowel contrast study (shows mucosal irregularity and narrowing).
- Crohn's colitis is diagnosed by endoscopy and biopsy.
- Perineal disease may require assessment by EUA, anal ultrasound, or MRI scanning.
- Upper GI endoscopy and biopsies may show features of Crohn's disease in gastric mucosa.

Treatment

Medical treatment

Principles are to reduce inflammation and control complications.

- Systemic (5-ASA) drugs are first-line acute and long-term treatment.
- Systemic steroids (prednisone) control acute exacerbations of inflammation, and steroids with very high first-pass metabolism (budesonide) can be used chronically.
- Immunosuppressive agents (azathioprine, 6-mercaptopurine) are used as maintenance therapy, and anti-TNF-α antibodies (infliximab) may be effective in fistulizing complications.
- Dietary manipulation (elemental diet) may reduce inflammatory factors.

Surgical treatment

Principles are to deal with septic complications, relieve significant bowel obstruction, and remove as little bowel as possible. Indications for surgery include the following.

- *Acute*: free perforation, severe hemorrhage, acute severe colitis, complete intestinal obstruction
- *Subacute*: inflammatory mass, subacute obstruction, abscess formation, symptomatic fistulation
- *Chronic*: steroid dependency or complications, growth retardation, cancer treatment or prevention

Extraintestinal manifestations of Crohn's disease

Associated with disease activity	*Independent of disease activity*
Pyoderma gangrenosum	Ankylosing spondylitis
Erythema nodosum	Polyarthritis
Primary biliary cirrhosis	

Other forms of colitis

Key facts and pathological features

Colitis may result from various insults of widely differing origin, other than idiopathic inflammatory bowel disease.

Acute infective colitis

- Typically caused by pathological variants of normal enteric organisms, e.g., enteropathogenic *Escherichia coli*. Only rarely does this form progress to acute severe colitis.
- Typhoid colitis (*Salmonella typhi*) is rare in the United States. It is typified by acute bloody diarrhea, with biopsy showing few if any neutrophils present in the colonic mucosa (due to bone marrow suppression by typhoid condition).

Pseudomembranous colitis

This form is caused by *Clostridium difficile* infection and is associated with antibiotic use, particularly third-generation cephalosporins (even as little as a single dose). Toxin produced by the organism causes acute, severe inflammation in the mucosa with rapid mucosal loss. Acute neutrophil infiltration, exudate, and slough form gray-white "plaques" of material on the denuded colonic surface called *pseudomembranes*. It may rapidly progress to acute severe colitis, especially in the immunocompromised or acutely unwell.

Neutropenic colitis

This form occurs in severely immunocompromised patients with neutropenia and/or neutrophil dysfunction. It is caused by multiple, normally nonpathogenic enteric organisms colonizing the colonic mucosa.

Radiation colitis

Acute, transient colitis is caused by mucosal injury secondary to external beam radiotherapy. It sometimes progresses to stricture formation after months or years.

Ischemic colitis

This form is most common at the splenic flexure, where collateral blood supply between the middle and left colic arteries is poorest. It is usually precipitated by an acute occlusion of part or all of the inferior mesenteric artery. Ischemic colitis may progress to infarction; otherwise it tends to settle spontaneously, although it may form an ischemic stricture.

Clinical features

Symptoms are broadly similar, independent of underlying cause. Typical features include vague abdominal pain, mild fever (absent in neutropenic colitis), and diarrhea (which may be bloody, especially in ischemic, radiation, severe pseudomembranous, and typhoid colitis). Cessation of diarrhea in the absence of treatment suggests that acute severe colitis is developing and should be investigated urgently.

Diagnosis and investigations

The diagnosis and investigation depend on the suspected cause:
- Stool sent for *C. difficile toxin*;
- Stool sent for ova and parasite (O&P) test
- Plain abdominal radiograph may show thickened colonic haustra.
- CT scan of abdomen often shows typical mucosal thickening in colitis.
- Flexible endoscopy (usually flexible sigmoidoscopy) with visualization of pseudomembranes and biopsy

Treatment

Medical treatment

- *Acute infective colitis*: antibiotics only if patient is severely symptomatic
- *C. difficile colitis*: vancomycin 250 mg po qid /metronidazole 500 mg po tid
- *Neutropenic colitis*: broad-spectrum antibiotics, bone marrow support
- *Radiation colitis*: symptomatic treatment only; antidiarrheals
- *Ischemic colitis*: supportive treatment. Anticoagulation may be appropriate if the underlying cause is thromboembolic.

Surgical treatment

▶▶ This is rarely indicated. Any form of colitis may progress to acute severe colitis and require emergency subtotal colectomy. Indications are as follows:
- Failure to respond to maximal medical therapy with life-threatening colitis
- Complications of colitis: uncontrollable bleeding, perforation (especially in ischemic or neutropenic colitis)

Clinical pearls—anatomy of the large bowel

The large bowel has several main arterial (and lymph node) territories that are used for resections for cancer:
- Ileocolic artery (from SMA): last terminal ileal loop, cecum, and ascending colon
- Middle colic artery (from SMA): transverse colon up to the splenic flexure
- Left colic (from IMA): splenic flexure and descending colon
- Superior rectal artery (from IMA): upper rectum

Colorectal polyps

Polyp is a purely descriptive term; any growth from the lining of the large bowel can be described as a polyp. Polyps may be predominantly raised with a stalk attachment (pedunculated), flat and spreading over the surface of the bowel wall (sessile), or, occasionally, a combination of the two.

Key facts and pathological features

Polyps may arise for many different reasons.

Juvenile polyps

These are mucin-filled cystic swellings of the lower rectal mucosa. Rarely, they may be part of a hereditary syndrome (juvenile polyposis) with multiple juvenile polyps throughout the colon—there is a slightly increased risk of colorectal cancer.

Hamartomatous polyps

These polyps contain excessive amounts of the normal architectural components of the bowel wall and are usually isolated. They may be part of a hereditary syndrome (Peutz–Jeghers syndrome) with polyps characterized by extensive branched growth of the muscularis mucosa—there is a slightly increased risk of colorectal and other GI cancers.

Hyperplastic polyps

Small, sessile polyps form from normal elongated mucosal crypts.

Adenomatous polyps

- True neoplastic polyps formed by excessive growth of the colorectal epithelium. They are divided according to morphology of the glandular tissue into tubular, tubulovillous, and villous types.
- They may be sessile, pedunculated, or mixed.
- This form is thought to be the precursor of most colorectal cancers. The risk of cancerous change within an adenomatous polyp increases with size (particularly over 5 cm), villous morphology, and sessile form.
- The majority are sporadic (either isolated or in small numbers), although occasionally these may be part of a hereditary syndrome.

Familial adenomatous polyposis (FAP)

FAP is caused by an autosomal dominant defect in the *APC* gene on chromosome 5. it is characterized by large numbers (between dozens and thousands) of adenomatous polyps in the colon and rectum and an increased risk of polyp formation in the stomach and duodenum. The risk of cancerous transformation in any given polyp is similar to that in normal polyps, but the overall risk is very high because of the vastly increased number present.

FAP is associated with the following:
- Sesmoid formation, particularly in the abdominal tissues
- Multiple osteomas, fibromas, and thyroid inflammation

A range of abnormalities of the mismatch repair (MMR) genes predisposes adenomas to acquire multiple genetic defects and thus progress more rapidly than normal to cancer, although the overall rate of adenoma formation is similar to that in general population.

Clinical features

Most polyps are asymptomatic, although symptoms may occur with increasing size and with proximity to the anus. Typical symptoms are as follows:

- Bleeding: usually low volume, dark red, often flecks or mixed with stool
- Mucus discharge: white, clear, or watery; most common with large villous adenomas. It may cause hypokalemia and hypoproteinemia if the villous adenoma is large with copious mucus discharge.
- Prolapse: if pedunculated and low in the rectum, polyps may prolapse out of the anus.

Diagnosis and tests

- Most polyps are diagnosed by colonoscopy.
- Most patients with polyps require further follow-up colonoscopies to keep them under surveillance for future polyp formation. The frequency and length of follow-up depend on the number, size, and histology of the polyp.[1]
- Hereditary polyposis syndromes may be investigated by genetic mutation analysis.

Treatment

Medical treatment

- Colonoscopic polypectomy is carried out for pedunculated polyps larger than 1–2 mm.
- Patients with FAP require regular gastroscopy and upper GI surveillance to identify premalignant polyps.

Surgical treatment

- Surgical excision is required for polyps that are too large or unsuitable for colonoscopic removal and in which there is a risk of current or future malignant change. For colonic polyps, this means either laparoscopic or open colonic resection.
- Rectal polyps may be removed by transanal endoscopic microsurgery (TEM), standard transanal exision, or a low anterior resection.
- FAP is usually treated by proctocolectomy (usually with ileoanal pouch formation) before early adulthood. Other polyposis syndromes may also be treated by prophylactic colectomy.

---

1 Atkin WS, Saunders BP (2002). Surveillance guidelines after removal of colorectal adenomatous polyps. *Gut* **51** (Suppl. V) v6–v9.

Colorectal cancer

Key facts

Colorectal cancer (CRC) is the second-most common tumor and the most common GI malignancy. One in 18 people will experience CRC. The peak age of incidence is 45–65, but incidence is increasing at younger ages.

Pathological features

The predominant type is adenocarcinoma (mucinous, signet ring cell, and anaplastic subtypes). CRC is classified as well, moderately, or poorly differentiated. Predisposing factors include the following:

- Polyposis syndromes (including FAP, HNPCC, juvenile polyposis)
- Strong family history of colorectal carcinoma
- Previous history of polyps or CRC
- Chronic ulcerative colitis or colonic Crohn's disease
- Diet poor in fruit and vegetables

Morphology

CRC may occur as a polypoid, ulcerating, stenosing, or infiltrative tumor mass. The majority (75%) lie on the left side of the colon and rectum (rectum, 45%; descending/sigmoid, 30%; transverse, 5%; right-sided, 20%); 3%–5% of patients have a synchronous carcinoma at time of diagnosis.

Clinical features

Rectal location

- Red blood per rectum
- Change in bowel habit: difficulty with defecation, sensation of incomplete evacuation, and painful defecation (tenesmus)

Descending-sigmoid location

- Red blood per rectum
- Change in bowel habit: typically increased frequency, variable consistency, mucus drainage, bloating, and flatulence

Right-sided location

Iron deficiency anemia may be the only elective presentation.

Emergency presentations

Up to 40% of colorectal carcinomas will present as emergencies.

- Large bowel obstruction (colicky pain, bloating, lack of flatus)
- Perforation with peritonitis
- Acute red blood per rectum

Diagnosis and tests

Elective presentation

Digital rectal examination or rigid sigmoidoscopy is used for rectal carcinoma. Flexible sigmoidoscopy should identify up to 75% of tumors (left-sided) but is unable to determine right-sided disease; colonoscopy should performed if the level of suspicion is high. Virtual colonoscopy is appropriate if colonoscopy is contraindicated or inappropriate. Tumor marker (CEA) is of no use as a diagnostic test but can be used to monitor disease if it is raised at diagnosis and falls to normal after resection.

Emergency presentations

These are commonly diagnosed by abdominal CT scan or urgent colonoscopy.

Staging tests

- To assess presence of metastases (liver, lung, or para-aortic; see Box 10.1): Most common is an abdominal CT scan and a chest X-ray.
- To assess local extent: CT scanning is adequate for colonic carcinoma. Pelvic MRI or transrectal ultrasound must be used for rectal cancer.
- Assessment of synchronous tumors: Colonoscopy or barium enema is usually performed (if it has not already been performed for the purpose of diagnosis) to identify synchronous tumors.

Box 10.1 Pathological staging: TNM

Tis	Carcinoma in situ
T1	Tumor invades submucosa
T2	Tumor invades muscularis propria
T3	Tumor invades through muscularis propria into subseros or perirectal fat
T4	Tumor invades organs
N0	No lymph nodes invaded
N1	Invasion in one to three nodes
N2	Invasion of four or more nodes
M0	No distant metastases
M1	Distant metastases present

Treatment

Potentially curative treatment

Such treatment is suitable for technically resectable tumors with no evidence of metastases (or metastases potentially curable by liver or lung resection).

- Surgical resection (with lymphadenectomy) is the only curative treatment. Typical operations include the following:
  - Right/transverse: right/extended right hemicolectomy
  - Left/sigmoid: left hemicolectomy
  - Rectum: low anterior resection or abdominoperineal resection (APR)
- Preoperative (neoadjuvant) chemoradiotherapy may be used in rectal cancer to increase the chance of curative resection.
- Adjuvant chemotherapy (5-FU based) is offered for tumors with positive lymph nodes or evidence of vascular invasion.
- Hepatic or lung resection may be offered to a few patients with suitable metastases and a clear resection of the primary tumor.

Palliative treatment

Such treatment is for unresectable metastases or unresectable tumors.

- Chemotherapy may effectively extend life expectancy with a good quality of life.
- Obstructing tumors may be endoluminally stented with self-expanding metal stents or transanally ablated if rectal.
- Surgery is reserved for untreatable obstruction, bleeding, or severe symptoms.

Restorative pelvic surgery

Key facts

For operations involving removal of part or all of the rectum or for tumors in the rectum, it is often desirable to avoid performing a permanent colostomy or ileostomy, and surgical techniques have been developed to help prevent this result. These techniques are commonly encountered on colorectal surgical wards and are associated with specific issues and complications.

Low or ultralow anterior resection

Anterior resection is the removal of part or all of the rectum. Remaining proximal colon is then brought into the pelvis and anastomosed to the remaining stump of tissue.

- *Low anterior resection* refers to an anastomosis that takes place below the level of the peritoneal reflection—i.e., a short stump of rectum remains that is used for the anastomosis.
- *Ultralow anterior resection* refers to an anastomosis that takes place on to the top of the anal canal—i.e., no native rectum remains. The anastomosis may be stapled or sewn by hand.

The lower the level of the anastomosis, the higher the risk of anastomotic complication, particularly anastomotic leakage. Most low and almost every ultralow anastomosis will have a temporary loop ileostomy formed with it. These are there to reduce the consequences of leakage by diverting the fecal stream from the large bowel. A loop stoma reduces the chance of major septic complications, but cannot prevent them.

Indications

- Rectal carcinoma
- Rectal adenoma untreatable by other means
- Severe or complex perineal sepsis (including rectovaginal fistula)

Ileoanal pouch formation

For operations in which all the colon and rectum is removed but removal of the anus is not required, a permanent stoma can be avoided by formation of an ileal pouch. This is usually a double fold of ileum joined side to side ("J" pouch). The pouch is joined either by hand or by staples to the upper anal canal (ileoanal anastomosis). A temporary loop ileostomy is often formed for the same reasons as for a low anterior resection.

Indications

- Ulcerative colitis not responding to medical management
- Familial adenomatous polyposis or multiple colorectal polyposis
- Multiple colonic tumors including the rectum

Complications of pelvic anastomosis (anterior resection and ileoanal pouch)

- Leakage occurs in up to 15% of cases; the rate is highest in the lowest anastomosis. Typically it presents as fever, abdominal pain, and tachycardia.
- Bleeding is uncommon, and usually settles with supportive treatment.
- Ischemia: the proximal bowel involved in the anastomosis may become ischemic. This may present as a leak, bleeding PR, or fever and tachycardia. It may resolve spontaneously; progressive ischemia (if not corrected by surgery) results in perforation and death.
- Stenosis. Narrowing of the anastomosis is an occasional late complication. It presents with difficulty in defecation and small-volume frequent stools. Treatment is dilatation under anesthetic; it very rarely requires reoperation.

Transanal endoscopic microsurgery (TEM)

Large adenomas and, less often, small carcinomas of the rectum are sometimes treated by a full-thickness local excision of the tumor from the rectum rather than excision of the rectum itself. This procedure avoids the risks of abdominal surgery and APR. If the tumors are too high to reach with retractors they may be reached by TEM, which involves use of laparoscopic instruments via a rigid proctoscope.

Complications

- Bleeding from the site of excision—this rarely requires active treatment.
- Infection in the pelvic tissues is rare, presenting with deep pelvic pain, fever, tachycardia, and disturbance of bowel habit. Treatment is usually by IV antibiotics.
- Rarely, free perforation when resecting tumors are above the peritoneal reflection

Diverticular disease of the colon

Key facts

Colonic diverticula are acquired outpouchings of colonic mucosa and overlying connective tissue through the colonic wall.

- They tend to occur along the lines where the penetrating colonic arteries traverse the colonic wall between the taenia coli.
- They are associated with hypertrophy of the surrounding colonic muscle with thickening of the colonic mucosa. This is probably due to the underlying pathological process, which is high-pressure contractions of the colon causing chronic pressure on the colonic wall.
- The peak age of presentation is 50–70 years, but diverticular disease is increasing in frequency and occurring at a progressively younger age.

Clinical and pathological features

Asymptomatic

The majority of diverticular disease is found incidentally.

Acute diverticulitis

In this form there is rapid onset of left lower quadrant pain, nausea, and fever, frequently with loose stools. The patient is usually febrile with moderate tachycardia and left lower quadrant tenderness. The colonic wall shows acute neutrophil infiltration around the inflamed diverticulum and in the subserosal tissues.

Bleeding diverticular disease

Usually spontaneous in onset with no prodromal symptoms, this type presents with large-volume dark red, clotted rectal blood. It is due to rupture of a peridiverticular submucosal blood vessel and is not typically associated with inflammation.

Complications

Pericolic or paracolic mass or abscess

▶ Acute diverticulitis may progress to persistent pericolic infection with thickening of surrounding tissues and formation of a mass. If this suppurates, a pericolic abscess forms. Enlargement and extension of this into the paracolic area leads to a paracolic abscess. The features are those of acute diverticulitis, with a swinging fever, fluctuating tachycardia, unresolving abdominal pain, and a tender left lower quadrant mass.

Peritonitis

▶▶ Perforation of a pericolic or paracolic abscess usually leads to purulent peritonitis. Direct perforation of the acute diverticular segment freely into the peritoneal cavity leads to feculent peritonitis. The features are those of acute diverticulitis, with high fever, severe abdominal pain, and generalized guarding and rigidity.

Diverticular fistula

Acute infection with paracolic sepsis may drain by perforation into adjacent structures. This is typically the posterior vaginal vault in women or the bladder in either sex. Colovesical fistula leads to recurrent UTI caused by enteric organisms with bubbles and debris in the urine. Colovaginal fistula leads to feculent vaginal discharge.

Stricture formation

Chronic or repetitive inflammatory episodes may lead to fibrosis and narrowing of the colon. A history of recurrent diverticulitis with recurrent, colicky abdominal pain, distension, and bloating suggests stricture formation.

Diagnosis and tests

- Colonoscopy is a relatively poor investigation to assess the number and extent of diverticula.
- WBC during acute episodes of inflammation
- CT scanning is the test of choice to identify complications including abscess formation and perforation.
- Colonoscopy or barium enema is required after an episode to rule out malignancy.

Treatment

Medical treatment

- High-fiber diet, high fluid intake, and stool softeners to reduce intracolonic pressure.
- IV antibiotics (levofloxacin 500 mg IV qd and metronidazole 500 mg IV tid) during acute infective exacerbations.
- po antibiotics if patient is able to tolerate them (e.g., ciprofloxacin 500 mg po qd).
- Significant paracolic abscesses may be drained by radiological guidance.

Surgical treatment

- ▶ Resection is indicated for acute inflammation failing to respond to medical management, undrainable paracolic sepsis, or free perforation. The affected region should be resected (segmental colectomy). The ends may be reanastomosed if they are healthy and the patient's general condition is suitable. If not, a proximal end colostomy and oversewing of the distal end is usual (Hartmann's type resection).
- Stricture may be treated by elective resection or intracolonic stenting.
- Diverticular fistula should be treated by elective resection to prevent recurrent infections.

Rectal prolapse

Key facts

Rectal prolapse may be partial thickness (usually just mucosa) or full thickness involving all the layers of the rectal wall. Full thickness may be contained within the rectum (internal prolapse is also called intussusception). It is most common in postmenopausal women and in women who have undergone multiple vaginal deliveries, and is associated with chronic straining and chronic disorders of defecation (which cause weakness of the pelvic floor and sphincter complex) and constipation due to pelvic-outlet obstruction. Occasionally it occurs in children suffering from constipation (usually self-limiting).

Pathological features

Mucosa involved in prolapse undergoes chronic changes.
- Typically glandular branching and occasional gland misplacement occur.
- Thickening of the muscularis mucosa and excess submucosal collagen deposition are found.
- Mucosal inflammation and focal ulceration may also occur. Extensive mucosal ulceration associated with mucosal prolapse may result in an appearance called "solitary rectal ulcer."

Clinical features

- *Mucosal prolapse*: discharge of mucus and small-volume fecal staining; pruritus ani; occasionally small-volume, bright red rectal bleeding
- *Internal full thickness prolapse*: sensation of rectal fullness or mass; incomplete defecation; dissatisfaction after defecation and repeated defecation.
- *External full-thickness prolapse*: external prolapsing mass after defecation (usually requiring manual reduction); mucus and fecal soiling; occasional bright red rectal bleeding (sometimes voluminous, particularly if prolapse becomes ulcerated)

Diagnosis

- Rigid sigmoidoscopy may show features of mucosal inflammation, particularly the anterior rectal mucosa.
- Prolapse may be demonstrable in the exam room upon straining.
- A defecating proctogram may be performed to confirm the diagnosis if it is unclear and if surgery is contemplated. A proctogram is required to confirm the diagnosis if internal prolapse is suspected. It may also demonstrate associated problems of the pelvic floor and rectocele.
- Colonic transit studies may be used if there is suspected slow-transit constipation and resection is possible.

Treatment

Medical treatment
- Avoidance of straining and adaptation of defecatory habit (biofeedback)
- Avoidance of constipation (stool softeners and bulking agents rather than stimulants)

Surgical treatment

Mucosal prolapse

- Recurrent banding or dilute phenol injection of excess mucosa
- Mucosal excision
- Stapled anopexy (also called procedure for prolapse and hemorrhoids [PPH]) is sometimes used.

Full-thickness prolapse

Surgery is indicated to prevent development of fecal incontinence. The choice of operation depends on the patient's age and the extent of prolapse (internal vs. external).

- Delorme's perineal rectopexy (mucosal excision with sutured plication of the excessively long rectal muscle tube in an effort to shorten it to prevent prolapse) is least successful, with the highest recurrence rate of all surgical procedures, but it may be used in the frail or elderly.
- Altmeier's perineal rectal resection (mucosal and rectal muscle tube excision with sutured perineal anastomosis) avoids an abdominal operation but has increased morbidity due to perineal anastomosis.
- Transabdominal rectopexy (mobilization of the rectum and suturing to the presacral fascia) may be done via laparotomy or laparoscopically. Most surgeons no longer use a prosthetic mesh, as it is associated with complications. This procedure has the highest success rate for prevention of recurrence of prolapse. It may be combined with a sigmoid resection if there is marked associated constipation.

Clinical pearls—anorectal physiology

- The internal anal sphincter is smooth muscle and under involuntary control of the pelvic autonomic system. Relaxants include nitric oxide donors (e.g., GTN) and calcium antagonists (e.g., diltiazem).
- The external anal sphincter is skeletal muscle and under voluntary control of the pudendal nerve (S2, S3, S4). Relaxation (by temporary partial paralysis) may be achieved by botulinum toxin injection.
- Defecation is a complex sensorimotor process that requires intact pelvic autonomics, sacral spinal nerves, and pelvic floor muscle function.

Pilonidal sinus disease

Key facts

Single or multiple sinuses ("pits") exist in the midline of the buttock clefts. These usually contain hair, inspissated secretions, and debris. They are most often seen in men and in dark-haired, hirsute people, especially of Eastern Mediterranean origin. They are probably caused by local trauma causing retention of hairs within initially normal midline pits. They may be precipitated by long periods of sitting, e.g., among truck drivers, computer operators.

Pathological features

This disease is typified by chronic inflammation. Once inflammation has started, sinuses often extend and may become interlinked. Lateral tracks may run out into the neighboring buttock tissue.

Clinical features

- *Irritative features*: Intermittent discharge and inflammation with pain and swelling.
- *Acute sepsis*. Acute abscess formation is common with swelling, pain, and erythema. It may discharge spontaneously or may cause fistulization with sinuses appearing in the lateral buttock tissue.
- *Chronic sepsis* usually follows unresolved acute sepsis either after spontaneous discharge or surgical drainage.

Diagnosis

- Very extensive sinus formation and fistulation may be assessed by MRI scanning of the buttocks.
- Ensure that the patient is tested for hyperglycemia.

Treatment

Medical and nonsurgical

- Most chronic irritation can be controlled by topical hygiene (shaving local hairs, washing accessible cavities), which usually requires a family member or partner to perform. Intermittent courses of antibiotics may be required for septic episodes.
- Developing acute sepsis may be suitable for antibiotic treatment, but once pus has collected, surgical drainage is required. This may be under local or general anesthetic.
- Recurrent acute sepsis or persistently symptomatic chronic sepsis usually requires surgical treatment.

Surgical

Principles of surgical treatments are
- Excision of all sinus openings
- Obliteration of all infected or chronically inflamed tissue.

Although a primary excision may be left open to close by secondary intention, this offers no better long-term solution than other strategies and requires daily dressings for many weeks or months. Primary closure of the excision wound requires
- Tension-free apposition of the skin edges (which may be by lateral flaps, e.g., Karyadakis or Bascom procedures, or by plastic surgical flaps, e.g., rhomboid, rotational, or Z plasty flaps)
- Obliteration of the natal cleft by flattening (thought to be most important in the prevention of recurrence by reducing the risk of further hair implantation)

Fistula in ano

Key facts

A *fistula* is an abnormal connection of two epithelial surfaces, and the two surfaces joined in fistula in ano are the anorectal lining and the perineal or vaginal skin. Fistulas are very common, especially in otherwise fit young adults. They may occur in the presence of Crohn's disease. There is a minor association with obesity and diabetes mellitus. Very rarely is a fistula due to trauma or ulceration of anorectal tumors.

Pathological features

The most common cause is sepsis arising in an anal gland that forces its way out through the anal tissues to appear in the perianal or, in women, vaginal skin (cryptoglandular theory of fistula in ano). The fistula often presents initially as an acute perianal abscess. The tissues through which the track pushes determine the classification of fistulas (see Fig. 10.1).

Clinical features

- *Acute perianal abscess.* Rapid onset of severe perianal or perineal pain. Swelling and erythema of the perianal skin with fever and tachycardia
- *Recurrent perianal sepsis.* Recurrent intermittent sepsis typified by gradual buildup of "pressure" sensation and swelling in the perianal skin and eventual discharge of blood-stained purulent fluid.
- *Chronic perianal discharge.* Persistent low-grade sepsis of the track with chronic discharge of seropurulent fluid via a point that is usually clearly identified by the patient.

Diagnosis

Confirm the presence of a fistula and attempt to determine the type of fistula by identifying the course of the track.

- Examination of the perineum and rectal examination may reveal a palpable fibrous track.
- Examination under anesthesia (EUA) with probing of any external opening can aid identification of the course of the track.
- Endoanal ultrasound (sometimes with hydrogen peroxide injected into the track) is used to identify the course of the track.
- MRI scanning is probably the most sensitive method of determining the course of the track and identifying any occult perianal or pelvic sepsis.
- Flexible sigmoidoscopy may be indicated if associated colorectal disease, e.g., Crohn's disease, is suspected.

Treatment

Medical treatment

- Antibiotics may reduce symptoms from recurrent sepsis but cannot treat the underlying fistula.
- Medical treatment of inflammatory bowel disease may dramatically reduce symptoms from associated fistulas.

Surgical treatment

Principles of surgical treatment are as follows.

- Drainage of any acute infection, if present
- Prevention of recurrent infection—usually by insertion of a loose seton suture, e.g., silastic sling
- Low fistula in ano. Lay open the track, remove all chronic granulation tissue, and allow to heal spontaneously (fistulotomy). There is little risk of impairment of continence because there is minimal division of sphincter tissues.
- High fistula in ano
  - Close the internal opening (endorectal flap advancement).
  - Slowly divide the sphincter tissue between the fistula and the perianal skin (cutting seton); this has a low risk of incontinence.
  - Fill the fistula with fibrin glue or an anal fistula plug.

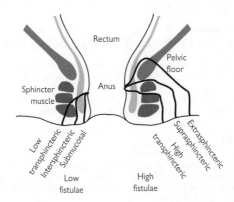

Fig. 10.1 Classification of fistula in ano.

Hemorrhoids

Key facts

Hemorrhoid is a broad term often used incorrectly to refer to any perianal excess tissue. True hemorrhoids are excessive amounts of the normal endoanal cushions that comprise anorectal mucosa, submucosal tissue, and submucosal blood vessels (small arterioles and veins). The most common age of onset is in young adulthood. It is associated with constipation, chronic straining, obesity, and previous childbirth. Hemorrhoids may become ulcerated and inflamed if recurrently prolapsing.

- If they are confined above the dentate line, hemorrhoids are referred to as "internal."
- If they extend below the dentate line, hemorrhoids are referred to as "external."
- Hemorrhoids typically occur in the same location as the main anal blood vessel pedicles (described as 3, 7, and 11 o'clock positions as seen in the supine position).

Clinical features

- Features of irritation. Pruritus ani, mucus discharge, and perianal discomfort
- Features of damage to mucosal lining. Recurrent post-defecatory bleeding: bright red, not mixed with stools; on paper or splashing in the toilet pan
- Features of prolapse. Intermittent lump appearing at anal margin, usually after defecation, which may spontaneously reduce or require manual reduction

Diagnosis

- Diagnosis is usually by anoscopy.
- Flexible sigmoidoscopy or colonoscopy may be appropriate if there is concern about the cause of symptoms. Remember: hemorrhoids rarely start over the age of 55 years. In these cases, it is often best to assume another cause until otherwise shown.

Treatment

Medical treatment

- Avoidance of constipation and straining: bulking or softener laxatives

Surgical treatment

- Banding is best for prolapse symptoms (this is not possible for external components because of excellent nerve supply of lower anal canal).
- Dilute phenol injections (5% in almond oil) are best for bleeding symptoms.
- Hemorrhoidectomy for large, external hemorrhoids or hemorrhoids that fail to respond to conservative treatment. This is associated with a small risk of impaired continence and anal stenosis.
- Stapled anopexy (also called procedure for prolapse and hemorrhoids [PPH]) is sometimes used for circumferential prolapsing hemorrhoids.

Clinical pearls—anatomy of the anus

- The lower third of the anal canal is somatic tissue in origin with stratified squamous epithelium. It is very sensitive (pudendal and distal sacral nerves) and has a relatively poor blood supply and healing ability.
- The upper third of the canal is visceral tissue in origin with columnar epithelium. It is insensitive and has an excellent blood supply and healing ability.

Acute anorectal pain

Causes and features

Fissure in ano

Acute severe, localized, "knife-like" pain is felt in the anus during defecation. Fissure in ano is often associated with deep, throbbing pain for minutes or hours afterwards due to pelvic-floor spasm. There is blood on the paper when wiping (small-volume, red-pink streaks or spots).

Hemorrhoids

Hemorrhoids are usually acutely prolapsed and inflamed, with associated perianal lump, soreness, and irritation. They may bleed, often profusely and bright red.

Perianal abscess

There is a gradual onset of constant, localized perianal pain. Associated swelling involves tenderness and possible discharge. The abscess may have associated systemic features of fever, malaise, and anorexia.

Perianal hematoma

This is usually of sudden onset; it is acutely painful with associated perianal swelling (dark red colored).

Rectal prolapse

Acute, full-thickness rectal prolapse occasionally causes pain. There is an obvious large, perineal lump that is dark red-blue with surface mucus and occasionally some surface ulceration.

Emergency management

Establish diagnosis

- Good inspection and careful digital rectal examination followed by anoscopy are usually all that is required.
- Rigid sigmoidoscopy may be painful and is often unnecessary.
- Flexible sigmoidoscopy is rarely indicated.

Early treatment

- Give adequate analgesia: opiates may be necessary.
- Topical treatment is highly effective: cool pads, and topical local anesthetic gels.

Definitive management

Fissure in ano

The mainstay of acute treatment is analgesia and anal sphincter muscle relaxants, e.g., topical glyceryl trinitrate (GTN) 0.2% ointment, diltiazem 2% ointment. Local anesthetics are helpful early in treatment. Sometimes the fissure requires a lateral sphincterotomy.

Hemorrhoids

These may require bed rest with continued topical treatment until swelling resolves and spontaneous reduction begins. Acute hemorrhoidectomy is almost always best avoided because of the risk of overexcision of anal tissue.

Perianal abscess

Incision and drainage is a surgical emergency, particularly if the patient is diabetic or immunosuppressed.

Perianal hematoma

Incision to allow decompression of acute hematoma may be necessary—this is often done under topical LA.

Rectal prolapse

Swelling may be reduced by cool packs and elevation. This condition very rarely requires emergency surgery.

Acute rectal bleeding

Causes and features

Acute rectal bleeding is broadly divided into regions of the colon from which it comes. The blood's appearance may differ according to origin.

Anorectal

Bright red blood, on the surface of the stool and paper, after defecation
- Hemorrhoids
- Acute anal fissure
- Distal proctitis
- Rectal prolapse
- Anal or rectal cancer
- Conduloma accuminata

Rectosigmoid

Darker red blood, with clots, in surface of stool and mixed
- Rectal tumors (benign or malignant)
- Proctocolitis
- Diverticular disease

Proximal colonic

Dark red blood mixed into stool, or altered blood
- Colonic tumors (benign or malignant)
- Colitis
- Angiodysplasia
- NSAID-induced ulceration

Upper GI bleeding occasionally produces dark red rectal bleeding, but it is usually associated with significant hemodynamic instability when sufficiently large.

Features: signs
- Tachycardia and hypotension suggest substantial loss.
- Left lower quadrant tenderness suggests diverticular inflammation with bleeding.

Emergency management

Resuscitation
- Establish large-caliber IV access. Give crystalloid fluid in 1000 mL increments if patient is tachycardic or hypotensive.
- Catheterize and monitor ins and outs if patient is hypotensive.
- Send blood for Hct, BUN, Cr, type and cross, and coagulation.

Establish a diagnosis
- Rigid or flexible proctosigmoidoscopy should be performed in all cases to exclude a simple anorectal cause.
- Urgent flexible sigmoidoscopy and colonoscopy may be undertaken. This procedure is higher risk than elective endoscopy but may confirm an origin and may allow therapeutic intervention (adrenaline injection, heater probe coagulation, argon plasma coagulation [APC]).

- Urgent selective mesenteric arteriography is used for obscure or persistent bleeding: active bleeding of 0.5 mL/min is required.
- Urgent gastroscopy should be used to exclude massive upper GI bleeding if suspected.

Early treatment
Consider a blood transfusion if there is a major bleed (persisting hemodynamic instability despite resuscitation, Hct <30).

Definitive management

Anorectal causes
Most of these can be controlled by local measures such as injection, coagulation, or packing.

Acute colitis
- IV or po metronidazole if thought to be effective, until organism is identified
- IV hydrocortisone if thought to be ulcerative or Crohn's colitis
- Surgery may be necessary—whatever the etiology—if bleeding persists (but source must be localized).

Diverticular disease
- IV antibiotics (levofloxin 500 mg qd + metronidazole 500 mg tid)
- Angiographic embolization is used if bleeding fails to stop and the patient is not critically unstable for time in radiology.
- Surgery is high risk but may be unavoidable. If the location is known, a directed hemicolectomy may be performed (on-table colonoscopy may be used). If not, a subtotal colectomy is safest.

Angiodysplasia
- Colonoscopic therapy (injection, heater probe, APC) is ideal.
- Angiographic embolization may be possible.
- Right hemicolectomy is occasionally unavoidable.

Undiagnosed source
Rarely, the patient remains unstable with active bleeding and no cause can be reliably confirmed. Surgical options to deal with this situation include the following:
- On-table colonoscopy with washout via colotomy to locate bleeding source
- Formation of mid transverse loop colostomy and subsequent targeted hemicolectomy
- "Blind" subtotal colectomy

Acute severe colitis

Causes and features

Any cause of colitis may progress to acute severity. Common causes include the following:

- Severe ulcerative colitis (UC; usually pan-colitis). Occasionally, acute severe colitis is the presentation of UC with no prior history.
- Acute infective colitis (e.g., salmonella, *C. difficile*, ameba, parasites)
- Neutropenic colitis
- Pseudomembranous colitis (*C. difficile* related)
- Progressive Crohn's colitis (usually with a clear prior history)

Symptoms

- Diarrhea (usually bloody with urgency and frequency). Constipation may be an ominous feature suggesting acute colonic dilatation.
- Abdominal pain (generalized)
- Malaise, anorexia, and fever (systemic inflammatory features)

Signs

- Fever, tachycardia, possible hypotension
- Abdominal tenderness. Peritonitis suggests perforation.

Complications

Any acute severe colitis may develop any of these complications.

- Hemorrhage
- Hypokalemia
- Hypoalbuminemia
- Perforation (localized or generalized)

Toxic dilatation is a term used to describe the situation of acute, severe colitis with colonic dilatation usually associated with reduced bowel frequency and impending perforation.

▶ *Fulminant severe colitis* is defined as tachycardia >120 bpm or stool frequency >10×/24 hr or albumin <25 g/dL.

Emergency management

Resuscitation

- Establish large-caliber IV access. Give crystalloid fluid in 1000 mL increments if patient is tachycardic or hypotensive.
- Catheterize and monitor ins and outs if patient is hypotensive.
- Send blood for Hct, BUN, Cr, type and cross, and coagulation.

Establish a diagnosis

- Stool for *C. difficile*, Gram stain and culture, and microscopy for cysts, O&P
- Plain abdominal X-ray (looking for colonic dilatation) and erect chest X-ray (looking for free gas)
- Rigid or flexible sigmoidoscopy and biopsy only if patient is not unstable

Early treatment
- Give IV hydrocortisone if the diagnosis of UC is likely. If infective colitis is suspected, consider withholding steroids until the *C. difficile*, Gram stain, and culture results are back.
- Give blood transfusion if patient is anemic.
- Perform surgery if peritonitis or free gas is found on chest X-ray. (The operation for any acute colitis is usually total abdominal colectomy and end ileostomy formation).

Definitive management
Acute ulcerative colitis
- IV hydrocortisone, converted to oral prednisone if responding to treatment
- Infliximab if no evidence of abscess or perforation
- Surgery for failure to respond to medical treatment or acute complications of hemorrhage or perforation
- Regular blood investigations and plain abdominal radiography to monitor treatment

Infective colitis
- IV or po metronidazole until organism is identified
- *Salmonella*, *C. difficile*: metronidazole
- Surgery for failure to respond to medical treatment or acute complications of hemorrhage or perforation

Neutropenic colitis
- IV antibiotics
- Bone marrow support
- Surgery for failure to respond to medical treatment or acute complications of hemorrhage or perforation

Postoperative anastomotic leak

Causes and features

Any intra-abdominal anastomosis may leak (see Box 10.2). The highest risk of leak occurs with esophageal and rectal anastomosis. The lowest rate of leak occurs with small-bowel anastomosis.

Anastomotic leak may present as one of several clinical pictures.

▶▶ Peritonitis

Acute, severe generalized abdominal pain with generalized guarding and rigidity. Fever, tachycardia, and tachypnea are common. Diagnosis is usually clinical but may also require a CT scan.

Intra-abdominal abscess

Fever and tachycardia, commonly around 5–7 days postoperatively. Localized tenderness related to the anastomosis may be present. Diagnosis should be sought by CT scan.

Enteric fistula

A fistula may occur between the anastomosis and the wound or another organ. This is usually the result of a subclinical leak and abscess formation that discharges through a pathway of low resistance. It often presents late as an apparent wound infection that discharges with enteric content. Diagnosis is made by CT scan or, occasionally, fistulography, if the fistula presents very late.

▶ Cardiovascular complications

⚠ Sepsis originating from an initially subclinical leak may present with apparent cardiovascular complications, e.g., AF, supraventricular tachycardia, chest pain, and sinus tachycardia. A wise precautionary rule is as follows: Any acute postoperative disturbance of physiology in a patient with an intra-abdominal anastomosis is due to a leak until proven otherwise.

Emergency management

Resuscitation

- Establish large-caliber IV access. Give crystalloid fluid in 1000 mL increments if patient is tachycardic or hypotensive.
- Catheterize and monitor ins and outs if patient is hypotensive.
- Send blood for Hct, BUN, Cr, type and cross, coagulation.
- Give appropriate analgesia if patient is not on an epidural or PCA.

Establish a diagnosis

- Acute peritonitis needs no diagnostic investigation. Emergency re-look laparotomy should be organized immediately.
- CT scanning with IV and oral contrast is the investigation of choice for all other suspected leaks.
- For rectal anastomoses, a water-soluble contrast study may delineate a leak.

Box 10.2 Risk factors for increased risk of leak

- Chronic malnutrition
- Immunosuppression
- Unprepared bowel, e.g., obstruction
- Poor blood supply or bowel ends
- High-dose steroid use
- Diabetes mellitus
- Local or generalized sepsis
- Metastatic malignancy
- Tension on bowel ends

Early treatment

- Give IV antibiotics (e.g., IV levofloxacin 500 mg qd + metronidazole 500 mg tid).
- Monitor fluid balance hourly.

Definitive management

▶▶ Peritonitis

- This always requires surgical intervention unless the patient is deemed unfit.

Once the leak has been identified, options for management include the following:
- Dividing the anastomosis, closing the distal end, and forming the proximal end into a stoma;
- Emptying the bowel (lavage) and forming a proximal diversion
- Re-forming or repairing the anastomosis (only suitable for fit patients with minimal contamination and an otherwise healthy anastomosis); this should be done with proximal diversion

Intra-abdominal abscess

- Radiologically guided drainage and antibiotics, provided the patient does not develop peritonitis or show signs of secondary complications. May still ultimately require diversion
- Open surgical drainage, if abscess is inaccessible or unresponsive to radiological drainage

Enteric fistula

- Usually managed by antibiotics. May close spontaneously. If it fails to close, surgical repair may be required.
- May need earlier intervention if abscess or peritonitis develops.
- Open surgical drainage, if abscess is inaccessible or unresponsive to radiological drainage.

Enteric fistula

- Usually managed by antibiotics. May close spontaneously. If fails to close, surgical repair may be required.
- Treat for abscess or peritonitis if either develop.

Pediatric surgery

Daniel P. Doody, MD

Principles of managing pediatric surgical cases

Key facts

- Infants and children are not small adults.
- Children come in different sizes. Always obtain a weight before starting treatment.
- Fluids and drug doses depend on body weight.
- Babies and children have different differential diagnoses from those of adults.
- Children often differ from adults in physiology and anatomy (see Table 11.1).
- Babies and young children have difficulty communicating symptoms.

Special problems with babies

- Thermoregulation is impaired.
  - Immature sweating
  - High surface area to body weight increases rate of heat loss
  - Prone to hypothermia
- Minimal glycogen stores in newborns make them prone to acute hypoglycemia.
- The principal breathing pattern is diaphragmatic.
  - More prone to breathing difficulties, with abdominal distension
- Immature body physiology
  - Less biological functional reserve than adults
  - Acute disturbances of physiology are more serious, with less room for error.
- Babies may not metabolize drugs as expected.
  - Intravenous fluids
  - Maintenance fluids

Box 11.1 Pediatric fluid regimen

4 mL/kg/hr total fluid for each of the first 10 kg of weight (0–10 kg)
2 mL/kg/hr total fluid for each of the next 10 kg of weight (11–20 kg)
1 mL/kg/hr total fluid for each subsequent kg of weight (over 21 kg)

- Always calculate fluid and sodium requirements according to weight.
- Remember to add glucose, especially for neonates.
- Adjust the fluid regimen (Box 11.1) according to clinical setting for neonates and premature babies.
- Resuscitation fluids
  - Crystalloids should be given as primary resuscitation fluids.
  - Mild dehydration: 10 mL/kg bolus. Repeat as necessary.
  - Moderate dehydration: 20 mL/kg bolus. Repeat as necessary.

Table 11.1 Basic physiological parameters in children

	Neonates	Adolescents
Blood volume (mL/kg)	100	75-80
Oral fluid intake (mL/kg/day)	150	30–50
Daily Na^+ intake (mmol/kg)	2–3	1–2
Daily K^+ intake (mmol/kg)	2–3	1
Systolic BP (mmHg)	40–50	100–120
Resting pulse rate (bpm)	120–160	70–80

Congenital diaphragmatic hernia

Key facts

- Incidence: 1:2200 conceptions and 1:4000 live births
- Fetal loss with severe diaphragmatic hernia is common.
- Posterolateral congenital diaphragmatic hernia (CDH) with newborn respiratory distress is among the deadliest of newborn anomalies.
- Mortality in the current era still approaches 50%.

Types

Bochdalek hernia (posterolateral hernia)

- With newborn distress (80%–85% left; 10%–15% right; 1%–3% bilateral)
- 10% of posterolateral hernias will be discovered beyond the newborn period. There is equal distribution of left- and right-sided hernias with late presentation.

Morgagni hernia

This anterior diaphragmatic hernia into anterior mediastinum may be associated with other cardiac and abdominal wall anomalies.

Central hiatal hernia

Mortality from a congenital diaphragmatic hernia defect is almost solely associated with Bochdalek hernia. Mortality from Morgagni hernia may be associated with complex cardiac anomalies.

Factors associated with greater mortality

- Prematurity
- Low birth weight
- Large diaphragmatic defects
- Associated cardiac defects

Pulmonary pathology associated with Bochdalek posterolateral hernias:
- Pulmonary hypoplasia with decreased bronchiolar and alveolar end units
- Anatomically immature with pseudoglandular stage of development
- Physiologically immature with surfactant deficiency
- Pulmonary vascular hypoplasia associated with increased pulmonary vascular reactivity (persistent pulmonary hypertension of newborn [PPHN])

Treatment

- Immediate intubation with minimal mask ventilation (lessens gastric and small bowel distention)
- Passage of nasogastric tube (NGT)
- Appropriate lines for arterial monitoring and intravenous access
- Ventilation strategies:
  - Gentle ventilation with permissive hypercapnia
  - High-frequency oscillating ventilation
  - Inhaled nitric oxide may stabilize infant (but is unlikely to improve mortality or need for ECMO).

- Extracorporeal membrane oxygenation (ECMO) for those infants failing ventilation strategies
  - The International Registry of Extracorporeal Life-Support Organization (ELSO) shows a 52% survival rate among infants with CDH who require ECMO support.
- At this time, other pulmonary vasodilators have not been shown to consistently help with the pulmonary hypertension associated with CDH.

Surgery

- Delayed until infant is stable (usually a few days) and has shown improvement in pulmonary hypertension.
- A large defect should be closed by patch with 1 mm Gore-Tex as the preferred replacement.
  - Higher mortality is associated with larger defects requiring a patch.
  - A higher risk of late recurrent hernia occurring outside of the critical newborn period is associated with patch repair.
- Returning viscera to the small peritoneal cavity may require the use of silo or patch repair on the anterior abdominal wall.
- Fetal surgery has not been shown to improve the mortality associated with CDH.

Outcome

- Delayed pulmonary mortality is seen after survival in the newborn period but there is often ongoing severe chronic lung disease of the newborn.
- Many long-term survivors of CDH repair will have reactive airway disease and asthma.
- Many infants benefit by early intervention and physical therapy.
- Infants with CDH have a higher incidence of severe gastroesophageal reflux disease and many will need surgery for correction.

Other congenital thoracic anomalies

Bronchogenic cysts

Incidence
Although a rare lesion, it is the second-most common cystic lesion of the mediastinum in children.

Presentation
- It may be associated with infections and respiratory compromise of the airway, particularly if located in the subcarinal position.
- It may be associated with pneumonias, tracheal compression, and SVC compression in adults.
- Complications of cysts include fistulization into airway, hemorrhage, ulceration, infection, and possible malignant degeneration.

Evaluation
CT imaging is usually most accurate in defining the extent of the lesion and location. It is typically found in the tracheoesophageal groove and may be found in the neck as well as the mediastinum.

Pathology
This may include cartilage but most frequently includes respiratory epithelium.

Treatment
- Surgical resection is definitive.
- Marsupialization or less definitive procedures (i.e., aspiration) may temporize but will not prevent recurrence.

Congenital cystic adenomatoid malformations (CCAM)
Incidence: 1:25,000 conceptions

Features
- Hamartomatous malformation of lung with cystic proliferation of bronchiolar-like structures
- Type I: Macrocystic lesions measuring up to 2–10 cm
- Type II: Smaller cystic lesions measuring 0.5–2 cm
- Type III: Microcystic lesions that present a solid mass and may be associated hydrops fetalis, fetal demise, premature birth, and severe newborn respiratory distress
- ~50% of antenatally diagnosed cases will disappear by birth and will not be seen on postnatal chest X-ray.

Anatomy
- Normal connection of tracheobronchial tree and pulmonary vasculature

Clinical presentation
If not recognized antenatally, typical presentation before age 2 years is most frequently in the radiographic evaluation of respiratory compromise and presumed pulmonary infection.

Treatment

Elective surgical resection of involved lobes can be performed if the malformation persists at birth.

Pulmonary sequestration

Lung tissue has no identifiable bronchial communication.

- Extralobar sequestration lies outside the visceral pleura and typically abuts the mediastinum. This may be located in the diaphragm or occasionally in the upper abdomen.
- Intralobar sequestration is located in the normal pulmonary parenchyma.

Distinguishing feature

- There is usually no connection to tracheobronchial tree.
- Systemic arterial blood supply is typically from the thoracic or abdominal aorta.
- Blood supply may traverse the diaphragm.
- Blood supply may return through pulmonary veins or through systemic veins.

Associated anomalies

- Diaphragmatic hernia, congenital cystic adenomatoid malformation, foregut anomalies

Presentation

Extralobar sequestration is typically found incidentally. Intralobar sequestration may be associated with recurrent pulmonary infections and high-flow arteriovenous shunts leading to congestive heart failure.

Congenital lobar emphysema

Incidence is rare: 1:10,000 to 1:30,000.

Presentation

- Typically in newborn period with worsening respiratory distress and evidence of emphysematous lobar enlargement on routine chest X-ray
- Left upper lobe (40%) or right upper (20%) or right middle lobe (35%)
- The first X-ray in a newborn may show a fluid-filled lobe.
- In the first week, the fluid is absorbed and the air expansion of the abnormal lobe is more apparent

Pathology

This condition is ascribed to bronchial cartilaginous weakness and air trapping.

Treatment

- In most affected newborns, thoracotomy and lobar resection is appropriate and life saving.
- For premature infants with acquired lobar emphysema associated with chronic lung disease of the newborn, selective intubation of the contralateral bronchus has been shown to be helpful and may make surgery unnecessary.

Acute abdominal emergencies— overview

Key facts
- The child may have subtle symptoms until late in the disease course.
- Such emergencies are often ascribed to a nonsurgical problem, e.g., colic, gastroenteritis, or constipation.
- Features of peritonitis are often difficult to elicit in babies.
- Cardinal features of obstruction are as follows:
  - Vomiting
  - Abdominal distension
  - Failure to pass meconium in newborns
  - Pain

Vomiting in children
Vomiting is common in newborns and is often entirely benign. It may be due to the following:
- Overfeeding
- Rapid feeding
- Regurgitant reflux
- Air swallowing (inadequate burping)
- Metabolic causes (inborn errors of metabolism, acidosis)
- Infections (UTI, chest infection, meningitis)
- Bile-stained vomiting is a surgical emergency until proven otherwise.

Abdominal distension
- Most pronounced in distal obstruction and less so in proximal causes of obstruction
- Failure to pass meconium
- Term babies should pass meconium within 24 to 36 hr.
- Babies with proximal obstruction or atresia may still pass meconium.

Pain
Pain may be difficult to assess in infants. Typical features are
- Irritability
- Decreased oral intake
- Lethargy
- Pallor
- Diaphoresis
- Erratic heart rate.
- Grunting

Diagnostic features
History
- Family or genetic history for cystic fibrosis: meconium ileus
- Premature birth: necrotizing enterocolitis
- Timing of onset related to birth
  - The more proximal the obstruction, the earlier the presentation.

Examination
- Blood in vomit or stool may indicate necrotic bowel.
- Degrees of distension: most pronounced with distal obstruction

Tests
- Plain abdominal X-ray may show diagnostic features:
    - "Double bubble sign": duodenal atresia or malrotation
    - "Ground glass": meconium ileus
    - Multiple loops of small bowel: distal obstruction
    - Intramural gas (pneumatosis intestinalis): necrotizing enterocolitis
    - In newborns it is difficult to distinguish small bowel distention from large intestine distention.
    - Free air: intestinal perforation
- Abdominal ultrasound
- Abdominal mass: intussusception, tumor, duplication cyst

Esophageal atresia

Key facts

- This congenital abnormality of the formation of the upper aerodigestive tract results in partial or complete interruption of the esophageal lumen.
- Esophageal atresia is often associated with other congenital abnormalities (VACTERL association: Vertebral, Anal, Cardiac, TracheoEsophageal, Renal, Limb anomalies).

Clinicopathological features

- May be diagnosed on prenatal ultrasound. Features include maternal polyhydramnios, absent stomach bubble, and associated abnormalities.
- Postnatal diagnosis relies on features of the following:
  - Persistent salivary drooling
  - Regurgitation of all feeds
  - Cyanosis with feeding.
- Failure to pass NGT into stomach
- H- or N-type tracheoesophageal fistula is unusual: it presents with recurrent aspiration or chest infections typically as an infant or toddler.

Diagnosis and treatment (see Fig. 11.1)

- Plain X-ray abdomen and thorax: NGT coiled in esophagus
- Presence of stomach gas suggests tracheodistal esophageal fistula.
- Plain X-ray spine: associated vertebral abnormalities
- Echocardiography: associated cardiac abnormalities

Medical treatment

- Keep head of bed elevated.
- Keep patient npo and use oro-esophageal tube to continuous low wall suction.
- Give antibiotics for possible aspiration pneumonia.

Surgical treatment

Isolated atresia

- Gastrostomy for feeding + continuous drainage of upper pouch or cervical esophagostomy.
- Delayed closure of defect (may require interposition graft if a long segment is involved, i.e., >4 vertebral bodies)

Atresia with tracheoesophageal fistula

- Closure of fistula and primary anastomosis of esophageal defect
- If infant is premature or presents with pneumonitis:
  - Gastrostomy with retropleural ligation of fistula
  - Later transthoracic repa and ir of esophageal defect

Isolated tracheoesophageal fistula

- Ligation of fistula (typically through low cervical approach)

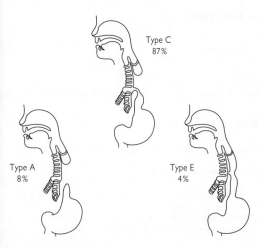

Fig. 11.1 Classification of esophageal atresia. Type C (III), distal fistula; type A (I), atresia without fistula; type E (V), H-type fistula. Reproduced with permission from McLatchie G, et al. (2008). *Oxford Handbook of Clinical Surgery*, 3rd ed. Oxford: Oxford University Press.

Pyloric stenosis

Key facts

- Incidence: 3/1000 live births
- Higher male:female incidence (4:1)
- Increased familial risk
- It often occurs in first-born boys.
- Hypertrophy of circular muscle of pylorus presents at 3–6 weeks of age.

Clinical features

Classical

- Persistent nonbilious vomiting becoming increasingly forceful to projectile
- Baby usually looks well in early state
- Secondary gastritis may cause blood-staining or coffee-ground emesis.
- There is often a history of positioning, multiple formula changes, and treatment for gastroesophageal reflux.
- The baby appears active and hungry, especially after vomiting.
- Small, bright green "starvation stools" are passed infrequently.
- Weight gain is poor.
- Dehydration with hypochloremic alkalosis supervenes in an untreated, established condition.
- Dehydration, pallor, and weight loss are seen in advanced cases.
- Epigastric fullness with left-to-right gastric peristaltic wave
- A test feed is usually performed to palpate a pyloric "tumor" (see Box 11.2).

Diagnosis and investigations

- If pyloric "tumor" is felt, no radiological investigations are necessary prior to surgery.
- Ultrasound shows thickened (>3 mm), elongated (>15 mm) pyloric muscle with decreased movement of fluid through a narrow canal (term infants).
- Barium meal (rarely necessary) shows an enlarged stomach, increased gastric peristalsis, and elongated, narrowed pyloric canal with "shouldering" of tumor on antral and duodenal lumens.
- Electrolytes and capillary blood gases: ↓ Na^+, ↓ K^+, ↓ Cl^-, base excess, and ↑ pH
- Paradoxical aciduria with hypochloremic alkalosis

Treatment

Resuscitation with IV rehydration

- Correct initial hypovolemia with bolus 0.9% saline 10 mL/kg.
- Correct hypochloremic alkalosis and hypokalemia (which may take 12–24 hr) with 0.45% sodium chloride/5% dextrose with added potassium chloride (2–4 Meq/dL) at a rate of 120–150mL/kg per day.
- The NGT, if not passed preoperatively, needs to be passed before intubation.
- Rapid-sequence intubation is required to minimize risk of aspiration.

Surgical treatment
- Pyloromyotomy (division of pyloric muscle fibers without opening of bowel lumen)
- Done via right upper quadrant or periumbilical incisions, or laparoscopically
- Use caution not to open mucosa (1% risk) and avoid the prepyloric vein ("vein of Mayo").

Start feeding within 4–6 hr postoperatively and increase to full volume by 24 hr. Small regurgitations should be expected in the early postoperative course.

Box 11.2 How to perform a test feed

- Undress baby in warm room and place on caregiver's lap with head elevated.
- Sit opposite baby and caregiver; position baby so head is to examiner's right.
- Begin feeding (breast or bottle). With active suckling the abdominal wall relaxes.
- Palpate with left hand (middle finger).
- Begin above umbilicus and feel into right upper quadrant under liver edge.
- Wait to feel appearance of olive-sized, firm, mobile lump in angle between liver edge and upper right rectus muscle (the pyloric 'olive').
- If stomach is distended, pylorus becomes more difficult to feel—aspiration of NGT may help.

Malrotation and volvulus

Key facts and clinical features (neonates)

Malrotation

- This can present at birth or soon after, and symptoms are due to failed or partial rotation of the foregut and hindgut, leading to duodenal obstruction.
- "Ladd's bands," crossing the second portion of the duodenum, are occasionally the cause of the intestinal obstruction.
- Duodenal obstruction beyond the ampulla of Vater leads to bile-stained vomiting.
- The cecum may be in an abnormally high or midline position.

Volvulus

Twisting, in clockwise direction, of nonfixed midgut on its narrow-based mesentery through more than 360°. results in obstruction of the superior mesenteric blood vessels.

Signs

- Sudden onset of abdominal pain
- Bile-vomiting
- Sometimes rapid progression to shock
- Passage of blood per rectum
- Presentation may be less dramatic with chronic intermittent pain.

These conditions are most dangerous in the newborn period because of delay in diagnosis and rapid development of gut ischemia.

Older children may present insidiously or with sudden onset of symptoms with rapid onset of shock.

Diagnosis

If in doubt, operate. Viability of twisted bowel is very time dependent—delays in diagnosis can be catastrophic.

Plain abdominal X-ray

- Gastric distention or "double bubble" sign with some distal gas
- Often a nonspecific bowel gas pattern is seen despite volvulus.

Barium meal

- Obstruction of second part duodenum
- Non-rotation of duodenum/jejunum
- Corkscrew appearance of proximal small bowel loops
- Absent C loop of duodenum.

Ultrasound scan

- Reversed relation of superior mesenteric artery and vein

Doppler ultrasound

- Absent or abnormal small bowel blood flow

Treatment

- Aggressive fluid resuscitation including decompression with NGT
- Emergent surgery to avoid irreversible bowel ischemia in cases of volvulus
- Ladd's procedure
  - Counterclockwise untwisting of volvulus
  - Division of Ladd's bands to open mesenteric plate
  - ± Fixation of right colon to left colon
  - Appendectomy
- Laparotomy may reveal the following:
  - Obstructed but viable bowel
  - Patchy ischemic changes that may or may not recover after reduction of volvulus
  - Established necrosis
- Initial resection of all apparent ischemic gut risks short bowel syndrome.
- Second-look laparotomy (24–48 hr) allows reassessment prior to resection.

Intussusception

Key facts
- Incidence: ~2/1000 live births
- Age at presentation: 3 months to 3 years with peak age of presentation at 6–12 months
- M:F = 2:1
- Fewer than 10% of pediatric cases have a clear focal pathological cause that starts the intussusception ("apex"; children older than 3 years of age and adults are more likely to have surgical lead point).

Clinicopathological features
- Invagination or telescoping of the proximal bowel (called the *intussusceptum*, e.g., terminal ileum/ileo-cecal valve) into the distal bowel (called the *intussuscipiens*, e.g., cecum/ascending colon)
- Idiopathic intussusception may be due to enlargement of submucosal lymphoid follicles (Peyer's patches).
- Pathology at the apex may be
  - Meckel's diverticulum
  - A polyp
  - Lymphoma
  - Enteric cysts

Clinical features
The classic triad of features is
- Abdominal pain (associated with pallor, screaming, arching, and restlessness)
- Palpable sausage-shaped mass (mid-abdominal or right upper quadrant)
- Passage of "red-currant jelly" stool in 40%–50% of cases (rectal examination may reveal guaiac-positive stools even if not obviously bloody)

Typically the infant is relatively settled between bouts of pain. Signs of shock (lethargy, poor feeding, hypotonia) require urgent fluid resuscitation. Features of obstruction (distension and vomiting) may occur.

Diagnosis
- Ultrasound (initial diagnostic test of choice): intussusception
  - Cross-section "doughnut" or "target" sign
  - "Pseudokidney sign" in longitudinal section
- Plain X-ray
  - May show right-sided soft tissue mass
  - Small bowel obstruction
  - Free air indicating perforation
- An air or water-soluble contrast enema is diagnostic and may be therapeutic.

Treatment

- Immediate IV fluid resuscitation to correct fluid losses and to restore fluid, electrolyte, and acid–base balance
- Maintenance fluid replacement and replacement of continued losses (vomiting or nasogastric losses)
- Reduction is only attempted once infant is resuscitated.

Methods of reduction

Radiological reduction

- A moribund infant or an infant with intra-abdominal air should go to the operating room without attempts at radiographic reduction.
- Contrast enema reduction (air or contrast) is therapeutic in 75% of cases, but success varies by center (40%–90%).
- Performed in radiology department under fluoroscopic control
- The surgeon should be notified before reduction is attempted.
- Evidence of irreducible obstruction or perforation mandates emergent surgery; classically, three attempts are made.
- Some centers report that partial or incomplete reduction may be successfully reduced by repeat contrast enema 4–8 hr after the initial attempt.

Surgical reduction

- Manual reduction by retrograde squeezing and gentle proximal traction
- Resection and anastomosis if bowel viability is in doubt (~10% require resection)
- Post-reduction shock may occur with release of bacterial products from viable but damaged bowel segment.
- Fever, sometimes >102.5°, may occur in the early postoperatiove period without evidence of bacteremia.
- Most patients recover rapidly with resumption of oral feeding in 12–24 hr and are discharged home in 1–3 days (recovery to discharge will be delayed if intestinal resection is required).

Complications

- Perforation during radiographic or surgical reduction
- The tecurrence rate is 5%–10% in radiologically reduced cases and about 3% even after operative reduction.
- Morbidity is low, but delayed diagnosis, inadequate resuscitation, and failure to recognize ischemic or perforated bowel account for a 1% mortality rate.

Appendicitis

Key facts

- This is the most common surgical cause of abdominal pain in the pediatric age group.
- Lifetime risk of appendicitis leading to appendectomy is ~8%–10%.
- There is an annual incidence of 4:1000 children.
- The most common age group is 5–17 years.
- The incidence of perforation seems to be diminishing, but 15%–30% of children will have gangrene or perforation.
- Perforation and gangrene occur more commonly in children under 5 years of age.
- Mortality is rare in the current era.

Diagnostic features

Symptoms

- Anorexia, nausea, or vomiting will occur in 95% of children with appendicitis.
- Most of the children will have all symptoms.
- Diarrhea is frequently seen with pelvic appendicitis.
- If complicated appendicitis develops, the child will begin to experience fever.

Classical description of pain

- Mid-abdominal to epigastric pain with migration to the right lower quadrant
- McBurney's point (1/3 the distance from the anterior superior iliac spine in a direct line to the umbilicus)

A thorough examination should include cardiac and pulmonary exams.

- It should be performed in a warm room and with warm hands.
- Ask the child to point to the area of greatest tenderness.

Examine abdominal fields away from the right lower quadrant to start the abdominal examination.

- Rovsing's sign is pressure in the left lower quadrant resulting in pain in the right lower quadrant.
- Obturator and psoas signs
  - Seen with retroileal or retrocecal appendices
  - Irritation of iliopsoas or obturator muscles

Rectal examination should be performed by at least one of the examiners and the stool should be tested for blood.

- Tenderness may localize to the right side of the rectum with pelvic appendicitis.
- The anterior and right-sided swelling or fullness into the rectum may indicate a pelvic abscess.

Laboratory evaluation

Obtain CBC with differential, urinalysis, and electrolytes, and coagulation profile.

- WBC >15,000 may indicate gangrene or perforation.
- 95% of children with appendicitis will have an elevated WBC and left shift unless they are being seen within 12 hr of the onset of symptoms.
- A small number of red blood cells on urinalysis may indicate bladder or ureteral irritation from right lower quadrant phlegmon.

Radiographic studies

Most plain abdominal radiographs are not helpful in evaluation for appendicitis.

- Ultrasound is helpful but lacks sensitivity.
  - Often technician-dependent
  - Less sensitive or specific than CT imaging
  - Helpful if clinician suspects ovarian pathology
- CT imaging
  - Very sensitive and specific
  - Significant radiation exposure

Treatment

Appendectomy

- May be performed by open or laparoscopic procedure, even in small children
- Laparoscopic procedures are often associated with shorter hospital stays and quicker return to activities of daily living.
- Small children have smaller abdominal domains and specialized instruments may be necessary for laparoscopy.
- Most surgeons agree that perioperative antibiotic coverage for enteric flora is indicated even in uncomplicated appendicitis.

Abscess associated with appendicitis

- A stable child with a chronic abscess complicating appendicitis with several days' history before presentation
  - Radiologic drainage of abscess, if appropriate
  - Initial IV antibiotics with transition to oral antibiotics
  - Interval appendectomy 8–12 weeks after acute event
- Septic or critically ill child with an intra-abdominal abscess complicating appendicitis
  - Early definitive surgery
  - Postoperative antibiotics with appropriate monitoring

Hirschsprung's disease

Key facts
- Incidence: 1 in 4500 live births
- More common in males

Pathological features
This disease is due to incomplete migration of neural crest cells into the hindgut, resulting in distal aganglionosis.
- Failure of coordinated peristaltic waves
- Abnormal anorectal relaxation
- Loss of rectoanal inhibitory reflex (RAIR)

Symptoms may involve the following:
- Anorectal sphincter (ultrashort segment)
  - Often presents as chronic constipation in the toddler or older child
  - Rectal biopsy will show ganglion cells.
- Rectum and rectosigmoid (short segment; 75%–85%)
  - Presents in infancy or early childhood
  - Transition zone may not be seen during contrast enema in first month of life
- Extensive colonic involvement (long segment; 10%)
- Total colonic disease (~10%)
  - May present with abdominal distention and diarrhea despite total colonic aganglionosis
  - Often extends some distance into distal small intestine

The proximal (normal) bowel becomes progressively distended as it tries to propel waste through the aganglionic and non-relaxing distal bowel.

Clinical features
- There is failure to pass meconium within 24–48 hr, abdominal distension, and bile vomiting.
- Infants with trisomy 21 have a greater incidence than that of the general population.
- It may present outside of the newborn period with poor weight gain, offensive diarrhea, or enterocolitis.

Diagnosis
- Plain films show features consistent with distal intestinal obstruction.
- Contrast enema shows less distensible rectum and may indicate a transition zone.
- Suction rectal biopsy confirms diagnosis: thickened nerve fibers (↑AChE) and aganglionisis
- Anorectal manometry (in older children) shows failure of anal relaxation on intraluminal rectal balloon distension (loss of RAIR).

Treatment

- Resuscitation
- Decompression of the colon with regular saline rectal washouts (irrigation and aspiration; NOT an enema).
- If decompression is not achieved or there is total colonic involvement, a diverting stoma is necessary. The stoma site must be confirmed by presence of ganglion cells (leveling stoma; i.e., level where ganglion cells are present).
- Definitive surgery is to remove the aganglionic bowel and bring normally innervated bowel to the anus (pull-through technique—Soave, Swenson, or Duhamel types).
- It may be performed as a one-stage procedure without a covering stoma.
- The pull-through can be performed transanally or transabdominally.
- Laparoscopy assists in establishing the level of aganglionosis and mobilizing the colon or rectum.

Complications

- Pelvic infection: infrequent
- Urinary incontinence: rare
- Retrograde ejaculation: rare
- Constipation: common
- Toilet-training is often delayed; common
- Enterocolitis can affect 20%–50% of children pre- and postoperatively (this is uncommon over 5 years of age unless an obstructive component persists after surgery).

Anorectal malformations

Key facts

- Incidence: ~1 in 5000 live births
- Such malformations are caused by failure of the correct septation of the hindgut cloaca or failure of formation of the anorectal canal (and associated pelvic floor structures).
- Low anomalies traverse a normal levator muscle.
- High anomalies end above the levator and are commonly associated with a fistula (bladder, urethra, vagina).
- Malformations may be part of VACTERL association or linked to chromosomal abnormalities.

Diagnostic features

Condition should be noted at the neonatal check.
- Recognition of an absent or abnormally placed anus
- Failure to pass meconium
- Abdominal distension if a diagnosis has been missed
- It may take up to 24 hr before meconium passes through the fistula.

Investigations and management

- Lateral prone X-ray of pelvis at 24 hr (assists in level assessment)
- Wagensteen-Rice view (supine invertogram to determine level of rectal pouch)
- Perineal ultrasound to visualize rectal pouch
- Renal ultrasound and echocardiography (for associated abnormalities)

Surgical treatment

- Low lesions (perineal fistula): single-stage perineal approach (anoplasty or dilatation)
- All other lesions
  - Initial diverting colostomy; typically in proximal sigmoid colon
  - Posterior sagittal anorectoplasty (PSARP) or Kiesewetter-Rehbein procedure at 1–6 months
  - Colostomy closure 4–6 weeks after procedure
- Contrast loopogram 1 week after stoma formation (position of fistula or renal anomalies)
- Regular blood work for electrolytes; if large fistula is present, check for a metabolic hyperchloremic acidosis
- Give prophylactic oral antibiotics if vesicoureteric reflux is demonstrated.

Prognosis

- Low anomalies often have relatively good function with a tendency toward constipation in later life.
- High anomalies often have impaired function with up to an 80% lifetime chance of soiling, incontinence, or severe constipation.

Rare causes of newborn intestinal obstruction

Duodenal atresia
- Caused by failure of development or canalization of the embryologic foregut
- May be complete (i.e., entirely separate proximal and distal duodenum) or partial (web obstruction in the second part of the duodenum)

Diagnostic features
- Bile-stained vomiting occurs from birth.
- Epigastric fullness on examination
- Look for features of associated trisomy 21.
- Plain abdominal X-ray: "double bubble" sign with no distal gas
- Must exclude malrotation with volvulus

Management
- Resuscitation
- Surgical bypass (duodenoduodenostomy)

Annular pancreas
- Presentation is similar to duodenal atresia
- Persistence of pancreas as ring around duodenum following rotation of ventral pancreas to form uncinate process

Surgical treatment
- Do not divide pancreatic ring as this may lead to acute pancreatitis and pancreatic fistula.
- Duodenoduodenostomy is similar to procedure for duodenal atresia.

Jejuno-ileal atresia
- Caused by probable in utero vascular insult to mesenteric vessels
- This may occur in a single segment or multiple segments and short segments or long stretches of small bowel may be involved.

Diagnostic features
- Bile-stained vomiting from birth
- Prominent abdominal distension, especially with more distal atresia
- Features of small intestinal obstruction on plain radiographs

Management
- Resuscitation
- Contrast enema may demonstrate "microcolon" and be helpful to exclude other diagnoses (e.g., Hirschsprung's disease, meconium ileus).
- Surgical anastomosis between atretic ends, occasionally with resection or tapering of dilated proximal segment

Meconium ileus

- Caused by the presence of impacted, abnormally thick meconium within the normal lumen of the small bowel
- Pathognomonic of cystic fibrosis (CF) but only 15% of infants with CF present with meconium ileus

Diagnostic features

- May be identified during antenatal ultrasound examination ("bright spots" in bowel) or with antenatal testing if there is a family history
- Presents in neonatal period with features of distal obstruction:
  - Bile-stained vomiting
  - Distension
  - Failure to pass meconium
  - Doughy mass in the right iliac fossa (meconium-obstructed bowel loops)

Management

- Resuscitation, IV fluids, NGT
- Plain abdominal X-ray
- Contrast enema may be diagnostic and therapeutic.
- Surgical removal of meconium (may involve a temporary ileostomy)
- Immunoreactive trypsin and commonly associated CF genes (**D**F508 mutation in *CFTR* gene)

Biliary atresia

Key facts
- Incidence: 1:8000 to 1:20,000 births
- Pathology: progressive inflammation of uncertain etiology involving biliary tract

Types and manifestation
- Most typically extrahepatic and intrahepatic involvement (90%)
- Occasionally intrahepatic without extrahepatic involvement (~10%)
- Rarely extrahepatic involvement without intrahepatic disease
- May be associated with other congenital defects (asplenia, polysplenia, situs inversus) (~3%–10%) (biliary atresia splenic malformation syndrome [BASM])
- Etiology unknown

Diagnostic features and evaluation
- Conjugated hyperbilirubinemia in early infancy with acholic stools
- Must exclude other neonatal cholestatic syndromes
    - Alagille syndrome (dysmorphic facies, chronic cholestasis, pulmonic stenosis, mild growth and mental retardation)
    - Metabolic causes: galactosemia, tyrosinemia, disorders of lipid metabolism
    - α_1-antitrypsin deficiency
    - Neonatal hemachromatosis
    - Parenteral nutrition-associated cholestasis
    - Neonatal hepatitis

Evaluation
- Laboratory evaluation to exclude α_1-antitrypsin deficiency and metabolic disorders
- Ultrasound evaluation of the liver and bile ducts
- HIDA scan with phenobarbital preload (5 mg/kg per day for 5 days)
- ERCP or MRCP, if available for infants
- Liver biopsy although shared findings with biliary atresia and neonatal hepatitis

Treatment
- Kasai portoenterostomy as urgent procedure once diagnosis is established
- Intraoperative cholangiogram to evaluate biliary tree as initial part of procedure
- Successful bile drainage is achieved when portoenterostomy is performed as early as possible.
    - Procedure performed by 60 days: ~70%
    - Procedure performed by 70 days: ~40%
    - Procedure performed by 90 days: ~25%
    - Procedure performed beyond 90 days: <20%

- Success may be predicted by serum bilirubin level achieved at 3 months postoperatively.
- There may be a role for perioperative steroids at the time of portoenterostomy
- Liver transplantation is appropriate for worsening liver disease complicating failed portoenterostomy.

Choledochal cyst

Key facts
- Incidence varies according to location and genetic background.
  - Western countries: 1:15,000 births
  - Japan: 1:1000 births
- Female:male = 4:1
- Uncertain etiology
  - Likely genetic and environmental factors
  - Abnormal pancreatic-choledochus junction
  - Distal displacement of ampulla of Vater
- Types
  - I—fusiform ductal dilatation involving common bile and common hepatic duct
  - II—isolated diverticulum from bile duct
  - III—cystic dilatation of the intrapancreatic portion of common bile duct
  - IV—cystic dilatation of the extrahepatic and intrahepatic bile ducts
  - V—cystic dilatation of intrahepatic bile ducts without extrahepatic disease (Caroli's disease)
- Lifetime malignancy risk of cholangiocarcinoma is 10%–30%.
  - May occur in children and young adults
  - May have synchronous and metachronous presentation
  - Rarely occurs in intrahepatic ducts
  - Risk remains if the cyst is not completely excised; there is a definite role for opening the cyst and performing mucosal resection in a cyst with severe inflammation involving porta hepatis.

Diagnostic features and presentation
- Classic triad: abdominal pain, jaundice, right upper quadrant mass
  - Seen in 20%–40% of cases
  - Less frequently seen in pediatric patients
- May present with fever and cholangitis
- May be associated with pancreatitis
- Choledochal cyst presenting in infancy with conjugated hyper-bilirubinemia may be associated with biliary atresia.

Evaluation
- Routine evaluation of liver function (hepatic enzymes, total and direct bilirubin, alkaline phosphatase, γ-glutamyl transferase [γGT]), hepatitis serology, CBC with differential, pancreatic enzymes
- Ultrasound of liver
- ERCP or MRCP

Treatment

- Initial treatment of cholangitis, if present
- Cyst excision and hepaticojejunostomy
- Partial cyst excision, mucosal resection, and hepaticojejunostomy if severe inflammation involves porta hepatis
- There is a very limited role for hepatic resection with intrahepatic ductal disease.
- Endoscopic sphincterotomy is used for small type-III cyst (choledochocele) (≤3 cm).
- Transduodenal resection and sphincterotomy are used for large type-III cyst (choledochocele) (>3 cm).

A persistent lifetime risk of cholangiocarcinoma, even after cyst excision, requires lifetime monitoring (CEA; CA 19-9).

Abdominal wall defects

Omphalocele (exomphalos)

Key facts
- Incidence: 1:7000 births

Clinicopathological features
- Failed formation of the anterior abdominal muscular wall covered by a membrane (unless ruptured)
- Hernia of the umbilical cord: presence of intestine in the base of the umbilical cord. Typically there is normal abdominal wall musculature.
- Omphalocele minor: the defect is <5 cm and only the bowel is present.
- Omphalocele major: the defect is >5 cm and bowel, liver, and other abdominal organs lie in the omphalocele sac.
- May be detected antenatally with an abnormal scan or raised maternal serum α-fetoprotein (AFP).
- In postnatal presentation there is an obvious defect.
- ~30% of infants will have other significant anomalies.

Diagnosis
- Investigations are directed at identifying associations (see Box 11.3). Check blood sugar; as some infants will have profound hypoglycemia.
- All newborn babies should have cardiac imaging prior to further management.

Treatment
- Parents may opt for termination in antenatally detected defects with associated major cardiac or chromosomal anomaly (mortality ~80%).
- Postnatal management involves protection of the sac, insertion of an NGT, IV access, and fluid management.
- Minor omphalocele should be suitable for reduction and primary closure of abdominal wall defect in the first days of life.
- Major omphalocele may be associated with an underdeveloped abdominal cavity, precluding primary reduction.
- In infants with other complex anomalies, epithelialization of the sac is encouraged with application of silver sulfadiazine paste, which results in a large ventral hernia suitable for delayed closure at ~1 year of age.
- Infants without other complex anomalies are likely better served by placing a silo and gradually reducing the viscera over 7 to 10 days. With reduction, the surgeon must be concerned about kinking the hepatic veins, worsening respiratory distress, and creating an abdominal compartment syndrome.

Surgical treatment
- Primary reduction of smaller defects: excision of sac, closure of defect (linear or purse-string), and closure of umbilical skin
- If the sac is ruptured or with larger defect:
  - Initial application of silo
  - Gradual reduction of intestinal content into abdominal cavity over 3–10 days

Box 11.3 Associations of omphalocele

- Chromosomal abnormality (trisomy 18, 13, 21)
- Cardiac and renal anomalies are found in up to 40% of cases.
- Beckwith–Wiedemann syndrome: omphalocele, macroglossia, gigantism, hyperinsulinism in infancy, renal or hepatic tumors
- Pentalogy of Cantrell: epigastric omphalocele, sternal cleft, ectopia cordis, anterior diaphragmatic hernia, ventricular septal defect
- Cloacal exstrophy (elephant's head deformity): lower abdominal omphalocele, bladder extrophy, microphallus, ileal intussusception through cloacal plate, imperforate anus, duplicated appendix or cecum

Gastroschisis
Key facts
- Incidence: 1:7000 births

Clinicopathological features
- There is a defect to the right of the umbilicus with protrusion of the stomach, small bowel, and large bowel.
- Associated with young maternal age and antenatal smoking or recreational drug use
- Most present antenatally with an abnormal antenatal ultrasound or raised maternal serum AFP.
- Antenatal diagnosis allows planned delivery (no evidence to recommend Cesarean section).
- Extraintestinal associated anomalies are uncommon.
- Intestinal atresia is found in 10%–20% of cases and may result in extensive in utero intestinal loss. This may lead to short bowel syndrome.

Diagnosis
- Associated anomalies are rare; no specific preoperative tests are required.

Treatment
- Planned vaginal delivery as close as possible to neonatal surgical unit
- Standard neonatal resuscitation (clean, dry, stimulate, facial oxygen)
- Insertion of NGT to decompress stomach
- Fluid balance must include considerable evaporative losses from the gut (generally 150%–200% maintenance).
- Broad-spectrum antibiotics
- Sterile film wrap to protect herniated bowel against trauma, contamination, heat loss, drying, and fluid loss
- Intestines should be placed on central abdomen or infant placed in right lateral decubitus position to ensure that the mesenteric root is not on stretch.

Surgical treatment
- If possible, delineate and close the defect.
- If herniated contents cannot be reduced, apply a silo to cover the gut and delay closure until the gut is reduced (7–10 days).

Necrotizing enterocolitis (NEC)

Key facts
- Intestinal inflammation ranges from mild mucosal injury to full-thickness necrosis and perforation.
- Perforated NEC is associated with 40% mortality in neonates.

Clinicopathological features
NEC is associated with the following:
- Premature delivery
- Intraluminal substrate (breast feeding may provide a protective benefit to premature infants)
- Hypoxia
- Systemic sepsis
- Significant cardiac lesions
- "Micro-epidemic" outbreaks in neonatal units
- Typically, NEC affects premature babies on ventilatory support.
- Features of bilious vomiting or aspirates, abdominal distension, bloody mucus passing per rectum.
- Patient may quickly show signs of severe sepsis/ or shock (tachypnea, tachycardia, hypotension, poor perfusion, temperature instability).

Diagnosis
Plain abdominal X-ray shows the following:
- Pneumatosis intestinalis
- Portal venous gas
- Free intraperitoneal air with perforation
- Dilated, thick-walled (edematous) bowel

Medical treatment
- Fluid resuscitation
- Broad-spectrum IV antibiotics
- Bowel rest and TPN
- Serial examinations, abdominal films, and platelet counts

Surgical treatment
Surgical treatment is indicated by complications:
- Perforation
- Failure to respond to medical treatment
- Abdominal mass
- Systemic sepsis

Surgical treatment may include the following:
- Peritoneal drainage in critical-conditon premature infant but followed by exploratory celiotomy in 24–48 hr
- Initial aspiration with bowel resection (usually with stoma formation)
- With extensive or near-total intestinal necrotizing enterocolitis, initial exploration with second-look exploration in 24–48 hr

Complications

- Septicemia
- Enteric fistulization
- Peritonitis
- Adhesions
- Wound infections are common in these extremely premature infants with severe abdominal infection.
- Enteric stricture (usually in colon)
- Short gut syndrome
- Irreversible sepsis and death

Inguinal hernia and scrotal swellings

Inguinal hernia

Key facts

- Childhood inguinal hernias derive from a persistent processus vaginalis and are almost invariably indirect.
- Male:female = 7:1
- Right-sided hernias (60%) are more common than left ones (25%); 15% are bilateral.
- There is a higher incidence of incarceration in infants with hernias than in adults.

Clinical features

- Usually noticed as a painless swelling, variable in size in the inguinoscrotal or labial area
- More prominent when the baby cries and may disappear intermittently
- Bowel entrapment causes pain and irreducibility leads to strangulation, intestinal obstruction, perforation, and peritonitis.
- Ovarian entrapment is common in females.
- Bile vomiting in a young infant should always prompt examination of the inguinoscrotal area.
- A cardinal feature is swelling in the groin above which the examining fingers cannot define the inguinal canal ("cannot get above").
- Asymmetrical thickening of the spermatic cord in the presence of a history compatible with a hernia is strongly suggestive of the diagnosis.
- Inguinal hernia is often hard to demonstrate during examination in the young pediatric patient and in infants.
- A history of inguinal swelling, often described when the child is straining or crying, is associated with an inguinal hernia in 90% of the children who present with such a history but an inconclusive office examination.

Treatment

- Prompt surgical treatment (first available date) is important in premature or young infants to avoid risks of complications.
- Herniotomy alone is adequate—there is no need to repair the walls of the canal. Usually this is a simple, straightforward day-case procedure.
- Acute surgery can be very difficult when the hernia is irreducible or strangulated and in very premature infants.
- Infants under 52 weeks postconceptual age are at risk for postoperative apnea following anesthesia and require overnight monitoring.
- The risk of postoperative apnea is lessened but not eliminated by use of spinal anesthesia.

Hydrocele

Key facts

- Congenital fluid-filled processus vaginalis and tunica vaginalis
- Hydroceles communicating with the peritoneal cavity in children are hernia–hydrocele complexes and should be treated as hernias with surgical repair in a timely fashion.

- The scrotum is usually smoothly enlarged, sometimes bluish in color, and the testis is often surrounded by the hydrocele.
- Occasionally hydrocele is acquired from trauma, infection, or a testicular tumor.
- Congenital hydroceles may resolve spontaneously up to age 18 months. Surgical intervention is deferred until 18 months if there is no evidence of a concomitant hernia.
- At operation, ligation of the patent processus vaginalis and drainage of the fluid are adequate. There is no need to excise the hydrocele wall.

Varicocele

- Due to a dilated pampiniform venous plexus of the spermatic cord.
- Onset is usually after puberty.
- Has the feel of a "bag of worms" during palpation of the cord
- Beware of any varicocele in childhood that may be due to obstruction of the renal vein by tumor (nephroblastoma).

Treatment

- Indications
  - Discomfort (aching)
  - Loss of testicular volume >15% of contralateral testis
  - Cosmesis
  - Concern about fertility
- Treatment of the varicocele may be surgical ligation either in the inguinal canal or in the retroperitoneum.
- Radiologically guided embolization has been used by some groups but does not seem to have an equivalent success rate to that of surgical ligation.

Idiopathic scrotal edema

- The etiology is unknown; it is possibly due to an acute allergic reaction.
- Characterized by painless, red, unilateral scrotal swelling extending to the groin and the perineum
- Rapidly resolves spontaneously—the clinical diagnosis precludes the need for investigation.

Other hernias in childhood

Umbilical hernia

Key facts
- Persistence of the physiological umbilical defect beyond birth
- These usually close spontaneously (especially in premature infants)
- They have a low incidence of complications (incarceration or strangulation).

Clinical features
- Usually noticed as a painless, intermittent swelling at the umbilicus

Treatment
- Will close spontaneously in >50% of cases
- As complications are infrequent, delay repaired until at least age 3 unless
  - Defect is markedly protuberant and in a period of observation becomes even more protuberant
  - Defect has an easily defined fascial ring and measures >1.5 cm, as these are unlikely to close spontaneously

Epigastric hernia

Key facts
- Defect in the midline linea alba between the umbilicus and the xiphoid process
- Does not close spontaneously

Clinical features
- Often noticed as midline supraumbilical "bump" when the child is shirtless.
- Often presents with incarcerated preperitoneal fat and mild local tenderness

Treatment
Simple sutured closure of the defect is required.

Prepuce (foreskin) and circumcision

Key facts

- This is one of the most common reasons for referral to a pediatric surgical clinic (see Box 11.4 for examination procedure).
- Prepuce (foreskin) is initially fused to the glans penis.
- Preputial "adhesions" lyse spontaneously as part of normal development.
- Separation of the prepuce from the glans is gradual.
  - 80% of newborns
  - 50% of 1-year-olds
  - 10% of 5-year-olds will have an incompletely retractable prepuce.
- Non-retractable foreskin

Clinical features

Only rarely does this condition cause problems.

- Dysuria
- Frequency
- Spots of blood
- Ballooning
- Urinary spraying.
- It occasionally causes recurrent balanitis with foreskin redness, soreness, and cellulitis.

Preputial "cysts" are often present—these are collections of subpreputial smegma and are part of normal development.

Treatment

- Often only reassurance and advice are needed.
- Leave the foreskin alone if asymptomatic.
- Frequent bathing and hygiene and gentle attempts at retraction
- 0.05% betamethasone cream topically applied tid may relieve symptoms and speed separation.
- Give topical or, rarely, oral antibiotics for balanitis.
- Persistent symptoms may warrant retraction and separation of adhesions under general anesthesia or circumcision.

Phimosis

This is defined as a non-retractable foreskin with associated scarring that will not resolve spontaneously.

Clinicopathological features

- May be congenital or acquired to inflammation from recurrent balanitis
- Phimosis is the most common cause of balanitis xerotica obliterans— the foreskin looks pale, thickened, and scarred.
- Additional symptoms to those of a non-retractable foreskin may include the following:
  - Retention of urine
  - Paraphimosis
  - Obstruction
  - Rarely, back pressure on the upper urinary tract

Consider an ultrasound scan for ascending urinary tract infection, in which case antibiotics are indicated.

Treatment
- Circumcision
- Dorsal slit of foreskin
- Preputioplasty (prepuceplasty), although excision of the fibrotic portion of foreskin may be complicated by scarring and recurrent phimosis

---

Box 11.4 How to examine a child's foreskin

- Try to ensure that the boy is happy and relaxed, lying on the examination couch or the parent's knee.
- Normal foreskin often appears long and "redundant."
- Gently hold the tip of prepuce between your fingertips, lift forward, and spread wide open. The preputial orifice is usually demonstrated.
- If retraction is attempted, perform gently to show pouting of mucosa
- Blanching of skin below the preputial opening is normal.
- A tight, white, contracted preputial orifice indicates fibrotic phimosis ("muzzling").

Undescended testis

Key facts

- Testicular descent from the fetal abdomen into the scrotum is normally complete by 6 months postnatally.
- Absence of a scrotal testis (cryptorchidism) may be due to
  - Agenesis (rare)
  - Intra-abdominal arrest of testicular descent
  - Incomplete descent (intracanalicular) or ectopic descent (inguinal, perineal, crural, penile)
- Incidence: 2%–4% of newborn boys, falling to 1.5% at 6 months as testicular descent is completed
- More common on the right side

Clinical features

- Undescended testis can be noted at the postnatal check, by parents, or by the pediatrician.
- It rarely presents acutely as torsion (tender mass in inguinal region).
- A retractile testis is one that can be brought down into the scrotum with gentle manipulation but retracts into the superficial inguinal pouch either spontaneously or with minor pressure (see Box 11.5 for excluding retractile testis).

Diagnosis

- No tests are required in palpable undescended testis.
- Chromosomal studies and an HCG stimulation test may be requested in bilateral impalpable testes.
- Ultrasound may help locate an impalpable testis.
- Diagnostic laparoscopy is helpful in defining the location and may initiate treatment if the testis is intra-abdominal.

Treatment

- Testis should be brought to the scrotum before 2 years of age to avoid secondary damage due to trauma, torsion, and increased ambient temperature.
- Hormone manipulation is ineffective in true undescended testis.
- Intracanalicular or ectopic testis should be managed by single-stage orchidopexy (see Box 11.6).
- Intra-abdominal testis can be brought down by one- or two-stage orchidopexy (with 50%–90% success).
- Laparoscopy for bilateral impalpable testes
- The scrotal position facilitates self-examination to detect signs of neoplastic change (~4x normal in an abdominal testis).

Complications

- Postoperative atrophy of the testis (<2%) unless there is intra-abdominal position (10%–50%)
- Retraction

Box 11.5 How to exclude retractile testis

- A cooperative, relaxed little boy is essential. Examine the boy on the caregiver's knee or while he is lying down.
- Control the inguinal canal with finger pressure (this prevents retraction of testis).
- Palpate tissues superficial to the external inguinal ring, working down to scrotum.
- Try to manipulate testis into the scrotum—then release.
- True retractile testis should remain in the scrotum briefly.
- ~95% of true retractile testes descend spontaneously before puberty and require no follow-up (~5% apparently retractile testes become "ascending" and require orchidopexy).

Box 11.6 Indications for orchidopexy

- Maximize sperm production.
- Prevent testicular torsion.
- Repair associated inguinal hernia.
- Cosmesis
- Reduce chance of undetected malignancy development and improve self-examination success.

Scrotal pain in pediatric patients

Testicular torsion

Key facts

The most important diagnostic study is ultrasound of the scrotum.

- Current imaging modality has high sensitivity and specificity in identifying etiology of scrotal pain, even though testicular blood flow may be difficult to image in preschool children.
- Testicular perfusion study is rarely indicated in current era.

There are two peak age groups, but this pain can occur at any age.

- Newborn
- Early adolescence

Newborn torsion

- Noted in newborn exam as a reddish, edematous, and swollen scrotum
- Spermatic cord torsion is extravaginal, involving tunica vaginalis and testis
- The testicle is rarely salvageable.
- Orchiectomy of the torsed testicle is indicated if the testicle is infarcted.
- Contralateral testicular fixation is recommended because synchronous and metachronous testicular torsions have been reported in infants.

Adolescent torsion

- Acute onset of testicular pain, typically in the early morning or after athletic activity
- High-riding testis often with scrotal edema and erythema
- Cremasteric reflex is not present.
- Bell clapper deformity
- The problem should be treated as a surgical emergency, as testicular salvage is greatest with surgical correction performed within 6 hr of pain onset.
- If clinical features and examination are highly suggestive of torsion, surgery rather than imaging is indicated.
- Testicular salvage occurs rarely if pain present for more than 24 hr.
- Orchiectomy is indicated for infarcted testis
  - For pain relief
  - Possible immunologic trigger for anti-sperm antibody
- A prosthesis should not be placed at the time of the orchiectomy procedure as this can result in a greater risk of complications.
- There is theoretical concern about subfertility or infertility from anti-sperm antibodies complicating testicular torsion if orchiectomy is not performed.

Torsion of appendix testis

- This is a common problem in prepubescent males, often associated with several hours' to several days' history of moderate testicular pain.
- Cremasteric reflex is present.
- Erythema may be seen on scrotum.

- A "blue dot" sign (indicative of infarction of testicular appendage) is seen in 10% of the cases.
- Reactive hydrocele is frequently found.
- Typically responds well to scrotal elevation and anti-inflammatories
- If pain is persistent and severe, it is appropriate to perform surgery for removal of infarcted appendage.

Incarcerated inguinal hernia

- Subtle incarceration at internal inguinal ring may lead to moderate testicular pain without clearly evident inguinal swelling.
- Careful examination with the child lying down may reveal a mass in upper inguinal canal.
- Reduction of hernia results in almost immediate relief of testicular pain.

Epididymoorchitis

- This is typically seen in later adolescence and in sexually active males.
- Ultrasound imaging demonstrates increased blood flow with edema of epididymis.
- Epididymitis alone may be seen in prepubescent males, secondary to viral infection.
- Orchitis may complicate mumps viral infection.
- Henoch-Schönlein purpura may be present with an epididymoorchitis even before skin lesions are seen.

Testicular trauma

- History typically indicates moderate to severe trauma as a direct blow to the scrotum. Trauma may occur following straddle injuries.
- Often tender and swollen with ecchymosis involving scrotum.
- Ultrasound imaging helps to define the extent of testicular injury.
- If hematoma is confined to soft tissues of the scrotum
  - No surgery is indicated
  - Provide scrotal support
  - Give anti-inflammatories and pain medication
  - Application of ice packs may be helpful in the first 24–48 hr.
- If imaging shows fracture of tunica albuginea, urgent surgical repair is indicated.

Infantile pyocele

- Typically seen outside the newborn period but in the first year of life
- The infant often has hydrocele and presents with a sudden onset of erythematous scrotum.
- Ultrasound reveals complex fluid around the testis, occasionally with septation, and may mimic torsion.
- If flow is well demonstrated in testis, a short course of IV antibiotics to cover gram-positive and gram-negative aerobic organisms (nafcillin/gentamicin or clindamycin/gentamicin) is appropriate.
- If there is no significant improvement in 24–48 hr, scrotal exploration is indicated for drainage of infected hydrocele.
- If there is any question about testicular flow and possible testicular torsion, surgical exploration of the scrotum is indicated, even though testicular torsion is unusual in this age group.

Solid tumors of childhood

Neuroblastoma

Key facts

- This is the most common solid abdominal tumor of childhood.
- Incidence: 12.3 per 1,000,000 children under age 15 years
- There is a spectrum of tumors derived from neuroblasts found in the adrenal gland, along the sympathetic chain, or extra-adrenal sympathetic tissues.
- This is an aggressive tumor with early spread to lymph nodes, liver, bone (cortex or marrow), orbits, and skin.
- It often presents as a painless large, abdominal mass in children <2 years of age.
- It may present as weight loss, hypertension, proptosis, or metastatic disease.
- Urinary VMA, HVA are elevated.
- CT scan provides optimal investigation for suspected neuroblastoma.
- Treatment is with a combination of chemotherapy, surgery, and radiotherapy.
- There may be a role for bone marrow transplantation in infants and children with neuroblastoma and indicators predicting poor outcome.
- Survival is between 30% and 90% depending on the site and stage at presentation.

Nephroblastoma (Wilms' tumor)

Key facts

- Incidence: 10.3 per 1,000,000 children under age 15 years
- Most common renal tumor in children
- Fast-growing tumor of the kidney
- Ranges from benign mesoblastic nephroma of infancy to poorly differentiated, malignant nephroblastoma in the older child
- Malignant tumors frequently metastasize to regional lymph nodes, the liver, and lungs.
- Presentation varies
  - A large, relatively painless abdominal mass in an otherwise well child is found incidentally.
  - Hematuria
  - Mild hypertension
  - Evidence of significant renal injury following minor trauma

Treatment

- Combination of chemotherapy, surgery, and radiotherapy according to histology and spread at diagnosis
- 5-year survival:
  - Early stage (favorable histology), 90%
  - Disseminated disease (favorable histology), 70%

Rhabdomyosarcoma

Key facts

- Incidence: 4.9 per 1,000,000 children under age 20 years
- Tumor of striated muscle origin from the bladder, vagina, prostate, or parameningeal tissue, and/or a soft tissue mass on limbs
- Pathology: embryonal or alveolar variants
- Hematuria, vaginal bleeding, and the appearance of grape-like cysts (sarcoma botryoides) at the vaginal introitus
- Histology influences the prognosis.
- Survival is up to 70% from treatment with surgery and chemotherapy.

Hepatoblastoma

Key facts

- Incidence: 1.5 per 1,000,000 children under age 15 years
- Most common hepatic malignancy in childhood
- AFP serum marker is typically elevated.
- Usually presents as a right hypochondrial mass extending across the midline
- Surgical resection is the goal.
- Chemotherapy may render initially inoperable tumors resectable.
- Depending on staging, size, and histology, survival of up to 70% is possible.

Neck swellings

Key facts

- Childhood neck lumps may be due to embryological abnormalities as well as to the same spectrum of conditions in adults (see Box 11.7 and Box 11.8).
- Embryological abnormalities may relate to the following:
  - Descent of the thyroid from the foramen cecum of the tongue (thyroglossal duct cysts)
  - Formation of 2nd, 3rd, and 4th branchial arches and clefts (branchial cleft cyst and sinuses)
  - Formation of lymphatic vessels and veins (cystic hygroma and complex vascular malformations)
- Lymphadenopathy is very common in children but typically waxes and wanes.
- If lymphadenopathy persists for longer than 2 months and measures more than 2 cm diameter, it should be biopsied.

Causes and clinicopathological features

Lymphadenopathy

The neck contains large numbers of lymph glands draining areas of potential infection in the mouth, nose, pharynx, and ears. Common causes of lymphadenopathy include URI, middle ear infections, tonsillitis, parotitis, dental abscess, and atypical mycobacterial infection.

- Malignant lymphadenopathy occurs but is less common; most commonly, lymphoma occurs.
- There can be metastatic nodes, e.g., from neuroblastoma or upper abdominal malignancies (uncommon).

Salivary gland swelling

- Swelling may be due to duct obstruction (stones or duct stenosis), infection (mumps), autoimmune disorders (recurrent parotitis), or neoplasia (adenoma).
- It is most common in the submandibular, sublingual, and parotid glands.

Skin and soft tissue lesions

- Dermoid cysts are usually in the midline above the hyoid bone and are infrequently infected.
- Sebaceous cysts are of epidermal origin with a small central punctum. They may occur anywhere but most commonly are on the scalp or back of the neck.

Lymphovascular lesions

- Hemangiomas can be mixed capillary or cavernous hemangiomas or hemangioendotheliomas within the neck and parotid area.
- Lesions may grow rapidly in size and lead to high-output cardiac failure or even carotid steal syndrome.
- Cystic hygroma (lymphangioma) is commonly in the posterior triangle of the neck but may involve extensive fields including the mediastinum, supraclavicular fossa, axilla, submandibular, and submental areas.

Treatment

- Excision of dermoid cysts, sebaceous cysts, thyroglossal cysts, thyroid neoplasms, salivary gland enlargements, and lymph gland enlargements (see Box 11.9)
- Incisional biopsy may be necessary and appropriate to establish diagnosis in a poorly defined mass in which cervical anatomy may be distorted.
- If secondary to mycobacterial lymphadenitis, chronic sinuses may develop and near-complete excision of the lesion will likely be required.
- Hemangioma requires supportive measures (intubation, steroids, interferon, and emergency surgical intervention).
- Cystic hygroma:
  - Sclerosant injection (OK 432—streptococcal derivative) is effective in lymphangiomas with few large cysts.
  - Surgical excision may be needed for extensive disease, particularly if there is evidence of respiratory compromise.

Box 11.7 Differential diagnosis of neck lump

Neck lumps may be lateral or midline.

Lateral	*Midline*
Lymph node	Submental lymph nodes
Branchial sinuses and cyst	Thyroglossal cyst
Cystic hygroma	Thyroid swelling
Torticollis (benign sternocleido-mastoid fibrosis)	Dermoid cyst
Hemangioma	
Lymphangioma	
Submandibular gland	
Parotid gland	
Neoplasm	

Box 11.8 Neck swellings by cause

Congenital	*Acquired*
Thyroglossal cysts	Reactive lymphadenopathy
Branchial cyst	Infective lymphadenopathy
Cystic hygroma	Secondary tumor deposits
Hemangioma	Lymphoma
Dermoid cyst	

Box 11.9 Anatomy related to neck lump surgery

- Incisions should be parallel with skin creases (Langer's lines).
- Subcutaneous closure should be meticulous (e.g., 4/0, 5/0, or 6/0 continuous subcuticular monofilament).
- The facial nerve passes between the two lobes of parotid gland.
- The lingual nerve swerves around the submandibular duct.
- The marginal mandibular branch of the facial nerve passes below and slightly anterior to the angle of the mandible.
- The thoracic duct enters the junction of left subclavian and jugular veins.

Major trauma

Marc A. de Moya, MD

Management of major trauma

Key facts

- Trauma is the leading cause of death in the first four decades of life, and for every person killed, three people are permanently disabled.
- Death from injury occurs in one of three time periods (trimodal).
  - First peak—within seconds to minutes. Very few patients can be saved because of the severity of their injuries.
  - Second peak—within minutes to several hours. Deaths occur due to life-threatening injuries.
  - Third peak—after several hours to weeks. Deaths are from sepsis and multiple-organ failure.
- The "golden hour" refers to the period when medical care can make the maximum impact on preventing death and disability. It indicates the urgency and not a fixed time period of 60 min.

The Advanced Trauma Life Support (ATLS) system

- ATLS is accepted as a standard for trauma care during the "golden hour" and focuses on the second peak.
- Injury can lead to death in certain reproducible time frames in a common sequence: loss of airway; inability to breathe; loss of circulating blood volume; and expanding intracranial mass.
- The primary survey following these areas (airway, breathing, circulation, disability, exposure [ABCDE]) with simultaneous resuscitation is emphasized.

Pre-hospital care and the trauma team

- Effort is made to minimize scene time, emphasizing immediate transport to the closest appropriate facility ("scoop and run").
- The hospital is informed of the impending arrival of the casualty.
- Triage is the process of prioritizing patients according to treatment need and the available resources (those with life-threatening conditions *and* with the greatest chance of survival are treated first).
- The trauma team consists of people familiar with care of the trauma patient, including trauma surgeons, emergency physicians, and nurses.
- The trauma team requires the support of orthopedic surgery, neurosurgery, radiography (including interventional radiology), and anesthesiology.

Management—primary survey

Identify and treat life-threatening conditions according to priority (ABCDE).

Airway maintenance with cervical spine protection

- Protect the spinal cord with immobilization devices or using manual in-line immobilization. Protect it until cervical spine injury is excluded.
- Access the airway for patency. If the patient can speak, the airway is not immediately threatened.
- Perform jaw thrust and avoid chin lift, maintaining c-spine stabilization. Consider an oropharyngeal airway.
- If the patient is unable to maintain airway integrity, secure a definitive airway.
- Definitive airway = oral endotracheal intubation or cricothyroidotomy

Breathing and ventilation
- Administer high-flow oxygen using a non-rebreathing reservoir.
- Inspect for chest wall expansion, symmetry, respiratory rate, and wounds. Auscultate the chest.
- Look for tracheal deviation, subcutaneous emphysema, or jugular vein distension (JVD).
- .Identify and treat life-threatening conditions: tension pneumothorax, open pneumothorax, massive hemothorax, or obvious flail chest.

Circulation with hemorrhage control
- Look for signs of shock.
- Hypotension most commonly = blood loss. Think: "blood on the floor and four more": external loss, and that from chest, abdomen, retroperitoneum, or muscle compartments. Do not underestimate losses from the scalp.
- Control external bleeding with pressure or suture/staple if from scalp.
- Obtain IV access using two 14-16G cannulae. Send blood for type and cross-match early.
- Commence bolus of warmed Ringer's lactate solution; use unmatched, O-negative or positive blood only for immediate life-threatening blood loss.
- Consider the need for surgical control of hemorrhage (laparotomy, thoracotomy).
- **IMPORTANT**: Fluid and blood resuscitation is NOT a surrogate for definitive hemorrhage control

Disability
- Perform a rapid neurological evaluation including pupils, Glasgow Coma Scale, and movement in extremities (upper and lower).
- After excluding hypoxia and hypovolemia, consider changes in level of consciousness to be due to head injury.

Exposure and environment control
- Remove clothing for thorough examination.
- Prevent hypothermia by covering patient with warm blankets or warming device and having a warm ambient temperature in the room. Use warm IV fluids.

Adjuncts to primary survey
- Monitor noninvasive BP, ECG, and pulse oximetry.
- Urinary catheter after ruling out urethral injury
- Diagnostic studies: X-rays (anteroposterior [AP] chest, and AP pelvis), ultrasound scan (focused assessment sonography for trauma [FAST]), CT scan, diagnostic peritoneal aspiration/lavage

Management—secondary survey
Begin only after primary survey is complete and resuscitation is continuing successfully.
- Take history: AMPLE (allergy, medication, past medical history, last meal, events of the incident)
- Perform a head-to-toe physical examination.
- Continue reassessment of all vital signs.
- Perform specialized diagnostic tests that may be required.

Thoracic injuries

Key features
- Thoracic injuries account for 25% of deaths from trauma.
- 50% of patients who die from multiple injuries also have a significant thoracic injury.
- The most common cause of these injuries is motor vehicle collisions.

Management—primary survey

Identify and treat major thoracic life-threatening injuries.

Tension pneumothorax
- Clinical diagnosis. There is no time for X-rays.
- Patient has respiratory distress, is tachycardic, and hypotensive.
- Look for tracheal deviation, decreased movement, and absent breath sounds over affected hemithorax.
- Treat with immediate decompression. Insert a 14G cannula into the second intercostal space in the mid-clavicular line. Follow this with insertion of a 28-36 Fr chest tube (C-T) into the fifth intercostal space between the anterior and mid-axillary line.

Open pneumothorax
- Occlude with a three-sided dressing.
- Follow by immediate insertion of a C-T through a separate incision.

Flail chest
- Results in paradoxical motion of the chest wall. Hypoxia is caused by restricted chest wall movement and underlying lung contusion.
- If segment is small and ventilation or oxygenation is not compromised, it is OK to closely observe with adequate analgesia (consider early thoracic epidural). Encourage early ambulation and vigorous physiotherapy. You may consider noninvasive positive-pressure ventilation.
- In more severe cases, endotracheal intubation with adequate PEEP is required.

Massive hemothorax
- Accumulation of more than 1500 mL of blood in pleural cavity
- Suspect this when shock is associated with dull percussion and absent breath sounds on one side of chest.
- Simultaneously restore blood volume and carry out decompression by inserting a 36-40 Fr C-T. Consider a second C-T if >300 cc is drained.
- The patient will need emergent thoracotomy to control bleeding if there is continued brisk bleeding, need for persistent blood transfusion, or persistent hypotension.

Cardiac tamponade
- Most commonly this results from penetrating injuries but can occur after blunt rupture of cardiac wall (right atrium > right vent >> left vent/atrium).
- Recognize by hemodynamic instability: hypotension, tachycardia, jugular venous distention, pulsus paradoxus, and faint heart sounds.
- The most sensitive and specific way to diagnose is with a pericardial view during FAST exam 95%–100% negative predictive value.

- Treatment is emergent surgical decompression and repair of cardiac injury (may consider pericardial window in the OR to confirm hemopericardium).
- The incision of choice for penetrating cardiac injury is median sternotomy

Management—secondary survey

Perform a further in-depth examination: in penetrating injuries, expose the patient fully and position them so that you can assess the front, back, and sides of the chest for any wounds missed in the primary survey.

Perform an erect chest X-ray, looking for the following injuries.

Simple pneumo- or hemothorax

Treat with a C-T if large or symptomatic.

Pulmonary contusion

There is a risk of worsening associated consolidation and local pulmonary edema. Treat with analgesia, physiotherapy, and oxygenation. Consider invasive or noninvasive respiratory support for a patient with significant hypoxia.

Tracheobronchial rupture

- Suspect this when there is a persistent large air leak or expanding subcutaneous emphysema after chest tube drainage.
- Thoracic CT scan and bronchoscopy are diagnostic.

Blunt cardiac injury (myocardial contusion or traumatic infarction)

- Normal initial 12-lead ECG effectively rules out significant contusion
- If the ECG is abnormal (the most common abnormality is sinus tachycardia), observe on telemetry x24 hr.
- If patient is unstable, perform echocardiogram.

Aortic disruption

- Suspect with history of decelerating force and evidence of mediastinal hematoma on chest X-ray (e.g., widened mediastinum >8 cm)
- Thoracic CT-angiogram is diagnostic.
- Consider initiation of IV short-acting beta-blocker followed by vasodilators to minimize dP/dT until definitive repair is done.
- Consider endovascular stenting vs open repair.

Diaphragmatic rupture

- Usually secondary to blunt trauma in restrained vehicle occupants (seat belt compression causes "burst" injury, most commonly on left side).
- Suspect in a patient with suitable history and raised left hemidiaphragm on chest X-ray.
- Penetrating trauma below the fifth intercostal space (roughly nipple-line) can injure the diaphragm.
- Thoracoabdominal CT scan can be diagnostic for large injuries.
- Penetrating small injures may require laparoscopy for diagnosis or repair.
- Treatment is primary repair with non-absorbable suture.
- Large defects may require prosthetic mesh.

Abdominal trauma

Key features

- Abdominal injuries are present in 7%–10% of trauma patients. These injuries, if unrecognized, can cause preventable deaths.
- Blunt trauma: the most frequent injuries are spleen (45%), liver (40%), and retroperitoneal hematoma (15%). Blunt trauma may cause
  - Compression or crushing, causing rupture of solid or hollow organs
  - Deceleration injury due to differential movement of fixed and non-fixed parts of organs causing tearing or avulsion from their vascular supply, e.g., liver tear and retrohepatic vena caval rupture.
- Blunt abdominal trauma is very common in MVCs in which
  - There have been fatalities.
  - Any casualty has been ejected from the vehicle.
  - Speed is greater than 35 mph.
- Penetrating trauma
  - Stab wounds cause damage by laceration or cutting. Stab wounds commonly involve the liver (40%), small bowel (30%), diaphragm (20%), and colon (15%).
  - Gunshot wounds transfer more kinetic energy, causing further injury by cavitation effect, tumble, and fragmentation. Commonly they involve the small bowel (50%), colon (40%), liver (30%), and vessels (25%).

Management—primary survey

- Any patient persistently hypotensive despite resuscitation for whom no obvious cause of blood loss has been identified by the primary survey can be assumed to have intra-abdominal bleeding.
- If the patient does not have an obvious operative indication, an abdominal or pelvic CT scan is routine in those with positive physical findings or who are unexaminable.

Management—secondary survey

History

- Obtain history from patient, other passengers, observers, police, and emergency medical personnel.
- Mechanism of injury: seat belt usage, steering wheel deformation, speed, damage to vehicle, ejection of victim, etc., in automobile collision; velocity, caliber, presumed path of bullet, distance from weapon, etc., in penetrating injuries
- Pre-hospital condition and treatment of patient

Physical examination

- Inspect anterior abdomen, which includes lower thorax, perineum, and log roll to inspect posterior abdomen. Look for abrasions, contusions, lacerations, penetrating wounds, distension, and evisceration of viscera.
- Palpate abdomen for tenderness, involuntary muscle guarding, rebound tenderness, and gravid uterus.
- Percuss to elicit subtle rebound tenderness.
- Assess pelvic stability.
- Conduct penile, perineum, rectal, or vaginal examinations, and examination of gluteal regions.

Investigations

Urinalysis
Frank hematuria may indicate bladder or kidney injury; microhematuria may indicate renal laceration.

Plain radiography
Supine chest X-ray is unreliable in the diagnosis of free intrabdominal air. Pelvic X-ray may demonstrate fractures.

Focused assessment sonography for trauma (FAST)
- Consists of imaging of the four Ps: pericardium, Morrison's pouch, perisplenic, and pouch of Douglas (or pelvic).
- FAST is used to identify the peritoneal cavity as a source of significant hemorrhage, with sensitivity of 85% and specificity of 100%.

Diagnostic peritoneal lavage
- Mostly superseded by FAST for unstable patients and CT scanning in stable patients. This procedure is useful when these modalities are inappropriate or unavailable, and for identification of the presence of free intraperitoneal fluid (usually blood).
- Aspiration of blood, gastrointestinal contents, bile, or feces through the lavage catheter indicates laparotomy; further lavage is not necessary (referred to as diagnostic peritoneal aspiration [DPA]).

Computerized tomography
- CT is the investigation of choice in hemodynamically stable patients in whom there is no apparent indication for an emergent laparotomy.
- It provides detailed information relative to specific organ injury and its extent and may guide conservative management.
- The tract of gunshot wounds can be easily visualized to assess penetration of thoracoabdominal cavities. (CT is not great at visualizing the extent of stab wounds, given the lack of cavitation.)

Local wound exploration
- Stab wounds may be explored in the emergency department (ED) with local anesthesia to assess depth (if it penetrates fascia, the patient must be observed, but you may consider exploration if exam is unreliable).
- If an adequate exploration does not demonstrate penetration of the abdominal wall, you may consider early discharge.

Indications for emergent laparotomy
- Blunt or penetrating abdominal trauma: unresponsive hypotension or transient responders.

Indications for urgent laparotomy
- Blunt trauma with CT features of solid-organ injury not suitable for conservative management
- Clinical features of peritonitis
- Any penetrating injury associated with visible viscera, clinical features of peritonitis or sepsis
- Most gunshot wounds that penetrate the abdomen will need a laparotomy; however, some physicians have considered close observation and serial abdominal exams for stable patients with reliable exams.

Vascular injuries

Key features

- Wounds that involve vascular structures of the extremity are a significant cause of morbidity and mortality in the traumatized patient.
- MVCs and falls are the most common causes of blunt injury.
- Stab wounds cause most of the upper-extremity vascular injuries, while gunshot wounds cause the majority of lower-extremity vascular injuries in penetrating vascular injury.
- Blunt trauma causes more morbidity than penetrating injuries because of associated fractures, dislocations, and crush injuries to muscles and nerves.

Management—primary survey

- Hemorrhage control is the **TOP PRIORITY**.
- Apply direct pressure to the open hemorrhaging wound.
- Limit fluid and blood resuscitation until definitive vascular control is achieved.
- A rapidly expanding hematoma suggests a significant vascular injury.
- Realign and splint any associated fracture. Immobilize dislocated joint.

Management—secondary survey

- Begin only after primary survey is complete and resuscitation is continuing successfully.
- Identify limb-threatening injuries.
- Look for hard or soft signs of vascular injury.
    - *Hard signs* are massive external blood loss, expanding or pulsatile hematoma, absent or diminished distal pulses, and a thrill or audible continuous murmur.
    - *Soft findings* are history of active bleeding at the scene, proximity of penetrating or blunt trauma to a major artery, small nonpulsatile hematoma, and neurological deficit.
- Measure distal systolic Doppler pressures of the injured arm or leg and compare with uninjured brachial systolic pressure. An index of <1.0 is a predictor of arterial injury.
- The presence of hard signs requires immediate operative intervention or arteriography.
- Intraoperative arteriography may help plan the operative approach.
- Some minimal arterial injuries can be managed nonoperatively.
- Embolization or endovascular stenting can be used to manage selected arterial injuries.

Principles of operative management

- Obtain proximal and distal control prior to exposing the injury.
- Inspect the injured vessel and debride as necessary.
- Remove intraluminal thrombus by using a Fogarty catheter.
- Flush lumen with heparinized normal saline solution.
- Consider temporary intraluminal shunting if the limb is ischemic and a delay of revascularization is anticipated (damage control or orthopedic fixation is required).

- Techniques used are lateral repair, patch angioplasty, end-to-end anastomosis, interposition graft, or bypass graft.
- Consider intraoperative completion arteriography.
- Ensure completed vascular repair is free of tension and covered with viable soft tissue.
- In patients with combined vascular and orthopedic injuries, perform intra-arterial shunting first to restore circulation, before orthopedic stabilization if the limb is ischemic. If the limb is not threatened it is O.K. to allow the orthopedic team to stabilize it prior to definitive vascular repair.
- Where there is massive soft tissue injury, debride all nonviable tissue.
- Anticipate development of compartment syndrome. Consider prophylactic fasciotomies to decompress all four compartments of the leg if warm ischemic time is >4 hr.
- Closely monitor limbs for compartment syndrome postoperatively if fasciotomies are not performed.

Head and spinal cord injuries

Causes and features

- The most common reasons for head injuries are falls, MVC, and assaults.
- About 80% of head injuries are mild, 10% are moderate, and 10% are severe.
- Up to half of the deaths from trauma under the age of 45 are due to a head injury.

Management—primary survey

- Maintain adequate oxygenation and BP. This avoids potentially devastating secondary brain injury.
- Maintain spine immobilization for blunt trauma.
- Determine consciousness level with the Glasgow Coma Scale (GCS; see Table 12.1).
- Provide definitive airway management in patients with a GCS ≤8.
- Avoid systemic analgesia or paralysis until a full neurological assessment is made.

Management—secondary survey

- Fully assess the head and neck.
  - Look for signs of basilar skull fractures (hemotympanum, "raccoon" eyes, CSF otorrhea or rhinorrhea, "battle signs")
  - Repeated monitoring of vital signs
  - Repeated assessment of conscious level (GCS).
- Penetrating injuries involving the spinal column but without neurodeficits are **not** unstable.
- Neurogenic shock is usually the result of a cord injury above T4 and manifested by hypotension and relative bradycardia. Treatment is volume resuscitation and vasopressors.

See also Box 12.1, Box 12.2, and Box 12.3.

Table 12.1 Glasgow Coma Scale*

Feature	Scale	Score
Eye opening (E)	No response	1
	In response to pain	2
	In response to speech	3
	Spontaneous	4
Motor response (M)	No response	1
	Extension (decerebrate)	2
	Abnormal flexion (decorticate)	3
	Withdrawal from pain	4
	Localizes pain	5
	Obeys commands	6
Verbal response (V)	No response	1
	Sounds	2
	Inappropriate words	3
	Confused sentences	4
	Orientated fully	5

* Minimum score, 3; maximum score, 15; if intubated score of 1 given for verbal and suffix *t* is added to total score (max score is 11t).

Box 12.1 Indications for CT scanning in head injuries

- GCS <13 at any point since the injury; GCS equal to 13 or 14 at 2 hr after the injury
- Suspected open or depressed skull fracture
- Any sign of basal skull fracture
- Post-traumatic seizure
- Focal neurological deficit
- More than one episode of vomiting
- Amnesia for >30 min, of events before impact
- Age ≥65 years, coagulopathy, or dangerous mechanism of injury, provided that some loss of consciousness or amnesia has been experienced

Box 12.2 Indications for neurosurgical referral in head injuries

- Major intracranial injury (epidural hematoma, moderate or large subdural hematoma, intracerebral hematoma)
- Progressive focal neurological signs
- Definite or suspected penetrating head injury
- A CSF leak or skull fracture
- Persisting coma (GCS ≤8) after initial resuscitation or deterioration in GCS score after admission

Box 12.3 Indications for admission in head injuries

- Patients with new, clinically significant abnormalities on imaging
- Patient has not returned to GCS = 15 after imaging, regardless of imaging results
- Patient fulfils criteria for CT scanning, but this cannot be done within the appropriate period because either CT is not available or the patient is not sufficiently cooperative to allow scanning
- Continued worrying signs, e.g., persistent vomiting, severe headaches
- Other sources of concern, e.g., drug or alcohol intoxication, other injuries, shock, suspected non-accidental injury, CSF leak

Plastic surgery

Jonathan M. Winograd, MD

Suturing wounds

Principles of wound closure

A wound can be closed in the following ways:
- Direct apposition of skin edges by sutures, glue, or staples
- Skin grafts (📖 p. 430)
- Tissue flaps (📖 p. 432)

Key facts

A correctly oriented incision, adequate hemostasis, and minimal tissue handling are prerequisites for an ideal scar. When closing wounds, bear in mind the following:
- All wounds leave scars; you must warn your patient of this.
- Hypertrophic scars are more likely on the sternal and deltoid regions and in areas that are subjected to shear and friction.
- Keloids are more likely on ears and the sternum.
- Speed of healing depends on site: the face heals more quickly than the trunk and limbs.
- Children and young adults heal more quickly and achieve stronger scars than the elderly, the chronically ill, and those on steroids.
- Stitch marks ("train tracks") are caused by epithelial growth into suture tracks and occur when sutures are left in longer than 7 days.
- Cross-hatching is more common when tight sutures cause ischemia.
- If sutures are removed too early the wound may dehisce, leaving a worse scar.

Suture techniques

- Eliminate dead space with deep sutures or a drain, but avoid suturing fat, which contributes no strength and may lead to fat necrosis.
- Consider buried, interrupted dermal sutures to reduce skin tension.
- Dermal sutures can be combined with a subcuticular running suture or skin tapes to avoid suture marks.
- Use the finest suture possible to maintain wound closure: 5/0 or 6/0 for the face; 4/0 or 5/0 for the hand; 2/0 to 4/0 for the trunk.
- Evert the wound; if it looks inverted, it will leave a depressed scar.
- Approximate wound edges without strangulating the skin.
- Dressings can be used to splint a wound or immobilize a limb during healing.
- Elevation will reduce postoperative swelling, bleeding, and pain.
- In a low-tension wound closure sutures may be removed at 5–7 days on the face, 7–10 days on the arm and anterior trunk, and 14 days on the back and lower limb.
- Most wounds benefit from being splinted with skin tape after removal of sutures.

Interrupted skin suture (Fig. 13.1a)
- Use fine-toothed Adson forceps or a skin hook to evert the skin.
- Pass the needle perpendicular to the skin through its full thickness.

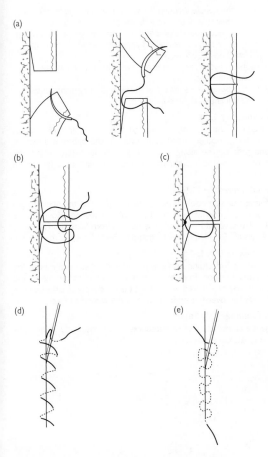

Fig.13.1 Types of suture. (a) Interrupted suture; (b) mattress suture; (c) deep dermal suture; (d) continuous suture; (e) subcuticular suture.

- Either remove the needle through the wound or continue in one sweep to the other side of the wound, using the forceps for counter-pressure so the needle passes perpendicular to the skin on its way out.
- Tie the knot so the skin edges are just apposed, bearing in mind the wound will swell postoperatively.
- Place the sutures evenly, approximately twice as far apart as they are from the wound margins.
- The distance between the suture and the wound margin should be similar to the thickness of the skin.

Mattress suture (Fig. 13.1b)

Pass the needle as above across the wound, then turn it around and pass it back as if doing another interrupted suture in the opposite direction. The second pass can be along the wound from the first (a horizontal mattress) or nearer the wound margin than the first pass (a vertical mattress suture).

Deep dermal suture (Fig. 13.1c)

Use the forceps or skin hook to evert the skin and pass the needle from deep to superficial on the dermal surface of the wound. Move to the other side of the wound and pass the needle from superficial to deep within the dermis. Tie a knot, which should be buried deep in the wound.

Subcuticular suture (Fig. 13.1d)

The suture is passed continuously within the dermis, usually near the dermoepidermal junction, from one end of the wound to the other, and pulled tight. It may be secured with a knot buried deeply at either end or with skin tapes laid over the suture ends and the wound surface.

Continuous suture (Fig. 13.1e)

This involves a combination of repeated interrupted-type sutures or inter-rupted, then mattress sutures.

Skin grafts

Definition

A **skin graft** is a piece of dermis and epidermis that is completely removed from its original bodily attachment (donor site). It is fixed to a recipient site and develops a new blood supply from underlying tissue.

- **Autograft**: transfer from one part of a person's body to another part
- **Isograft**: transfer between genetically identical individuals
- **Allograft**: transfer between individuals of the same species
- **Xenograft**: transfer between individuals of different species

Full-thickness skin grafts (Wolfe grafts) (Table 13.1)

- Contain epidermis plus the entire thickness of dermis
- Adnexal structures, e.g., hair, are included.
- Harvested by elliptical excision from sites of skin laxity, e.g., post-auricular skin crease, supraclavicular, preauricular, groin, or medial upper arm skin
- Graft is secured with a tie-over dressing, e.g., mineral oil-soaked soft cotton gauze wrapped in a nonadherent petrolatum-impregnated gauze, and inspected after a week.
- Donor site is sutured closed.

Split-thickness skin grafts (Thiersch grafts) (Table 13.1)

- Consist of epidermis plus a variable thickness of dermis
- Harvested by shaving off a layer of skin with a skin graft knife or dermatome. They can be taken from any area of the body (thigh skin is most often used, as it is plentiful and easy to access).
- The graft is often fenestrated (to stop blood or serous fluid collecting under it) or meshed (to expand the graft).
- The graft is secured with glue, sutures, or staples, then a nonadherent, compressive dressing. It is inspected after 5 days.
- Defect heals by re-epithelialization from epidermis within skin appendages in 2 weeks.

Graft healing

Stages of graft take

- Adherence (immediate): fibrin bond between graft and recipient bed
- Serum imbibition (days 0–4): graft absorbs fluid and nutrients from bed
- Revascularization (after day 4): blood enters the graft, either by flowing directly into the graft vessels (inosculation) or by new-vessel ingrowth (revascularization).

Reasons for graft failure

- Shearing: revascularization cannot occur if the graft is mobile.
- Infection of either the bed or the graft tissue
- Separation of graft from its bed by hematoma or seroma.
- Inadequate bed, e.g., bare cortical bone; tendon without paratenon
- Damage to the graft, e.g., poor surgical technique, excessive dressing pressure

Table 13.1 Split-thickness grafts versus full-thickness grafts

	Split skin graft	Full-thickness skin graft
Cosmesis	Thin, often hypertrophic scarring in graft	Good cosmesis, thicker
Contracture	Frequent, greatest with thin grafts	Rare
Availability	Plentiful; can reharvest after 14 days, at least twice per region	Limited by skin laxity and can never be reharvested
Take	Good—low metabolic needs and rapid take, 5–7 days	Needs optimal bed and take is slower, 7–14 days
Donor scar	Minimal—color change only, occasional hypertrophic scarring	Linear scar
Contraindications	Inadequate bed, e.g., exposed bone, tendon, cartilage (in which case flap is needed)	Large area to be covered
	Infected bed	Inadequate bed
	Areas where cosmesis is paramount	
	Functional requirements not adequately addressed with graft, e.g., area of the hand requiring movement	

Negative pressure dressings

These are dressings that apply negative pressure via a sponge placed in the wound cavity, covered with an airtight occlusive dressing, and connected to a vacuum pump. They increase the rate of granulation in a variety of wounds, including dehisced or infected sternotomy and laparotomy wounds, pressure sores, chronic open wounds, flaps, grafts, and burns. The dressing is changed every 48–72 hr. Exudate removed from the wound is collected in a disposable canister. Chronic wounds may heal completely with a negative pressure dressing by secondary intention. Alternatively, the negative pressure dressing may enhance wound granulation to the point where either a delayed primary closure or skin grafting may be possible. Please note that the V.A.C. name is proprietary to KCI and is not a generic term. The generic term is negative pressure dressing.

Surgical flaps

Definition

A **flap** is a unit of skin and other tissues that maintains its own blood supply while being transferred from donor to recipient site.

Classification of flaps (Fig. 13.2)

Blood supply

- *Random pattern.* Flaps survive on blood vessels in dermal and subdermal plexuses, which have no specific anatomical pattern. The length-to-breadth ratio is therefore limited.
- *Axial pattern.* At least one specific artery runs longitudinally within the flap, so the length-to-breadth ratio can be greatly increased. All composite flaps have an axial blood supply.

Transfer of local flaps

- *Advancement.* The base of the flap advances in the direction of the flap axis, e.g., V-Y flap of perianal skin into anal canal for anal stenosis.
- *Pivot.* Rotation or transposition. The flap rotates around a single pivot point, e.g., scalp rotation flap to cover a facial defect after tumor excision.
- *Interpolation.* The flap pedicle passes over or under adjacent skin to inset the flap into a nearby defect, e.g., paramedian forehead flap for nasal tip reconstruction.

Transfer of distant flaps

- *Direct.* Flap is moved directly to a nonadjacent area, e.g., cross finger flap.
- *Tubed.* Pedicle is curled inward to form a tube until the base of the flap is divided, e.g., tubed flap from upper arm for nose reconstruction.
- *Free.* Artery and vein to flap are completely divided, then reattached with microvascular anastomoses to a suitable artery and vein at the recipient site, e.g., radial forearm flap to release neck scar contracture.

Composition

- *Cutaneous.* Skin and subcutaneous tissue only, e.g., groin flap
- *Fasciocutaneous.* Includes deep fascia, making flap vascularity more reliable and allowing length-to-breadth ratio to be increased
- *Fascial or adipofascial.* The fascia (and subcutaneous fat) is transferred, but the skin, still attached, is replaced on the donor site, e.g., temporalis fascial flap. The transposed flap can then be skin grafted.
- *Muscle.* Useful for infected or traumatic wounds. The flap is skin grafted, e.g., gastrocnemius flap for exposed knee prostheses.
- *Myocutaneous.* Used in reconstructive surgery. The muscle carries the blood supply to the skin, e.g., latissimus dorsi myocutaneous flap.
- *Perforator flaps.* Modified myocutaneous flaps. A single artery and vein are dissected from skin, through muscle, to the parent vessels. The muscle is left at the donor site, so its function is retained.
- *Bone, osseocutaneous.* Bone with or without skin, e.g., fibular flap for reconstruction of mandible. Muscle may also be included.

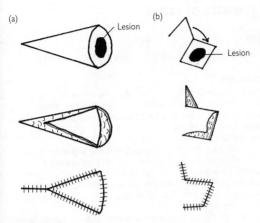

Fig.13.2 Types of random cutaneous flaps. (a) V-Y flap; (b) rhomboid flap.

Management of scars

Definition

A **scar** is an area of fibrous connective tissue, produced by healing.

Clinical features

A normal scar is initially flat and pale, then becomes red, itchy, and raised. Over months to years it settles back to a flat, pale, slightly shiny patch. Scarring is more pronounced if infection intervenes during healing, or in the presence of foreign bodies.

There are several types of abnormal scar.

- *Hypertrophic scars* are firm, red, itchy, and elevated above the skin surface, but within the boundaries of the injury. They are more common over presternal and deltoid regions, and regress with time.
- *Keloid scars* extend beyond wound boundaries. They do not regress spontaneously, and are painful and itch. They are common in dark skins, and in sites as above.
- *Stretched scars* are due to dehiscence of dermis under intact epidermis. They are common on the back and in areas of tension.
- *Scar contractures* are common over flexor surfaces of a joint. They occur when wounds heal by secondary intention, after spilt skin grafting, or when incisions cross a joint perpendicular to the flexion crease.

Treatment

Treatment aims to improve poor cosmesis, relieve local symptoms (pain, itch, irritation), or reduce restriction of associated joint movement.

Medical and conservative treatment

- *Observation.* "Benign neglect"
- *Massage.* The scar achieves a flat, pale state more quickly. Relieves itch.
- *Pressure.* Pressure garments are used for large areas, e.g., skin-grafted burns. Pressure devices, e.g., clip earrings for earlobe keloids, are also used. They are worn continuously until scars mature. Pressure reduces hypertrophy and contracture.
- *Silicone gel.* A sheet of gel tape is worn on the scar, up to 24 hr/day if tolerated. It reduces hypertrophy and relieves itch.
- *Lasers.* Pulsed dye lasers are used to reduce redness and hypertrophy. Carbon dioxide laser resurfaces depressed scars.
- *Intralesional injections.* Steroids and cytotoxics (e.g., bleomycin, 5-FU) reduce excess collagen formation; they are used to flatten hypertrophic and keloid scars and reduce pain and itch. Patients usually need repeated injections at 1- to 2-month intervals.
- *Radiotherapy* is occasionally given immediately postoperatively to wounds in patients known to be prone to hypertrophic or keloid scaring.

Surgical treatment

- *Excision and closure* is used for a stretched scar or a scar with "railroad tracks." Scars usually restretch to some extent. Keloid or hypertrophic scars are likely to recur if excised, and may be much larger than the original scar. Keloids should only be excised in combination with an intraoperative or postoperative course of steroid injections.
- *Z-plasty* (Fig. 13.3a) lengthens the scar. It can reorientate the scar into lines of relaxed skin tension, or break up the line of the scar and make it less noticeable.
- *W-plasty* (Fig. 13.3b) breaks up the line of the scar. It is used on scalp to avoid a hairless linear scar.
- *Scar release and resurfacing* is used when Z-plasty is inadequate for scar release, either because there is insufficient laxity adjacent to the contracture or adjacent skin is of poor quality. Resurfacing may include skin grafting, local flaps, or free tissue transfer.

(a)　　　　(b)

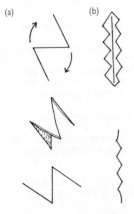

Fig.13.3 Surgical techniques for managing scars. (a) Z-plasty; (b) W-plasty.

Excision of simple cutaneous lesions

Planning

- Under good light, and before infiltration of anesthesia, mark the borders of the lesion. Mark the appropriate margin of excision: 2–5 mm for basal cell carcinoma (BCC); 4–20 mm for squamous cell carcinoma (SCC); 1–2 mm for biopsy of a pigmented lesion.
- Incision biopsies should include a border of the lesion and normal skin.
- For direct closure, convert the excision to an ellipse by using lines of relaxed skin tension as the long axis once the excision has allowed for tissue relaxation. Be guided by wrinkles and line of hair growth (hair generally grows in the direction of relaxed skin tension lines [RSTLs]).
- Wedge excisions are used on the borders of the ear, eyelid, and lip. Circular excisions are used where there is little skin laxity, using flaps or grafts to close the defect.

Anesthesia

- Calculate the maximum safe dose for your patient before you start infiltrating (📖 p. 572).
- Consider a mixture of bupivacaine 0.25% with lidocaine 1% to provide longer-acting anesthesia.
- Use of epinephrine with the infiltration reduces intraoperative bleeding and is safe even near anatomically "end" arteries (e.g., the digital arteries, penile artery) as long as there is no critical ischemia present already from trauma or arterial occlusive disease.
- In the face, nerve blocks (e.g., mental, infraorbital, supraorbital, and supratrochlear) may reduce the pain of infiltration, the volume of anesthetic needed, and distortion of the tissues by the anesthetic fluid.
- Check to ensure the anesthetic is working before starting excision.

Shave excision

This is used for benign, nonpigmented nevi and seborrheic keratoses. Use a number 10 blade to cut horizontally across the lesion at mid-dermal level.

Excision

- Be aware of underlying structures (e.g., the frontal branch of the temporal nerve when excising lesions from the temple). Ask your assistant to stretch the skin.
- Use a size 15 blade on the face; consider a larger size 10 blade on the thicker skin of the back.
- Cut the margins of the lesion perpendicular to the skin—this will aid closure.
- Cut away from the corners of the wound to avoid X-shaped overcuts. Cut the lower edge before the upper one—blood trickling down may obscure your view.
- Lift one corner of the lesion gently with a skin hook or fine-toothed (Adson's) forceps, and cut along the base of the lesion in horizontal lines at the level of the subcutaneous fat. Avoid traumatic handling of the lesion, which may compromise histological analysis.

- Perform accurate hemostasis.
- Close and dress the wound.

Postoperative care

- All lesions should be sent for histological analysis, clearly labeled (if necessary, with a marking stitch for orientation). **S**hort stitch, **s**uperior; **l**ong stitch, **l**ateral is a simple system to remember.
- Elevate the wound.
- Keep the wound dry until the skin is healed.
- Acetominophen, ibuprofen, and codeine are suitable analgesics; aspirin is best avoided because of the risk of bleeding.
- Patients should not drive on the day of surgery if the amount of discomfort will be a distraction and thus a safety hazard.

Burns—assessment

❶ Assessment and management of burns go hand in hand and are simultaneous in practice. They have been divided here only for ease of reading.

Causes

Most burns are due to flame or contact with hot surfaces; scalds are more common in children and the elderly. Chemical, electrical, irradiation, and friction burns are rare.

History

- Find out the exact mechanism, including temperature of water, duration of contact, concentration of chemical, or voltage.
- Record factors suggesting inhalation injury, e.g., burns in a confined space, flash burns.
- Inquire about other injuries.
- Document first aid given so far.
- Document timing of (1) injury, (2) first aid, and (3) resuscitation.

Examination

Estimate area of burn (see Box 13.1)
Do not include areas of unblistered erythema.

- Use the rule of nines (Fig. 13.4).
- Patient's hand is approximately 1% total body surface area (TBSA).
- The Lund and Browder chart (Fig. 13.5) is the most accurate method.
- Subtract % unburned skin from 100% to check calculation.
- Draw a picture, ideally, filling in the Lund and Browder chart.

Box 13.1 Estimating depth of burn

- *Epidermal*: erythema only
- *Superficial dermal*: pink, wet or blistered, sensate, blanches, refills
- *Deep dermal*: blotchy red, wet or blistered, no blanching, insensate
- *Full thickness*: white or charred, leathery, no blanching, insensate

Signs of inhalation injury

- Singed nasal hair
- Burns to face or oropharynx. Look for blistered palate.
- Sooty sputum
- Drowsiness or confusion due to carbon monoxide inhalation
- Respiratory effort, breathlessness, stridor, and hoarseness are signs of impending airway obstruction and require immediate intubation.

Features of non-accidental burn injury
Refer patient to pediatric burn unit if abuse is suspected in a child. Features include the following:
- Delayed presentation
- History inconsistent or not compatible with injury
- Other signs of trauma
- Suspicious pattern of injury, e.g., cigarette burns, bilateral "stocking" or "glove" patterns, genital involvement consistent with forced immersion. It is very rare for even the youngest child not to immediately react defensively and protect body parts when being burned or scalded.

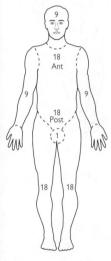

Fig. 13.4 Rule of nines.

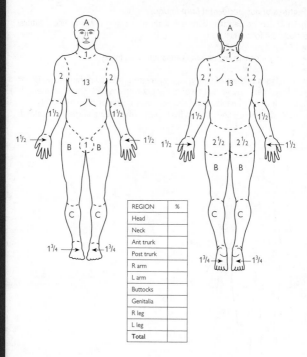

REGION	%
Head	
Neck	
Ant trunk	
Post trunk	
R arm	
L arm	
Buttocks	
Genitalia	
R leg	
L leg	
Total	

AREA	0	1	5	10	15	Adult
A = $\frac{1}{2}$ of head	$9\frac{1}{2}$	$8\frac{1}{3}$	$6\frac{1}{2}$	$5\frac{1}{2}$	$4\frac{1}{2}$	$3\frac{1}{2}$
B = $\frac{1}{2}$ of one thigh	$2\frac{3}{4}$	$3\frac{1}{4}$	4	$3\frac{1}{2}$	$3\frac{1}{2}$	$4\frac{3}{4}$
C = $\frac{1}{2}$ of one lower leg	$2\frac{1}{2}$	$2\frac{1}{2}$	$2\frac{3}{4}$	3	$3\frac{1}{4}$	$3\frac{1}{2}$

Fig. 13.5 Lund and Browder chart.

Burns: management

Immediate first aid

- Stop the burning process (do not endanger yourself).
- Cool the wound: use running water at 8°–25°C for 20 min except for some chemical burns.

Resuscitation

A. Airway maintenance with C-spine control. Intubate if there is suspected inhalation injury; airway edema can be rapidly fatal.
B. Breathing and ventilation
C. Circulation with hemorrhage control
D. Disability and neurological status
E. Exposure and environmental control
F. Fluid resuscitation: child, >10% TBSA; adult, >15% TBSA burned

- Start two peripheral IV lines, as large caliber as possible, preferably through unburned skin.
- Send blood for CBC, SMA 7, clotting, amylase, carboxyhemoglobin.
- Give 4 mL Ringers lactate solution/kg/%TBSA burned. Half of this is given over the first 8 hr following injury, half over the next 16 hr.
- Children also need maintenance fluid.
- Monitor resuscitation with urinary catheter (aim for urine output >1 mL/kg/hr).
- Consider ECG, pulse, BP, respiratory rate, pulse oximetry, and arterial blood gases (ABGs).

Perform secondary survey.

Referral to a burn unit (see Box 13.2)

Intubate patient before transfer if inhalation injury is suspected. Give humidified 100% oxygen to all patients. Wash the burn and cover with topical antibiotic and burn dressing. Give IV morphine analgesia. Place a nasogastric tube. Give tetanus prophylaxis if required.

Box 13.2 Criteria for referral to a burn unit

- >10% TBSA burn in adult; >5% TBSA in child
- Burns to face, hands, feet, perineum, genitalia, major joints
- Full thickness burns >5% TBSA
- Electrical or chemical burns
- Associated inhalation injury – always intubate before transfer
- Circumferential burns of limbs or chest
- Burns in very young or old, or patients with significant comorbidity
- Any burn associated with major trauma

Management of the burn wound

- Superficial dermal burns will heal without scarring within 2 weeks as long as infection does not deepen the burn.
- For small burns, outpatient treatment with simple, nonadherent dressings and twice-weekly wound inspection is sufficient.
- Wash burns with normal saline or chlorhexidine.
- Debride large blisters. Elevate limbs to reduce pain and swelling.
- Dress hands in plastic bags to allow mobilization.
- Topical silver sulfadiazine is used on deep burns to reduce risk of infection (but should not be applied until the patient has been reviewed by burns unit staff, as it makes depth difficult to assess).

Escharotomy

This is performed for circumferential full-thickness burns to the chest that limit ventilation or to the limbs that limit circulation. Loss of pulses or sensation is a late sign. In the early stages, pain at rest or on passive movements of distal joints indicates ischemia. Patients may also need fasciotomies if compartment syndrome is present, particularly in electrical injuries.

Excision and skin grafting

This procedure is performed for deep dermal or full-thickness burns that are too large to heal rapidly by secondary intention.

Electrical injuries

- *Low voltage* (<1000 V). Domestic electrical supply. Causes local contact wounds but no deep injury. It may cause cardiac arrest.
- *High voltage* (>1000 V). High-tension cables, power stations, lightning. Voltage at this level causes cutaneous and deep tissue damage with entry and exit wounds.
- Order ECG on admission for all injuries; continuous cardiac monitoring is required for 24 hr for significant injuries.
- In high-voltage injury, muscle damage may require fasciotomy. Deep injury is often far greater than suggested by external entry and exit sites.
- Myoglobinuria can cause renal failure: urine output >75–100 mL/hr. Alkalinization of the urine may be necessary.

Chemical burns

Treat with copious lavage for at least 30 min until all of the chemical has been removed and skin pH is normal.

- *Acid* causes coagulative necrosis; it penetrates skin rapidly, but is easily removed.
- *Alkali* (includes common household chemicals and cement) causes liquefactive necrosis, so it needs longer irrigation (>1 hr).
- *Hydrofluoric acid.* Fluoride ions penetrate burned skin, causing liquefactive necrosis and decalcification. A 2% TBSA burn can be fatal.
  - Irrigate with water.
  - Trim fingernails.
  - Topical calcium gluconate gel, 10%.
  - Give local injection of 10% calcium gluconate.
  - Start IV calcium gluconate.
  - The patient may need urgent excision of burn.
- *Elemental Na, K, Mg, Li.* Do not irrigate initially: they ignite in water. Cover in oil, remove pieces, then wash with water.
- *Phosphorus.* Irrigate with water, then debride particles, which will otherwise continue to burn. Apply copper sulphate, which turns particles black so they are easier to identify.
- *Bitumen.* Burns by heat; treat by cooling with water. Remove cold bitumen with peanut or paraffin oil.
- *Tar.* Burns by heat and phenol toxicity. Treat by cooling with water; remove with toluene.

Soft tissue hand injuries

History

- Mechanism of injury
- Dominant hand, occupation, hobbies
- Medical and smoking history, previous hand injuries, social history

Examination

Use local anesthetic block if needed for pain (check sensation first).

Look

Examine posture of hand and digits. Locate site of laceration(s) and tissue loss.

Feel

Check perfusion of hand and digits, pulses, as well as sensation in distribution of radial, ulnar, median, and digital nerves. Determine if there is pain over bones.

Move

- Long extensors extend metacarpophalangeal joints (MCPJs).
- Extensor pollicis longus (EPL) extends the thumb dorsal to plane of hand (i.e., up off a table).
- Flexor digitorum profundus (FDP) tendons flex distal interphalangeal joints (DIPJs). Isolate DIPJ by holding other finger joints in extension.
- Flexor digitorum superficialis (FDS) tendons flex proximal interphalangeal joints (PIPJs). Isolate FDS by holding all digits except the one under examination extended.
- Testing wrist flexors and extensors is unreliable as finger flexors and extensors may mimic function, but pain on movement suggests injury.
- Examine intrinsics, hypothenar, and thenar muscles, particularly abductor pollicis brevis (supplied by the median nerve) and abductor digiti minimi (ulnar nerve).
- Check stability of joints. Pain or abnormal movement on lateral deviation suggests collateral ligament damage.

Investigations

Obtain X-ray for fractures or foreign bodies. Review X-ray for suspected collateral ligament injuries before testing stability. Take photographs.

Treatment

- *Finger pulp injury.* Debride under tourniquet. If there is no bone exposed, it will heal by secondary intention. Exposed bone may need shortening or a local flap.
- *Subungual hematoma* is a painful bruise under the nail. Trephine nail with sterile needle to evacuate hematoma.
- *Nailbed injury* often occurs with distal phalanx (DP) fracture. Remove nail under tourniquet, irrigate wound, and repair nail bed with absorbable 7/0 suture using loupe magnification. Replace fenestrated nail as splint for eponychial fold.

- *Mallet finger.* Immobilize in a Stack splint for 6–8 weeks unless a large bony fragment is present, which may require fixation.
- *Foreign bodies.* Remove organic matter and painful foreign bodies.
- *Lacerations and puncture wounds*
  - Always explore with anesthetic and tourniquet to determine underlying structural damage.
  - Irrigate wounds and debride as necessary.
  - Tetanus prophylaxis
  - Amoxicillin/clavulanic acid for bites
  - Repair tendons, ideally primarily. Postoperative regimes typically involve splinting for 3 to 6 weeks, and 12 weeks without heavy lifting. Early motion protocols are instituted for tendon repairs under ideal conditions and allow for better functional outcomes, particularly for flexor tendon injuries in zone 2 (within the tendon sheath proximal to the insertion of the FDS tendon).
  - Repair nerves under magnification. Axonal regeneration progresses at 1 mm/day after 1 month from the time of repair.
  - Thoroughly irrigate open joints against the risk of septic arthritis. Collateral ligaments may need to be repaired, and are splinted for ~2–4 weeks post-repair.
- *Complications* include hematoma, infection, tendon or ligament rupture, stiffness, painful scars, neuroma, complex regional pain syndrome, scar contracture, and cold sensitivity.

Hand infections

Causes and features

Such infections are usually caused by penetrating injury (which may seem insignificant) or a bite. Hematogenous spread of infection (e.g., gonorrhea, septic emboli from endocarditis) to the hand is rare.

- *Infecting organisms.* After penetrating injury, *Staphylococcus aureus* is the most common, followed by streptococci. Human bites are often also contaminated with *Eikenella corrodens*. Viruses (hepatitis B and C, HIV) are rarely transmitted. *Pasteurella* spp. are common in infected cat and, less commonly, dog bites.
- *Paronychia* is infection of the nailfold. Acute infections are usually *Staphylococcus aureus*. *Candida albicans* causes chronic paronychia and may require excision of crescent of epinychium and topical antifungals. *Herpes simplex* causes whitlow with vesicles or bullae around the nail, but no pus. Multiple fingers may be involved. Avoid surgery in these cases.
- *Felon* is finger pulp infection. The fibrous septae must be divided to allow for egress of pus from within the pad with any drainange procedure.
- *Palmar space infection.* There are four fascial compartments in the palm (web space, hypothenar, mid-palm, and thenar). They usually confine infection initially. Pain, swelling, and reduced movement are features. Swelling is often more prominent on the dorsal surface of the hand.
- *Flexor sheath infection.* Kanavel's four cardinal signs are flexed posture of finger, pain on passive extension, fusiform swelling, and pain along the flexor sheath. Infection often requires continuous saline irrigation for 24–48 hr post-drainage after operative drainage of the sheath.
- *Bites* have a high risk of infection, so always irrigate, give antibiotic prophylaxis (amoxicillin/clavulanic acid), and refer patient for surgical exploration if there is no improvement within 24–48 hr.

Treatment

Delay can be disastrous, resulting in stiffness, contracture, and pain. Early cellulitis (24–48 hr after onset) may be treated by elevation, splinting, and antibiotics. Any collection of pus must be drained urgently.

Initial treatment

- Tetanus prophylaxis if indicated
- Elevation and splinting
- Start IV ampicillin/clavulanic acid, unless patient is allergic to penicillin, until sensitivities of infecting organisms are known.
- A plain X-ray may be useful to exclude associated fractures, foreign bodies, underlying osteomyelitis, and evidence of gas-forming infection.

Surgical treatment

- Use a tourniquet, but elevate rather than exsanguinate the limb.
- Send pus swabs and tissue samples for culture.
- Debride and irrigate wounds; fully explore pockets of pus.
- Leave wound open for delayed primary closure.

Postoperative care
- Continue elevation.
- Daily saline soaks or irrigation of the wound
- Splint for comfort with the wrist extended, MCPJs flexed, and interphalangeal joints (IPJs) extended. Mobilize hand with aid of physiotherapists.
- Give antibiotics until infection is resolved.

Dupuytren's disease

Key facts

This disease is a progressive thickening of the superficial palmar and digital fascia that may lead to contractures. The etiology is unknown, but there is a higher incidence among relatives of affected patients. Associated conditions include diabetes and epilepsy. Alcoholism, TB, HIV, hand trauma, and tobacco use have all also been implicated, although less clearly. Incidence is 1%–3% of northern Europeans, but it is uncommon in Africa and Asia. Incidence increases with age.

Pathogenesis

- The disease is classified by Luck into three phases: proliferative, involutional, and residual.
- In the proliferative phase, immature fibroblasts, many of which are myofibroblasts, produce extracellular matrix containing type IV collagen. This resembles a healing wound histologically.
- Mechanical tension appears to play a role in contractures.

Clinical features

- Thickened palmar and digital fascia forms nodules and cords.
- The condition progresses to contractures of the MCPJs and PIPJs of the affected rays.
- It tends to affect digits in order: ring, little, thumb, middle, index.
- Normal fascia is referred to as *bands*; diseased bands are called *cords*.
- A spiral cord may be a feature, wrapping around the neurovascular bundle (NVB) and displacing it to the midline and superficially, putting it at risk during surgery.
- The disease affects longitudinal fascial structures; the transverse palmar fascia is never involved and provides a landmark for dissecting NVBs.

Extrapalmar manifestations

- Garrod's pads: thickening over dorsal aspect of PIPJs
- Peyronie's disease: thickened plaques in the shaft of the penis
- Lederhosen's disease: thickened plantar fascia, but no contractures

Treatment

Indications for surgery

- >30° fixed flexion contracture at MCPJ, or any PIPJ contracture. Also any rapidly progressing contracture. Results are better for release of MCPJs than of PIPJs.
- Table-top test: surgery is indicated when the hand will not lie flat on the table.
- Pain in nodules or Garrod's patches: injection with steroid, or excision.

Many people with Dupuytren's disease never require surgery.

Surgical considerations
Skin

Typical incisions include the following:
- Linear incisions with Z-plasties
- Bruner incisions
- Multiple V-to-Y incisions
- Lazy "S" incisions
- Transverse palmar incision with longitudinal extensions
- Multiple short, curved incisions.
- Multiple Z-plasties may be used for operations requiring less access.

Closure may be direct, with skin grafts (split or full thickness), or with the palm left open to heal by secondary intention.

Fascia

This may be incised (fasciotomy) or excised (fasciectomy).
- Radical fasciectomy removes the entire palmar fascia (this is no longer recommended).
- Regional or limited fasciectomy removes only the diseased fascia.
- Segmental fasciectomy excises sections of the diseased fascia.
- Fasciotomy via a percutaneous approach using a needle provides temporary relief from contracture.
- Dermofasciectomy, or excision of fascia with overlying skin, is used for severe skin involvement and when the risk of recurrence is high.
- Collagenase injection for aid with cord rupture is currently in clinical trials with good reports of success.

Joint contractures

Release of fascia usually resolves contracture at the MCPJ. Fixed flexion at the PIPJ is more difficult to release. Consider releasing the check-rein and accessory collateral ligaments. DIPJs are rarely involved except in recurrent disease.

Postoperative care

The affected fingers are splinted in extension and active exercises begun in the first week, unless a skin graft has been used. Night splints are used for at least 3 months and may included dynamic extension splints.

Complications
- *Early*: damage to neurovascular structures (1%–3%), PIPJ hyperextension, hemorrhage
- *Intermediate*: infection, skin flap necrosis
- *Late*: complex regional pain syndrome; recurrence (25% of patients treated surgically will need further surgery for Dupuytren's disease)

Treatment of recurrence

Recurrence may be treated by repeat surgery, although this tends to be less successful and more extensive at each event. Amputation of a fixed flexed digit is occasionally an option, particularly if the digit hampers work or leisure activities.

Breast reduction

The aim is to reduce the volume and weight of the hypertrophied breast, while maintaining a blood supply to the nipple and creating an aesthetically pleasing breast.

Indications

- Neck, back, or shoulder pain
- Indentation of shoulder skin by bra straps (grooving)
- Persistent infections or soreness in the inframammary crease
- Restriction in activity, especially sport.
- Inability to find clothes that fit
- Psychological: embarrassment, low self-esteem

Operative considerations

Blood supply to the nipple

In order to lift the nipple, skin around it is de-epithelialized or excised. The base of the nipple is left attached to a mound of breast parenchyma (the pedicle) through which its blood supply travels. Because of the rich vascular anastamoses in the breast, numerous techniques are possible. Pedicles can be based inferiorly, superiorly, superomedially, laterally, or centrally. Alternatively, the nipple can be removed before the breast is reduced and replaced as a full-thickness graft. Nipple grafting is performed in breasts with extremely long pedicles with questionable nipple perfusion.

Skin excision and scars

An anchor shape (Wise pattern) excision leaves an inverted T-shaped scar. It runs around the areola, vertically down to the inframammary fold, and horizontally along the fold. Other options include periareolar incision only or periareolar incision with a vertical scar. These techniques limit the amount of breast tissue that can be resected. L-shaped and horizontal scar techniques are also possible but are more rarely used.

Postoperative care

The patient usually stays in the hospital overnight. She should wear a supportive bra and avoid heavy lifting for 4–6 weeks postoperatively.

Complications

- *Early*: Hematoma, infection, altered nipple sensation, skin loss or necrosis, fat necrosis, delayed wound healing, asymmetry
- *Late*: Unsightly scar, inability to breast-feed, pseudoptosis ("bottoming out"), recurrence (if done before breast is fully grown)

Most patients are nonetheless happy with the result, even if they do suffer complications.

Breast augmentation

The aim is to enhance breast size by placing an artificial implant beneath the breast.

Indications

This is performed for psychological reasons, e.g., self-consciousness or correction of asymmetry, either congenital or acquired. Inadequate breast volume may be due to hypoplasia, or to involution following childbirth or menopause.

Operative considerations

Incision

- *Inframammary fold*. Gives good visualization of the implant pocket, but leaves a visible scar
- *Peri-areolar*. Semicircular incision at the border of the areola. The scar fades well but access is limited. This approach is more likely to alter nipple sensation.
- *Transaxillary*. Eliminates scars on breast. Limited access is improved by using an endoscope.
- *Transumbilical*. Only used for saline-filled implants, inserted along a tunnel created superficial to rectus sheath. Endoscopy confirms position of the implant pocket. The implant is inflated once it is in position.

Position of implant

- *Submammary*. Under the normal breast
- *Subpectoral*. Under the pectoralis major (slightly less obvious upper border in the thin; has lower rate of capsular contracture but may move when the pectoralis contracts)

Type of implant

- *Size*. Depends on patient's choice
- *Shape*. Round implants are low or high profile (depending on how much they project forward); anatomical implants are teardrop shaped.
- *Shell*. Implants are made of a silicone shell that is smooth or textured. Textured implants have lower rates of capsular contracture but are typically less mobile within the implant pocket.
- *Implant filling*. Saline-filled implants allow for fine adjustment of volume, and can be filled or emptied postoperatively. Silicone gel–filled implants feel more like normal breast tissue. There is no current evidence to support implication in autoimmune diseases.

Postoperative care

- This is usually an outpatient procedure.
- A supportive bra is worn and heavy lifting avoided for 4–6 weeks.

Complications

- *Early*: Hematoma, infection, nerve injury (altering sensation to the nipple), incorrect position of implant.
- *Late*: Capsular contracture, rupture, or deflation; silicone gel bleed.
- Implants have a limited lifespan, up to about 20 years. The likelihood is that they will need to be removed or replaced at some time. Patients usually can breast-feed after augmentation. Patients are warned that mammography is technically more difficult, requiring different views.

Breast reconstruction

Aims
The principle aim is to recreate a breast mound resembling the contralateral breast, with minimal donor deficit, using a technique appropriate for the patient. After mastectomy, breast reconstruction is of psychological benefit. It is technically easier to perform it at the same time as mastectomy rather than as a delayed procedure, as there is no scarring in the site and original landmarks are present. It also reduces the number of operations required. However, there may be logistical difficulties if a combined breast surgery and plastic surgery team is needed. Also, some patients prefer to wait.

Surgical options
Tissue expander
The expander is placed in the subpectoral position and inflated with saline once the wounds are healed (2–4 weeks postoperatively) via a subcutaneous port. The skin is slowly stretched until a satisfactory size is reached. The implant can later be changed for a silicone gel–filled implant.

Latissimus dorsi myocutaneous flap
This is a pedicled flap based on the thoracodorsal vessels. The latissimus dorsi muscle, with an ellipse of overlying skin and fat, is tunneled under the intervening skin bridge into the breast defect. Depending on the size of the contralateral breast, an implant may be used under the flap.

Abdominal flaps
The transverse rectus abdominis myocutaneous (TRAM) flap consists of a transverse ellipse of skin on the lower abdomen, plus one of the two rectus abdominis muscles. This versatile flap may be based on either its upper (deep superior epigastric) or lower (deep inferior epigastric) vascular pedicles. The upper pedicle is used as a pedicled flap, tunneled under the abdominal skin into the breast. The lower pedicle is used as a free tissue transfer. If a sizeable muscular perforator vessel or group of vessels is identified, a deep inferior epigastric perforator (DIEP) flap can be used, leaving the muscle behind. This flap is usually large enough not to need an implant. A separate flap, based on the superficial inferior epigastric artery (SIEA), a branch of the femoral artery, can occasionally be used as the pedicle for a free tissue transfer of the abdominal adipose tissue and skin in this region. It does not require an incision in the abdominal fascia or the use of any muscle tissue. It is usually limited to the tissue on the ipsilateral side of the abdominal midline.

Nipple reconstruction
At a later stage, the reconstructed breast can be tattooed with a picture of a nipple, or a nipple formed with a combination of local flaps, skin graft, and grafts from the contralateral nipple.

Surgery to the contralateral breast
The opposite breast may be reduced, augmented, or lifted to improve symmetry.

Cardiothoracic surgery

Karen M. Kim, MD
Thomas E. MacGillivray, MD

Six common calls to the cardiothoracic ICU

Box 14.1 Atrial fibrillation (AF)

- Assess hemodynamic stability
- If patient is unstable (SBP <80 mmHg), perform synchronized cardioversion
- Physical exam: assess heart sounds, breath sounds, jugular venous distension
- Obtain chest X-ray, ABG, and ECG to assess mitigating causes (pneumothorax, volume overload, effusion, hypoxemia, acidosis, anemia, electrolyte imbalance, ischemia)
- Give KCl (10–20 mEq via central venous line) to maintain serum K^+ 4.5–5.0 mEq/dL
- Give magnesium sulfate 2 g IV
- Rate control with IV propranolol 1 mg q3–5 min and IV digoxin 0.25 mg q4hr for total dose 1.25 mg over 24 hr
- For refractory AF, give amiodarone 150 mg IV bolus (may repeat) followed by 1 mg/hr infusion for 24 hr

Box 14.2 Bleeding

- Get immediate help if chest drainage is >500 mL over 30 min
- Start fluid resuscitation (normal saline, lactated Ringer's, 5% albumin) to maintain CVP >10 mmHg, mean PAP >20 mmHg, SBP >100 mmHg
- Check Hb/Hct, platelets, PT, PTT, and fibrinogen
- Send for blood products: 4 units PRBC, 4 units FFP, 10 units platelets
- Give empiric protamine 25 mg IV
- Treat ongoing coagulopathic bleeding with transfusions to achieve Hb >8 g/dL, platelets >100,000/mm³, PTT <40 sec, fibrinogen >150 mg/dL
- Re-exploration for excessive bleeding (>500 mL/hr for 1 hr, >400 mL/hr for 2 hr, >300 mL/hr for 3 hr, >200 mL/hr for 4 hr)
- Abrupt cessation of bleeding is concerning for cardiac tamponade (assess clinically, check chest X-ray and echocardiogram)

Box 14.3 Hypotension

- Assess ABCs: **A**irway, **B**reathing, and **C**irculation
- Rate and rhythm management (defibrillation for VF/VT, atrial pacing for HR <90, atrioventricular pacing if AV block, treat AF as in Box 14.1, rapid atrial overdrive pacing for atrial flutter)
- If there is poor perfusion (cool periphery, low urine output <1 mL/kg/hr, metabolic acidosis), treat for low cardiac output (see Box 14.4)
- If patient is warm and well-perfused and has normal to high cardiac output (vasodilation), titrate vasopressors (norepinephrine, vasopressin, phenylephrine) to maintain MAP >65 mmHg, SBP >100 mmHg

Box 14.4 Low cardiac output

- Cardiac index (CI) <2.0 L/min/m^2
- Check ABCs
- Rate and rhythm management (defibrillation for VF/VT, atrial pacing for HR <90, atrioventricular pacing if AV block, treat AF as in Box 14.1, rapid atrial overdrive pacing for atrial flutter)
- Raise CVP >10 mmHg, mean PAP >20 mmHg with crystalloid (normal saline, lactated Ringer's) or 5% albumin
- Assess for tamponade, pneumothorax, ischemia
- Mixed venous oxygen saturation should be >60%
- Start milrinone 0.5 µg/kg/min or dopamine 2–5 µg/kg/min
- Insert intra-aortic balloon pump
- Consider ventricular assist device

Box 14.5 Impaired oxygenation or ventilation

- Get immediate help if O$_2$ saturation <85%
- Increase FIO$_2$ to 100% temporarily
- Check accuracy of O$_2$ sat probe
- Check position and patency of endotracheal tube (ETT)
- Assess for bilateral chest excursion, equal breath sounds
- Ensure that chest drains are patent and on suction
- Check PaO$_2$
- If you suspect pneumothorax, treat immediately with chest tube
- Disconnect patient from the ventilator and hand-ventilate the patient to assess compliance
- Suction ETT to clear mucous and to ensure patency
- Treat bronchospasm with albuterol nebulizer
- Check chest X-ray, looking for ETT position, pneumothorax, hemothorax, atelectasis, infiltrates, and edema and treat accordingly
- Suspect transfusion-related acute lung injury (TRALI) if new infiltrates are temporally related to transfusion

Box 14.6 Low urine output

- Check that the Foley catheter is patent
- Treat hypotension (see Box 14.3)
- Treat low cardiac output (see Box 14.4)
- Give furosemide 20 mg IV
- Start furosemide infusion 5–20 mg/hr, consider dose of chlorothiazide 500 mg IV
- Start dopamine 2 µg/kg/min

Basic cardiac physiology

Basic concepts

The circulatory system is a circuit that follows the principle of Ohm's law. Pressure is proportional to the flow and the resistance of a circuit. *Mean arterial blood pressure* (MAP) is calculated by adding a third of the difference between the diastolic and systolic pressures to the diastolic pressure. *Cardiac output* (CO) is the volume (flow) of blood pumped by the heart through the circulation (circuit) each minute. *Stroke volume* (SV) is the volume of blood ejected by the heart with each beat. Cardiac output is equal to the product of the heart rate and the stroke volume. *Cardiac index* (CI) is the cardiac output adjusted for patient size (cardiac output divided by body surface area) to more accurately reflect cardiac function. Stroke volume depends on *preload, contractility,* and *afterload* (see Table 14.1).

Preload

- *Preload* is the volume of blood in the left ventricle (LVEDV) resulting in left ventricular pressure (LVEDP) at end diastole.
- Because preload is difficult to measure directly in most clinical situations, indirect measures of preload can frequently be inferred from the measured "filling pressures" (i.e., central venous pressure [CVP], pulmonary capillary wedge pressure [PCWP], and left atrial pressure [LAP]).

Afterload

- *Afterload* is the force the myocardium and ventricle must overcome to shorten and contract, respectively.
- Afterload is a measure of the wall tension of the left ventricle during systole.
- The *systemic vascular resistance* (SVR) is a derived number that estimates whether the vascular bed is dilated or constricted. Although SVR is a component of afterload, the two terms are not synonymous.

Contractility and compliance

- *Contractility* is the intrinsic property of the muscle to shorten, which is not secondary to the preload or afterload.
- *Compliance* is a measure of the distensibility of the left ventricle in diastole; stiff, hypertrophied ventricles have low compliance.

Table 14.1 Important hemodynamic formulas and normal values

Cardiac output = HR × SV

Cardiac index = CO/BSA

Stroke volume index = SV/BSA

Mean arterial pressure = DBP + (SBP − DBP)/3

Systemic vascular resistance = [(MAP − CVP)/CO] × 80

Systemic vascular resistance index = SVR/BSA

Pulmonary vascular resistance = [(PAP − PCWP)/CO] × 80

Pulmonary vascular resistance index = PVR/BSA

	Normal value
Cardiac output (CO)	4.5–8 L/min
Stroke volume (SV)	60–100 mL
Body surface area (BSA)	2–2.2 m^2
Cardiac index (CI)	2.0–4.0 L/min/m^2
Stroke volume index (SVI)	33–47 mL/beat/m^2
Mean arterial pressure (MAP)	70–100 mmHg
Diastolic blood pressure (DBP)	60–80 mmHg
Systolic blood pressure (SBP)	110–150 mmHg
Systemic vascular resistance (SVR)	800–1200 dyne-sec/cm^5
Central venous pressure (CVP)	6–12 mmHg
Systemic vascular resistance index (SVRI)	400–600 dyne-sec/m^5/m^2
Pulmonary vascular resistance (PVR)	50–250 dyne-sec/cm^5
Pulmonary artery pressure (PAP)	20–30 mmHg
Pulmonary capillary wedge pressure (PCWP)	8–14 mmHg
Pulmonary vascular resistance index (PVRI)	20–125 dyne-sec/cm^5/m^2

Principles of cardiac surgery

Evidence

- Cardiac surgery has a stronger evidence base than many specialties. There are numerous randomized controlled trials, meta-analyses, and cohort studies published.
- Risk scoring systems (e.g., Society of Thoracic Surgeons, EUROscore) are well developed.
- There are clearly defined, evidence-based guidelines specifying exactly which surgery offers a better outcome than percutaneous catheter intervention (PCI) or medical therapies.

Preoperative preparation

Careful preoperative workup is essential. Attention to detail is paramount. Small abnormalities that would be of little consequence in other specialties can result in disaster in cardiac surgery.

- **History**. Quantify symptoms, previous myocardial infarction (MI) and/or stroke; note comorbidities (especially chronic obstructive pulmonary disease [COPD], renal dysfunction, peripheral vascular disease, bleeding or clotting disorders), MI less than 90 days prior (which increases mortality); drugs (aspirin, clopidogrel, and warfarin are normally stopped 5 days preoperatively to reduce bleeding); allergies; recent chest or upper respiratory tract infection. Valve patients should be cleared of dental infection by a dentist.
- **Physical exam**. Look for signs of heart failure (jugular venous distension, S_3 gallop, hepatomegaly, peripheral edema), carotid bruits, active infection, and conduit (varicose veins, vein stripping, Allen's test for the radial artery).
- **Labs**. CBC, electrolytes, BUN, creatinine, urinalysis and sediment, LFTs, PT, and PTT. Blood type and cross match 4 units PRBC.
- **Studies**. ECG and chest X-ray. Obtain carotid duplex scan in patients with history, symptoms, or signs of cerebrovascular disease or in any patient over the age of 65 years.
- **Echocardiography**. For patients undergoing structural heart disease surgery (e.g., valve reconstruction or replacement, congenital heart disease, etc.)
- **Coronary angiography**. All patients undergoing coronary artery bypass grafting and any patient older than 40 years having valve surgery
- **Consent**. Obtained by the attending surgeon or house staff

Postoperative management

The management of six common postoperative emergencies is outlined in Boxes 14.1–14.6. Most patients are stable enough to be extubated within the first 8 hr and leave the ICU within 24 hr, and are discharged home within 5 days.

First 6 hr

- Cardiac function will be impaired as much as 50% in the first 6–8 hr.
- Volume may be necessary to achieve higher filling pressures in order to maintain cardiac index.
- Pacing and inotropic support may be required.
- Aggressive blood glucose control (100–150 mg/dL) with insulin infusions has been shown to improve patient outcomes.
- Mediastinal bleeding should steadily decrease.
- Urine output is not an indicator of adequate cardiac output but should be maintained at >1 mL/kg/hr.

Postoperative days 1–2

- Inotropes and pacing are weaned and discontinued.
- Invasive monitoring lines are removed.
- Chest tubes are removed when drainage is <10 mL/hr for 2 hr.
- Patients with coronary artery disease should be started on an aspirin, beta-blocker, and HMG-CoA reductase inhibitor.
- Valve patients should be anticoagulated with warfarin depending on the prosthesis.
- The patient is mobilized out of bed.
- Diet is advanced as tolerated and analgesia is transitioned to oral medications.

Days 3–5

- Temporary pacing wires are removed if rate and rhythm are satisfactory.
- Valve repair patients should undergo baseline echocardiography.
- Medications are tailored and reviewed for discharge.
- Obtain chest X-ray and ECG prior to discharge.

Cardiopulmonary bypass

A main purpose of cardiopulmonary bypass (CPB) is to provide systemic circulation while the heart is being manipulated during cardiac surgery. CPB is used for any operation that involves opening the heart (e.g., valve surgery, repair of septal defects, pulmonary embolectomy), interrupting blood flow through the ascending aorta or arch (e.g., aneurysm repair, dissection), or resecting tumors invading the great vessels (e.g., renal cell carcinoma). CPB by itself does not stop the heart because coronary arterial blood flow continues, maintaining cardiac activity. CPB decreases myocardial O_2 demand by about 80% because although the heart continues to beat, it no longer has to perform the energy-expensive work of pumping blood.

- **Exposure.** Sternotomy with planned central cannulation. Minimally invasive incisions may require peripheral cannulation strategies.
- **Anticoagulation.** Systemic heparinization (3–5 mg/kg) to achieve ACT >400 sec prevents thrombus formation in the CPB circuit and consumptive coagulopathy.
- **Arterial cannulation.** Central (in the ascending aorta) or peripheral (in the axillary or femoral artery)
- **Venous cannulation.** Right atrial or bicaval (in the SVC and IVC)
- **Initiation of bypass.** Venous return by passive siphoning or by active suctioning flows to the venous reservoir. Blood is pumped through a membrane (where it is oxygenated and ventilated) and filtered (to remove bubbles and debris). A heater/cooler can be used to regulate blood and body temperature. Blood is returned through the arterial cannula to maintain systemic perfusion.
- **Separation from bypass.** Optimal conditions: T >35°C, regular heart rate and rhythm (sinus rhythm or paced), cardiac output (pump flow) and mean arterial pressure similar to pre-bypass, normal pH and K^+
- **Reversal of anticoagulation.** Protamine to return to baseline ACT (usually <120 sec)
- **Decannulation.**

Pathophysiology of cardiopulmonary bypass

CPB can be a double-edged sword. Although it maintains systemic circulation during cardiac manipulation, it can have a major impact on almost every organ system.

- **Coagulation.** Even with complete systemic anticoagulation, the coagulation and complement cascades are activated, resulting in consumption of platelets and coagulation factors and subsequent coagulopathy.
- **Inflammation.** CPB is associated with a significant systemic inflammatory response, resulting in increased capillary permeability (capillary leak syndrome).
- **Emboli.** Macro- and micro-emboli of atheroma, air, and clot can result from cannulation, clamping, and manipulation of the circulation, resulting in stroke, neurocognitive dysfunction, and end-organ ischemia.
- **Perfusion.** CPB can result in impaired renal, pulmonary, hepatic, and splanchnic perfusion.

Myocardial protection

If the surgeon wishes to operate on a still heart or if the operation requires interruption of coronary arterial blood flow, the heart can be mechanically and electrically arrested in several ways, given that provisions for myocardial protection are made. *Cardioplegia* is a term that describes many different solutions and approaches for myocardial arrest and protection. The solutions can be delivered antegrade via the aorta, retrograde via the coronary sinus, and directly to the coronary arteries via vein grafts. There are many components that constitute cardioplegia.

- **Temperature**. Cold solutions provide myocardial protection by decreasing myocardial metabolism. Cold cardioplegia is also a potent coronary vasodilator. Warm continuous cardioplegia can also be used to maintain myocardial viability but without the benefit of decreased metabolism afforded by hypothermia. Topical solutions or jackets are useful adjuncts.

- **Electrolytes**. Manipulation of the membrane potentials brings about electrical arrest and further decreases myocardial metabolism. Solutions rich in K^+ and Mg^{2+} and low in Na^+ and Ca^{2+} are among the most commonly used.

- **Blood vs. crystalloid**. Oxygenated blood solutions provide improved O_2 delivery at warmer temperatures. Although cold blood solutions have a higher affinity for O_2 (which is less desirable), they have beneficial effects on viscosity and buffering.

Coronary artery disease

Incidence

Based on the Framingham Heart Study, the lifetime risk for developing symptomatic coronary artery disease (CAD) after age 40 is 49% for men and 32% for women. CAD is the most frequent cause of death in American men and women, resulting in more than 1 in 5 deaths in the United States.

Risk factors

These include age, male gender, smoking, hypertension, diabetes, hyperlipidemia, obesity, and family history.

Presentation

CAD presents as angina, dyspnea, MI, or sudden death.

Pathophysiology

Atherosclerotic plaques can cause obstruction of blood flow in the coronary arteries (see Fig. 14.1), resulting in a spectrum of clinical consequences. The rate of progression is variable and unpredictable. Regression of plaques has been observed.

- >50% reduction in cross-sectional area can limit coronary blood flow in response to increased demand
- >90% reduction in cross-sectional area can result in MI at rest
- LV function normally *improves* with exercise. Patients with CAD may have a *decline* in LV function with exercise. The LV dysfunction can be regional in single-vessel stenosis or global in multivessel and left main stenoses.
- Acute MI is caused by sudden total or subtotal thrombotic occlusion of a vessel.

Diagnosis

- History and physical exam
- ECG may show evidence of old infarcts (Q waves or new bundle-branch block).
- Exercise treadmill test has 97% specificity for exertional angina.
- Myocardial perfusion studies increase specificity.
- Coronary angiography is diagnostic.

Indications for surgery

Despite a plethora of reports and trials comparing percutaneous catheter intervention with surgery for CAD, most of the studies are controversial and therefore confusing. Presently, the conventional wisdom recommends coronary artery bypass surgery for the following patient groups:

- >70% left main stenosis
- >70% left anterior descending (LAD) stenosis proximal to the first septal perforator
- >70% three-vessel disease
- Patients with less significant coronary disease who are having cardiac surgery for other reasons (e.g., valve replacement)

Coronary artery bypass surgery

The goal of coronary artery bypass grafting (CABG) is to revascularize myocardial territories rather than individual arteries.

- Sternotomy to obtain exposure
- Conduit (internal mammary arteries [IMA], greater saphenous veins, radial arteries) is harvested.
- Conduit is anastomosed to the coronary artery distal to the atherosclerotic lesion.
- Inflow (or proximal) can be derived from the ascending aorta or the mammary artery pedicles. The LIMA, when grafted to the LAD, has excellent long-term patency (>90% beyond 15 years), improves survival, and decreases the need for reoperation.
- Coronary artery bypass is performed with CPB ("on-pump") in 75% of patients.
- Coronary artery bypass without CPB ("off-pump," or OPCAB) may be of particular benefit in patients with pulmonary, renal, cerebrovascular, or hematologic diseases. Results of OPCAB are similar to those with on-pump CABG.

Complications

Complications are more likely to occur with advanced age, poor LV function, renal insufficiency, and COPD.

- Mortality 2.5%
- Stroke 2%
- Re-exploration for bleeding or tamponade 3%–5%
- Sternal wound infection, atrial fibrillation, renal failure

Prognosis

In untreated patients with symptoms severe enough to warrant coronary angiography, the risk of acute MI is 10% at 1 year and 30% at 6 years. Hospital mortality of MI is 7%–10%.

- In 3-vessel disease, 5-year mortality is 21% and higher if LVEF is <50%.
- In left main disease, mortality is 29% at 18 months and 45% at 5 years.

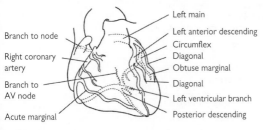

Fig. 14.1 Coronary artery anatomy.

Valvular heart disease

Mitral regurgitation (MR)

Incidence. Most common valve lesion, with prevalence of 2%

Etiology
- Myxomatous disease
- Ischemic heart disease
- Rheumatic disease
- Endocarditis
- Connective tissue disorders

Clinical features
- Pulmonary edema (acute MR)
- Exertional dyspnea (chronic MR)
- Pansystolic murmur radiating to the axilla
- Atrial fibrillation

Diagnosis
Chest X-ray shows cardiomegaly and pulmonary edema. Transthoracic echo is diagnostic for prolapse or restriction.

Indications for surgery
- Acute MR with pulmonary edema can be a surgical emergency.
- Chronic MR: severe MR with increasing left ventricular size
- The threshold for surgery declines when it is likely that the valve can be repaired rather than replaced.

Prognosis
- 1%–2% mortality for elective mitral valve repair
- 10%–15% mortality for emergent mitral valve replacement in acute MR

Mitral stenosis

Incidence. Prevalence is <1% in developed countries.

Etiology
- Rheumatic heart disease
- Congenital
- Rheumatoid arthritis
- Systemic lupus erythematosus (SLE)

Clinical features
- Dyspnea
- Atrial fibrillation
- Left parasternal heave
- Loud S_1
- Rumbling mid-diastolic murmur

Diagnosis. Transthoracic echo is diagnostic.

Indications for surgery. Mitral valve area <1 cm^2 (normal 3–4 cm^2)

Prognosis. Increased risk with worsening heart failure

Aortic stenosis
Incidence. Prevalence is <1%.

Etiology
- Senile calcific aortic stenosis
- Bicuspid aortic valve
- Rheumatic heart disease

Clinical features
- Triad of angina, syncope, and dyspnea
- Pulsus parvus et tardus
- Systolic murmur radiating to the carotid arteries
- Diminished S_2

Diagnosis. Transthoracic echo is diagnostic.

Indications for surgery. Symptoms, aortic valve area <0.8 cm^2

Prognosis
- Without aortic valve replacement (AVR): <5 years if there is angina, <3 years if there is syncope, <2 years if there is dyspnea
- Operative mortality is 3%–5%.

Aortic insufficiency (AI)
Incidence. Prevalence is <1%.

Etiology
- Bicuspid aortic valve
- Rheumatic heart disease
- Aortic dissection
- Endocarditis
- Marfan syndrome

Clinical features
- Dyspnea
- Wide pulse pressure
- Diastolic murmur

Diagnosis. Angiography or transthoracic echo

Indications for surgery
- Acute AI associated with pulmonary edema is a surgical emergency.
- Chronic AI is best treated before the LV dilates (>55 mm) and LVEF decreases (<55%).

Prognosis
Chronic AI is well tolerated until there is congestive heart failure (CHF). Operative mortality is 3%–5%.

Options for valve surgery
Valve repair
- Mitral valve repair for regurgitation has an excellent record for effectiveness and durability. Mitral valve repair is associated with improved short- and long-term survival compared with mitral valve replacement.
- Aortic valve repair techniques are improving.

Mechanical vs. tissue prosthesis
- Most mechanical valves consist of carbon disks or leaflets mounted on a cloth sewing ring (e.g., St. Jude, Carbomedics, Hall Medtronic). Tissue valves are porcine aortic valves or bovine pericardium mounted on a synthetic scaffold and cloth sewing ring.
- Decisions regarding mechanical vs. tissue valves revolve around durability and need for lifelong anticoagulation. Mechanical valves are more durable but require lifelong anticoagulation with warfarin. Tissue valves do not require warfarin but are more likely to require re-replacement.

Operative considerations
Exposure of any of the cardiac valves (see Box 14.7) can be achieved through a sternotomy or "less invasive" incisions (right thoracotomy, axillary incision, hemi-sternotomy).

Complications
- Stroke 3%–5% (increases with age)
- Wound infection, atrial fibrillation, heart block requiring a permanent pacemaker, renal failure

---

Box 14.7 Anatomy of the heart valves

- The aortic valve is a tricuspid valve (3% of the population has a bicuspid valve) attached to the coronal annulus within the aortic root. The aortic root has sinuses of Valsalva from which the left and right coronary arteries originate.
- The conduction system is located along the crest of the ventricular septum immediately below the commissure between the right and non-coronary cusps.
- The mitral valve has an anterior and posterior leaflet attached to a saddle-shaped annulus in the atrioventricular groove. The leaflets are attached to papillary muscles (anterolateral and posteromedial) by chordae tendinae.
- The circumflex coronary artery and non-coronary leaflet of the aortic valve are at risk of injury during mitral valve replacement.
- The tricuspid valve has three asymmetric leaflets (anterior, posterior, and septal).
- The AV node is located close to the anteroseptal commissure of the tricuspid valve and is at risk for injury during tricuspid valve replacement or annuloplasty.
- The left main coronary artery is immediately posterior to the pulmonic valve and is in jeopardy during pulmonary valve mobilization (Ross procedure) and pulmonary valve replacement.

Lung cancer

Key facts

Lung cancer is the most common cause of death from cancer in the United States (both men and women).

Risk factors

These include smoking, occupational factors (e.g., asbestos, polycyclic aromatic hydrocarbons, silica), radon exposure, genetic predisposition, and male sex.

Non-small cell lung cancer

Squamous cell carcinoma (SCC)

Some 30%–50% of all lung cancers are SCC, the most common type found in the United States. It often arises as an endobronchial mass, is slow growing, and metastasizes late.

Adenocarcinoma

Adenocarcinoma comprises 15%–35% of all lung cancers, and is the most common form of lung cancer in women. It is peripheral, shows moderate growth, and metastasizes early.

Large cell undifferentiated carcinoma

This carcinoma comprises 10%–15% of all lung cancers. It is peripheral and has two subtypes (clear cell and giant cell). Giant cell tumors are uncommon (<1% of lung cancers) and have a very poor prognosis.

Small cell lung cancer

Small cell undifferentiated carcinoma

Some 10%–25% of all lung cancers are this type; it is aggressive and not usually amenable to surgical resection. Response rates to chemotherapy are frequently in excess of 70% when disease is limited to the thorax, but many patients develop local recurrence.

Presentation

- Central tumors: hemoptysis, dyspnea, cough, wheezing, stridor, hoarseness, Horner's syndrome, SVC obstruction, postobstructive pneumonia, pleural effusion
- Peripheral tumors are often asymptomatic and can present with pleuritic chest wall pain from local invasion or progressive dyspnea from pleural effusion.
- Metastatic spread: weight loss, headache, bony pain and pathologic fracture, anorexia, jaundice, ascites, liver failure
- Physical exam: lymphadenopathy (e.g., supraclavicular Virchow's or scalene nodes), chest wall tenderness, clubbing, cutaneous lesions (e.g., acanthosis nigricans, hyperpigmentation), pleural effusion
- Paraneoplastic syndromes: PTH, ACTH, calcitonin, serotonin

Principles of management

- Treatment is determined after comprehensive staging (imaging, bronchoscopy, mediastinoscopy, and thoracoscopy).
- Surgery is normally offered to all patients with stage I and II disease, as well as specific patients with stage IIIa disease.
- Curative resection allows the best chance of long-term survival.

Survival

- Overall cure rate is low (~10%–13% of patients are alive at 5 years)
- Only 30% of patients present with stage I or II disease
- 5-year survival: stage I, 75%; stage II, 40%; stage III, <30%
- Perioperative mortality of lobectomy is 2%, pneumonectomy is 6%

Neoadjuvant and adjuvant therapy

- There is no proven benefit to radiation and chemotherapy over resection in treating stage I and II non-small cell lung cancer.
- Such therapy does improve survival in some patients with stage IIIa disease.

American Joint Committee for Cancer (AJCC) TNM classification (see Table 14.2)

Primary tumor (T)

- Tx: Primary tumor cannot be assessed, or tumor is proven by presence of malignant cells in secretions but is not visualized by imaging or bronchoscopy
- T0: No evidence of primary tumor
- Tis: Carcinoma in situ
- T1: Tumor ≤3 cm without invasion proximal to a lobar bronchus
- T2: Tumor >3 cm that is >2 cm from the carina, tumor of any size that has invaded the visceral pleura, or tumor of any size associated with atelectasis or obstructive pneumonia that extends to the hilar region but involves less than the entire lung *and* is not associated with a malignant pleural effusion
- T3: Tumor of any size with direct extension into contiguous structures (e.g., chest wall), without invasion of the heart, great vessels, trachea, esophagus, or vertebral body, *or* tumor involving a main bronchus <2 cm distal to the tracheal carina but not involving the carina
- T4: Tumor that involves the mediastinum, heart, great vessels, trachea, esophagus, or vertebral body *or* tumor associated with a malignant pleural effusion

Nodal involvement (N)

- Nx: Regional lymph nodes cannot be assessed
- N0: No demonstrable metastasis to regional lymph nodes
- N1: Metastasis or extension into ipsilateral peribronchial and/or ipsilateral hilar nodes, and intrapulmonary nodes including involvement by direct extension of the primary tumor
- N2: Metastasis to ipsilateral mediastinal and/or subcarinal lymph nodes
- N3: Metastasis to contralateral mediastinal, contralateral hilar, ipsilateral or contralateral scalene, or supraclavicular lymph nodes

Distant metastases (M)
- Mx: Distant metastasis cannot be assessed
- M0: No known distant metastasis
- M1: Distant metastasis present

Table 14.2 AJCC TNM staging for lung cancer

Stage	Tumor	Node	Metastasis
Occult carcinoma	Tx	N0	M0
Stage 0	Tis	N0	M0
Stage Ia	T1	N0	M0
Stage Ib	T2	N0	M0
Stage IIa	T1	N1	M0
Stage IIb	T2	N1	M0
	T3	N0	M0
Stage IIIa	T1	N2	M0
	T2	N2	M0
	T3	N1	M0
	T3	N2	M0
Stage IIIb	Any T	N3	M0
	T4	Any N	M0
Stage IV	Any T	Any N	M1

Pleural effusion

Physiology
A small amount of fluid normally exists in the pleural space secondary to Starling's forces (increased hydrostatic and decreased oncotic pressure in the parietal pleura compared to decreased hydrostatic and increased oncotic pressure in the visceral pleura). A pleural effusion is an increased amount of fluid in the pleural space (see Table 14.3).

Causes of transudates
- Congestive heart failure
- Cirrhosis
- Nephrotic syndrome
- Myxedema
- Pulmonary edema
- Meigs syndrome

Causes of exudates
- Neoplasms: bronchogenic carcinoma, breast cancer, mesothelioma
- Infections: pneumonia (parapneumonic effusion, which can progress to empyema), tuberculosis
- Hemothorax
- Chylothorax
- Subphrenic abscess
- Collagen vascular diseases: rheumatoid arthritis, SLE, Wegener's granulomatosis, Sjögren's syndrome

Clinical presentation
Symptoms
Cough, dyspnea, chest pain, dull sensation in the chest. Many cases are asymptomatic.

Signs
Signs include decreased breath sounds, dullness to percussion, crackles, and egophony.

Studies
A chest X-ray and CT scan can show blunting of the costophrenic sulcus with a meniscus, or a subpulmonic collection mimicking an elevated hemidiaphragm. Effusion in the fissure can mimic a tumor.

Table 14.3 Light's criteria

	Transudate	Exudate
Protein	≤3 g/dL	>3 g/dL
LDH	≤200 IU	>200 IU
Pleural/serum LDH	≤0.6	>0.6

Management

- Treatment of the underlying cause
- Tube thoracostomy
- Chemical pleurodesis (e.g., talc, tetracycline, bleomycin)
- Open or video-assisted thoracoscopic surgical abrasion pleurodesis
- Surgical pleurectomy
- Pleuroperitoneal shunt

Complications

- Infection, empyema
- Recurrence of effusion
- Injury to underlying lung parenchyma leading to bronchopleural fistula

Pneumothorax

Pneumothorax is the presence of air in the pleural space with secondary lung collapse.

Primary spontaneous pneumothorax

This type is commonly seen in tall male smokers, with 90% of cases being unilateral, more common on the right. It is usually caused by rupture of small subpleural blebs (air sac <2 cm) found in the apex of the upper lobe or superior segment of the lower lobe. It may also be caused by rupture of a bulla (air sac >2 cm).

Presentation

Cough, dyspnea, chest pain, dull sensation in the chest. Many cases are asymptomatic.

Studies

Listen for decreased breath sounds, dullness to percussion, crackles, and egophony.

Complications
• Tension pneumothorax
• Pneumomediastinum
• Recurrent pneumothorax

Conservative management
• Needle/catheter aspiration, tube thoracostomy ± chemical pleurodesis

Surgery

Surgery is indicated for the first episode only if there is prolonged air leak, tension pneumothorax at presentation, bilateral pneumothoraces, occupational hazard, or previous contralateral pneumonectomy. Surgery is indicated for second and subsequent pneumothoraces. The goal of surgery is to resect the blebs and bullae and obliterate the pleural space with adhesions or by parietal pleurectomy.

Recurrence rate

Recurrence is 2% following surgical pleurectomy, 5% following thoracoscopic procedures, and 5%–10% following chemical pleurodesis.

Secondary spontaneous pneumothorax

Causes
• Cystic fibrosis, COPD, asthma, interstitial lung disease, lymphangioleiomyomatosis
• Infections: AIDS, *Pneumocystis carinii*, tuberculosis, parasitic, mycotic
• Malignancy: bronchogenic carcinoma, metastatic lung cancer
• Collagen vascular disorders: Marfan syndrome, Ehlers-Danlos syndrome, scleroderma
• Catamenial
• Esophageal rupture (Boerhaave's syndrome)

Post-traumatic or iatrogenic pneumothorax

Causes
- Penetrating stab wounds
- Rib fractures
- Central line placement
- Endoscopy
- Radiographic biopsy

Pneumomediastinum

This condition is uncommon. It occurs following exertion or increased intra-abdominal pressure. Any disruption of the mediastinal visceral envelope from the aerodigestive tract can result in pneumomediastinum. It can be associated with cocaine or marijuana use.

Presentation
There is a sudden onset of chest pain, along with dyspnea, subcutaneous emphysema, dysphonia, and Hamman's crunch.

Studies
Chest X-ray can show air outlining the strap muscles of the neck and the cardiac silhouette. A CT scan is more sensitive for smaller volumes of air.

Evaluation
Bronchoscopy, esophagoscopy, nasopharyngeal endoscopy, and laryngoscopy can be used to exclude perforation of the aerodigestive tract.

Management
In the absence of perforation of the aerodigestive tract, nonoperative management is indicated.

Mediastinal disease

Box 14.8 Anatomy of the mediastinum

The **mediastinum** is the space between the pleural sacs, below the thoracic inlet, and above the diaphragm.
- **Superior mediastinum**
  - From the sternal notch to T5
  - Contains the great vessels, trachea, esophagus, phrenic nerves, vagus nerves, and thoracic duct
- **Anterior mediastinum**
  - Anterior to the pericardium
  - Contains sternopericardial ligaments, thymus, and lymph nodes
- **Middle mediastinum**
  - Contains pericardial cavity, heart, great vessels, and phrenic nerves
- **Posterior mediastinum**
  - Posterior to the pericardium
  - Contains esophagus, descending aorta, azygous veins, thoracic duct, lymph nodes, and sympathetic chain

Mediastinal masses
- **Anterior**. Thymoma, lymphoma, germ cell tumors, thyroid
- **Middle**. Mediastinal cysts (foregut, neuroenteric, pericardial), aneurysms of the great vessels
- **Posterior**. Neurogenic (ganglioneuromas, Schwannomas, neurofibromas, paragangliomas), aortic aneurysms

Thymoma
- May be benign or malignant
- Usually asymptomatic in adults, whereas children often present with thoracic outlet obstruction or upper airway compromise
- Appears as a smooth mass in the upper half of the chest X-ray
- Surgical resection via sternotomy is recommended
- Associated with myasthenia gravis; thymectomy may be effective treatment for myasthenia gravis, regardless of whether a thymoma is present

Superior vena cava syndrome
- Characterized by swelling of the face, neck, and arms; dyspnea, orthopnea, cough; cyanosis of the face and lips; distended and tortuous veins over the chest wall
- Malignant disease of the thorax occurs in 90% of patients with SVC syndrome.
- Chronic granulomatous fibrosing mediastinitis, histoplasmosis, *Nocardia*, tuberculosis, radiation, and sarcoid are some benign causes.
- Radiation is the most common modality to treat malignant causes of SVC syndrome. Chemotherapy is a reasonable alternative for sensitive lesions.
- Benign causes can be treated by replacement or bypass of the superior vena cava in selected cases.

Pericardial effusion

Key facts
- Abnormal fluid in the pericardial space (normal ~20–50 mL)
- May be acute or chronic
- Acute accumulation of fluid can cause cardiac tamponade (see Box 14.9)
- Causes: pericarditis, CHF, malignancy (metastatic lung and breast cancer, lymphoma, leukemia), uremia, infectious, autoimmune

Clinical features
- These depend on the time course. Acute accumulation of a small amount of fluid can cause life-threatening cardiac tamponade, whereas chronic accumulation of large volumes of fluid may be well tolerated.
- Chronic pericardial effusion may present with decreased exercise tolerance, atypical chest pain, dyspnea, orthopnea, and associated signs of CHF, as well as features of cardiac tamponade.

Management
- Medical management includes diuretics and pericardiocentesis ± catheter drainage.
- Pericardial window via thoracotomy, subxiphoid approach, or video-assisted thoracoscopic surgery (VATS)

Box 14.9 Cardiac tamponade

Signs and symptoms
- Beck's triad (hypotension, jugular venous distension, muffled heart sounds)
- Pulsus paradoxus: >10 mmHg decrease in SBP upon inspiration
- Tachycardia
- Oliguria
- Widened mediastinum on chest X-ray
- Equalization of CVP, pulmonary artery diastolic pressure, PCWP

Management
- Fluid resuscitation
- Emergency pericardiocentesis
- Pericardial window
- Emergency thoracotomy or sternotomy

Peripheral vascular disease

Mark Conrad, MD

Acute limb ischemia

Causes

Acute thrombosis in a vessel with preexisting atherosclerosis (60%)
- Predisposing factors are dehydration, hypotension, malignancy, polycythemia, or inherited prothrombotic states.
- Features suggestive of thrombosis are the following:
  - Previous history of intermittent claudication
  - Slow onset or incomplete occlusion
  - No obvious source of emboli (see below)
  - Decreased or absent pulses in the contralateral limb

Emboli (30%)
- 80% have a cardiac cause (AF, MI, ventricular aneurysm).
- Arterial aneurysms account for 10% of distal emboli and may be from the aortoiliac, femoral, popliteal, or subclavian arteries.
- Most emboli lodge at bifurcations of arteries as the diameter of the vessel suddenly reduces.
- The most frequent sites of impaction are the brachial, common femoral, popliteal, and aortic bifurcation ("saddle embolus").
- Features suggestive of embolism are the following:
  - No previous history of claudication
  - Rapid onset and complete occlusion
  - Cardiac arrhythmias (especially AF)

Rare causes
- Aortic dissection, trauma, iatrogenic injury, peripheral aneurysm (particularly popliteal), and intra-arterial drug use

Features

Symptoms and signs (any cause)
- Look for the six *P's*: pain, pallor, pulselessness, paresthesia, paralysis, and perishing cold.

Complications
- Death (20%)
- Limb loss (40%): ischemia leads to irreversible tissue damage within 6 hr in a previously normal limb.

Emergency management

Resuscitation
- Give 100% oxygen.
- Get IV access and consider crystalloid fluid up to 1000 mL if the patient is dehydrated.
- Take blood for CBC, troponin, clotting, glucose, and creatine phosphokinase (CPK) (to rule out myonecrosis).
- Request a chest X-ray and ECG (look for arrhythmias).
- Give opiate analgesia (5–10 mg morphine IM).

Establish a diagnosis

Patients will often have coexisting coronary, cerebral, or renal disease. The diagnosis is threefold:

- Type (embolism or thrombosis). A thorough history and examination is essential (see Causes, previous page).
- Limb viability assessment (see Box 15.1)
- Underlying cause, through echocardiography, 24-hr holter monitor, angiogram, hypercoaguable-state screening

Box 15.1 SVS/ISCVS criteria for limb viability

Category	Sensory loss	Motor loss	Doppler signals	Management
I	None	None	Positive	Elective
IIA	Minimal	None	Absent	Urgent
IIB	Major	Any	Absent	Emergent
III	Anesthesia	Paralysis	Absent	if <3 hr old

Early treatment

- Consider giving heparin (5000 U unfractionated heparin IV bolus and start an infusion of 1000 U/hr) if there are no contraindications (e.g., aortic dissection, multiple trauma, head injury).
  - Recheck activated partial thromboplastin time (APTT) in 4–6 hr.
  - Aim for a target time of 2–2.5 times the normal range.

Definitive management

This depends on the severity of ischemia. There are three broad categories:

- *Irreversible* (non-salvageable limb). Amputation is inevitable and urgency is important to prevent the systemic complications of muscle necrosis (hyperkalemia, metabolic acidosis, acute renal failure, cardiac arrest).
- *Complete* (acutely threatened limb). This condition requires expert vascular input: thrombolysis, angioplasty, embolectomy, or urgent arterial bypass may be required depending on the individual circumstances.
- *Incomplete* (viable limb). Heparinization is needed to prevent further propagation of thrombus, as well as urgent imaging, and consideration of intervention (thrombolysis, angioplasty, arterial surgery).

Principles of embolectomy

- May be performed under local anesthesia
- Facilities for angiography and vascular reconstruction must be available.
- Incisions should be over the site of access, not the site of suspected embolism (brachial artery, common femoral artery, popliteal artery).
- Expose and control (by vessel loops) all in- and outflow vessels.
- A 3–5 F Fogarty embolectomy catheter is passed proximally and distally.
- If good inflow and good backflow are achieved, then close with interrupted 6/0 Prolene sutures and confirm return of distal pulses.
- Completion angiography may be undertaken on table.
- On-table thrombolysis is required if there is residual thrombus in runoff vessels.
- Surgical reconstruction or bypass may be necessary if there is in situ thrombosis on an underlying critical stenosis.
- Fasciotomies (four compartments) may be necessary if the leg is tense or prolonged ischemia has occurred to prevent a postoperative compartment syndrome.
- IV heparin infusion: check APTT at 4–6 hr and daily thereafter. Also repeat APTT 4 hr after every change in dosage, keeping APTT at 2–2.5 times the normal range.
- Start warfarin once heparin is therapeutic.

Chronic upper limb ischemia

Key facts

Upper limb ischemia occurs less frequently than lower limb ischemia.

Causes

- Previous trauma or axillary irradiation leading to arterial stenosis
- *Buerger's disease* affects small vessels of the hands and feet, principally in smokers, and is associated with Raynaud's phenomenon. Mostly young men but also women may be affected. It presents with digital gangrene or ischemia and may present with acute limb ischemia in young people.
- *Subclavian steal syndrome.* There is reversed flow in the vertebral artery/diminished hindbrain perfusion (dizziness/syncope), and arm claudication.
- *Takayasu's arteritis* is uncommon in the United States; major arch and upper limb vessels are affected.
- *Thoracic outlet syndrome* (see Fig. 15.1)
  - This term is used to cover a spectrum of symptoms resulting from compression of the neurovascular bundle as it leaves the chest to enter the upper limb, in an area enclosed by the first rib, clavicle, and scalenus anterior.
  - It presents as a variable combination of neural, arterial, and venous symptoms exacerbated by elevation of the limb, with pain, paresthesia, weakness, or arm claudication. 95% of cases are neurogenic and 5% are due to an arterial or venous cause.

Clinical features

- Weakness, cramp, or exercise-related pain and digital ischemia or gangrene
- Examine bilateral upper limb pulses, BP in both arms (elevated and at sides), and wrist Doppler pressures.
- *Roos test.* The arm is abducted to 90°, hands up with elbows braced backward, chin elevated, hands serially clenched and opened for 1–2 min. The test is positive if there is pain or weakness in the hand or forearm.
- *Adson's test.* Pulse diminishes or is absent on elevation and abduction of arm with head turned to the contralateral side. Reliability is improved by using it in conjunction with arterial duplex.
- *Allen's test* assesses integrity of the palmar arch and dominant vessel (radial or ulnar).
- *Tinel's test* is used to exclude carpal tunnel syndrome.

Diagnosis and investigation

- Cervical spine and thoracic outlet X-rays; wrist Doppler pressures
- CT/MRI to exclude fibrous bands/cervical rib
- Arterial duplex or angiography to exclude proximal arterial lesions

Treatment

Thoracic outlet syndrome

- Mild neurogenic problem: simple analgesia, physical therapy and advice on risk factors

- Surgery has good results for those with arterial or venous symptoms and complications.
- Excision of the first rib/band will improve symptoms in over 90%.
- Careful evaluation is needed prior to surgery for pure neurological symptoms, e.g., nerve conduction studies.

Cervical sympathectomy in upper limb disease
Indications
- Palmar hyperhidrosis (*not* axillary)
- Buerger's disease or small vessel disease with digital gangrene

Approach
- The aim is to denervate the second and third thoracic ganglia.
- The approach is almost universally thoracoscopic and open approaches have been largely abandoned.

Complications
- Horner's syndrome
- Pneumothorax
- Hemorrhage
- Compensatory truncal hyperhidrosis
- Frey's syndrome (gustatory sweating)

Axillary hyperhidrosis
The treatment of choice is now SC botulinum toxin injections to the axillary sweat glands, repeated as necessary.

Anatomy of thoracic outlet

Several structures can compress the neurovascular structures:
- Cervical rib: articulates with C7
- Scalene muscle: aberrant anatomy or scarring or swelling from trauma
- Costoclavicular ligament

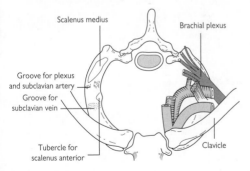

Fig. 15.1 Structures involved in thoracic outlet syndrome.

Chronic lower limb ischemia: introduction

- Atherosclerosis is a generalized disease and has a predilection for the coronary, cerebral, and peripheral circulations.
- In the lower limb it may affect the aortoiliac, femoral, or popliteal, and calf vessel levels singly or in combinations (see Box 15.2, Fig. 15.2).
- Single-level disease usually results in intermittent claudication (IC) and two-level disease in critical limb ischemia (CLI).

Box 15.2 Rutherford classification of lower limb ischemia

0 Asymptomatic
1 Mild claudication
2 Moderate claudication
3 Severe claudication
4 Ischemic rest pain
5 Minor tissue loss
6 Major tissue loss

Category 4–6 = critical limb ischemia (CLI)

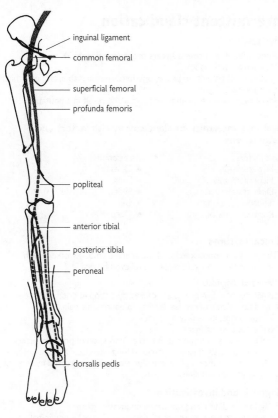

inguinal ligament

common femoral

superficial femoral

profunda femoris

popliteal

anterior tibial

posterior tibial

peroneal

dorsalis pedis

Fig. 15.2 The arterial supply to the leg.

Intermittent claudication

Key facts

- Affects 7% of men over 50 years of age (see Box 15.3)
- Male:female ratio is 2:1
- One-third of patients improve, one-third remain stable, and one-third deteriorate.
- 4% of cases require an intervention and 1% result in amputation.

Box 15.3 Intermittent claudication: risk factors and associations

Risk factors
- Hypertension
- Hyperlipidemia
- Diabetes mellitus
- Tobacco smoking
- Positive family history

Associations
- Obesity
- Diet
- Sedentary lifestyle
- Gender
- Occupation

Clinical features

- There is pain upon exercise of the affected limb: it worsens with increasing level of exercise, and is relieved by rest.

Differential diagnosis
- Spinal stenosis. Symptoms are caused by a drop in distal cauda equina blood flow due to exercise, leading to neurogenic pain.
- Osteoarthritis, especially hip joint
- Nerve root entrapment
- Popliteal artery entrapment due to compression of popliteal artery over medial head of gastrocnemius during exercise. Distal pulses are reduced or absent on plantar flexion alone. This is treated by surgical release after MRI defines anatomy.

Diagnosis and investigation

- Diagnosis is clinical and not based on invasive imaging.
- Serum fasting glucose, serum cholesterol, BP checked on initial presentation
- Imaging is only conducted for worsening symptoms, failure to respond to conservative management, or consideration of surgery.
  - Angiography (usually digital subtraction [DSA], perhaps CT angiogram [CTA], or magnetic resonance angiogram [MRA]).
- Abdominal ultrasound if aneurysmal disease suspected.

Treatment

Risk factor modification

Some 40% of patients with peripheral vascular disease have coronary or cerebral arterial disease. The mainstay of treatment is aggressive risk factor modification. The patient should stop smoking, receive oral statin treatment, increase exercise, and be aided in control of BP and serum glucose.

Endovascular treatment

- Angioplasty ± stent. This has excellent results in the aortoiliac segment (over 90% success) and good results in the superficial femoral segment (90% success and 60%–80% patency at 2 years).
  - Usually performed under local anesthesia, percutaneously
  - Rarely performed for claudication in the popliteal and tibial segments because of high risk of occlusion

Surgery

Indications for surgery are as follows.

- Failure or unsuitability for endovascular treatment in the aortoiliac segments. Procedures available are the following:
  - *Aortobifemoral graft*: 5-year patency of over 90% but carries a 5%–8% mortality rate and a risk of impotence; used for younger patients
  - *Femoral-femoral crossover bypass graft*: Used for isolated unilateral iliac disease. 90% 1-year patency
  - *Common femoral endarterectomy*: Used for isolated common femoral disease; good results and a low complication rate
- Short-distance claudication, severe lifestyle limitation, or failed medical therapy in infrainguinal (superficial femoral, popliteal, and distal) disease. Risks are significant. Procedures are the following:
  - Femoral-above-knee popliteal bypass: 80% 2-year patency with vein or prosthetic graft
  - Femoral-below-knee popliteal bypass: 70% 2-year patency with vein graft
  - Femoral-distal (below-knee) bypass: 5-year patency <35%. Usually reserved for critical ischemia; not recommended for claudication

Critical limb ischemia

Critical limb ischemia may be defined as ischemia that is likely to progress to limb loss or progressive tissue loss if it remains untreated.

Clinical features

- By Rutherford classification (Box 15.2), critical ischemia is present if there is
  - rest pain for >2 weeks not relieved by simple analgesia; *or*
  - resting ankle pressure <40 mmHg (toe pressures <30 mmHg if diabetic); *or*
  - tissue necrosis, i.e., the presence of gangrene or ulceration.
- Rest pain typically occurs at night and during elevation of the limb and is relieved by hanging the limb in a dependent position.
- Arterial ulceration is typically painful, shallow, and non-bleeding with few signs of healing.

Diagnosis and investigation

Diagnosis is clinical. Investigation should aim to do the following:
- Identify and treat risk factors: serum glucose, serum cholesterol, BP, smoking cessation.
- Identify location and severity of all arterial stenoses involved, through the following possible modalities:
  - Color duplex Doppler ultrasound: zero risk, non-interventional, best for proximal vessels, common femoral and iliac arteries are more difficult to assess
  - Angiography (usually DSA): interventional, carries risk of arterial injury and contrast nephropathy, best for popliteal and distal vessel assessment
  - Magnetic resonance angiography (MRA): low risk, avoids contrast

Treatment

- All efforts should be made to revascularize if possible (providing the general condition of the patient allows it).
- The general principle is to deal with the most proximal stenoses first and progress to distal disease only if critical ischemia is still present.

Medical care

- Nursing care, protect and float heels
- Analgesia: opiates

Endovascular treatments

Angioplasty ± stent for proximal stenoses (aortoiliac, common femoral, superficial femoral). This is less successful in popliteal and distal disease.

Surgery
- Femoral-distal bypass to popliteal or calf vessels
- Amputation
  - Usually below knee or above knee in smoking-related atherosclerosis
  - Distal amputations (toe, forefoot, ankle) may be appropriate in diabetic disease.
- There is little evidence for treatment with prostacyclin or sympathectomy (surgical or chemical).

Aneurysms

Key facts

- An *aneurysm* is an abnormal localized dilatation of a blood vessel.
- It may be associated with structural abnormalities of collagen and elastin in the vessel wall.
- Prevalence: 5% of men over the age of 65; increases with age
- Male:female ratio is 9:1.
- Associated with hypertension, tobacco smoking, and family history (all associated with atherosclerosis)

Pathological features

Types

- *True aneurysms* contain all three layers of artery wall. They may be fusiform (symmetrical dilatation) or saccular. The underlying cause is usually atherosclerosis related but may be associated with infective causes (mycotic aneurysm), Marfan syndrome, and Ehlers–Danlos syndrome (collagen and elastin abnormalities).
- *False aneurysms* do not contain all three layers of vessel wall and often are only lined by surrounding connective tissue or adventitia. They are often secondary to penetrating trauma, iatrogenic injury (e.g., femoral cannulation, surgery), or infection.

Sites

Sites include thoracoabdominal, abdominal, and peripheral (iliac, femoral, popliteal, visceral, carotid, or subclavian).

Clinical features

Thoracoabdominal

- Crawford classification types I–IV (dependent on involvement of descending thoracic or abdominal aorta)
- Often asymptomatic. These aneurysms present with symptoms of acute chest pain (angina/MI), back pain, acute aortic regurgitation, or cardiac failure due to complications (acute aortic syndrome).
- 50% are diagnosed by widened mediastinum on chest X-ray.
- Rupture has high mortality and is rare without prior symptoms.
- Surgery has up to 10% mortality and 10% risk of paraplegia. 10% of patients require dialysis after surgery.
- Endovascular stenting has become the procedure of choice in anatomically suitable patients.

Abdominal aortic

- 95% start below the origin of the renal arteries (infrarenal).
- 15% extend down to involve the origins of the common iliac arteries.
- Associated with other peripheral aneurysm (e.g., popliteal)
- 5%–10% are "inflammatory" (have gross connective tissue changes around the aortic wall in the retroperitoneum).
- Most are asymptomatic. 40% are detected incidentally (clinical examination, ultrasound, abdominal X-ray, CT, MRA)
- Ultrasound screening is recommended in male smokers age ≥55 years.

- 6-monthly scans for surveillance if size 4–5.4 cm (1% per annum risk of rupture)
- Mycotic aneurysms are rare but have a high rupture rate.
- The risk of rupture and mortality increases with increasing aneurysm diameter.
- Surgical intervention is indicated for
  - AP diameter >5.5 cm (may be less: related to age or body habitus)
  - Rapidly increased diameter on serial surveillance scans

Peripheral aneurysms
- *Iliac.* 2% of patients >70 years. These are mostly common iliac and often silent. They are rarely palpable, and rupture may be missed as acute abdomen or renal colic.
- *Femoral.* Mostly asymptomatic pulsatile groin swelling or pain (25%). They may present with lower limb ischemia.
- *Popliteal.* Many are asymptomatic and over half are bilateral. They may present with acute limb ischemia and have a high limb loss in thrombosis. They should be repaired if 2 cm and if thrombus is present.
- *Carotid.* Rare and may be bilateral. They may present with neurological or pressure symptoms, or simply as a pulsatile neck swelling. Diagnosis is with duplex scan and rarely presents with rupture.
- *Visceral.* Account for 1% of all aneurysms. These are generally small and often asymptomatic until rupture. The splenic artery is the most common, followed by hepatic and renal arteries. SMA aneurysm is associated with infection.

Treatment of abdominal aortic aneurysm
The aim is to prevent death, as 30%–80% of patients with ruptured abdominal aortic aneurysms will die even with surgery.

Elective surgery
- Open repair by inlay synthetic graft. This may be a "straight tube" if the aneurysm is confined to the aorta or "bifurcated" if there are common iliac aneurysms as well. There is a 3%–7% operative mortality.

Endovascular repairs
- Endovascular aneurysm repair with a stent graft (EVAR): femoral insertion of covered stent to reinforce the aneurysmal segment
- Advantages: less invasive technique; reduced early mortality
- Disadvantages: high early reintervention rate; requires lifelong surveillance. There is a 10% annual reintervention rate.

Ruptured abdominal aortic aneurysm

Causes and features

- Associated with hypertension (especially uncontrolled), smoking, family history, and atherosclerosis (p. 158).
- Rare in patients <55 years old
- Risk of rupture relates to maximum AP diameter:
  - 0.5% per year, <4.0 cm diameter
  - 1% per year, 4–5.5 cm
  - >3% per year, >5.5 cm
- Patients with a "contained leak" with initial hemodynamic stability proceed rapidly to rupture.
- Less than 50% of patients with a ruptured AAA reach the hospital alive and the overall mortality of the condition may be as high as 75%–95%.
- Outcome is best in the hands of an experienced vascular team (vascular surgeon, vascular anesthetist, experienced nursing team, two assistants, and ICU) and a rapid transfer from the ED to OR.

Symptoms

- Severe or sudden onset of epigastric or back pain
- History of sudden "collapse" often with transient severe hypotension
- Patient may have history of AAA under surveillance

Signs

- Cardinal signs are unexplained rapid-onset hypotension, pain, and sweating.
- A pulsatile abdominal mass is not always present and aggressive abdominal palpation may risk acute deterioration.

Emergency management

Resuscitation

- If the diagnosis is seriously considered, call for vascular surgical assistance immediately. Transfer to the OR may be required even as resuscitation continues.
- IV access via two large-bore cannulae, catheterize, cross-match blood (8 units blood, 8 units platelets), ECG
- High-flow oxygen via non-rebreathing mask
- *Do not* aggressively fluid resuscitate the patient. "Permissive hypotension" reduces the risk of worsening the rupture.
- Give modest doses of analgesia (morphine 5–10 mg).

Establish a diagnosis

- If the patient is stable and the diagnosis is uncertain, a contrast-enhanced CT scan of the abdomen is the investigation of choice.
- If the patient is going to CT, make sure that blood has been sent for cross-match and IV access has been established before they go.

Early management

Ruptures fall into three groups:

- Considered not a candidate for surgery but for analgesia and palliative care. Mortality is essentially 100%. The decision is based on age, status, comorbidity, expressed patient preference, and family wishes.
- Free rupture with collapse and critical condition: all candidates for surgery require emergency transfer to the OR.
- Contained rupture: may be stable after initial presentation but likely to progress to free or complicated rupture unless urgently surgically treated. Endovascular stenting has been used in this setting with success.

Principles of surgery for rupture

- If patient is unstable, muscle relaxation/anesthesia is not started until patient is prepared and draped and the surgical team is ready to go.
- If patient is hemodynamically stable, the central line and arterial line are sited while waiting for blood to arrive and for the surgical team to be ready.
- Give antibiotic prophylaxis.
- The proximal neck is controlled rapidly with aortic cross-clamping (if there is free rupture use a supraceliac clamp). Full fluid expansion with blood can now safely begin.
- Distal outflow of aneurysm is controlled. The proximal clamp should be moved infrarenally if possible.
- The sac is opened and lumbar vessels and inferior mesenteric artery are oversewn to control back-bleeding.
- A Dacron/Gore-Tex graft is sewn to the proximal neck and tested.
- Distal anastomosis is performed next and tested.
- Sequential reperfusion is undertaken, accompanied by volume expansion to minimize post-declamping shock. Ideally, the SBP should be maintained over 85 mmHg.
- Blood products at this stage may be required to correct coagulopathy (e.g., platelets and FFP). Make sure anesthesia stays ahead on volume status.
- The sac is closed over the graft to reduce the risk of aortoenteric fistula.

Postoperative care

- Transfer patient to ICU.
- Correct clotting and maintain hemoglobin >10 g/dL.
- Adequate analgesia and accurate fluid balance
- Attention to cardiac, renal, and pulmonary dysfunction

Complications

- Death
- Renal failure
- Lower limb embolism
- Gut ischemia or infarction

Vascular malformations

Key facts

Malformations are classified broadly into two principal groups.

Primary hemangiomas (with endothelial hyperplasia)

- All are congenital or idiopathic.
- They are mostly sporadic but may rarely be part of a familial syndrome, e.g., von Hippel–Lindau syndrome.
- Pulmonary hemangiomas commonly seen in hereditary hemorrhagic telangiectasia are linked to a deficiency in endoglin (endothelial growth factor).

True arteriovenous malformations (AVM)

AVMs have three main causes:

- *Congenital:* Origin or cause is unknown. These are mostly sporadic but may rarely be part of a congenital syndrome (e.g., Klippel–Trenaunay).
- *Traumatic* AVMs may follow relatively minor trauma.
- *Iatrogenic* AVMs follow a variety of surgical or interventional procedures.

Pathological features

Vascular malformations are histologically categorized as capillary, venous, lymphatic, or mixed in type, depending on the predominant vessel type affected, and are subdivided into low- or high-flow varieties.

Clinical features

- Congenital AVMs are usually evident at birth and the superficial lesion may only represent a part of the overall abnormality.
- Symptoms are dependent on the size, site, and type of vessel affected, and whether the AVMs are high or low flow.

Low flow

- These may result in considerable cosmetic deformity if large (e.g., Klippel–Trenaunay).
- Pain may be a feature due to spontaneous thrombosis of some or all of the venous elements.
- Classically, the symptoms are worse after exercise when blood flow is maximized.

High flow

- These are largely asymptomatic but there may be a detectable venous thrill or bruit.
- They may result in local hyperhidrosis, heat, or ulceration or present with profuse bleeding.
- They may lead to high-output cardiac failure if large and untreated.

Diagnosis and investigation

- Color duplex diagnoses the lesion, can estimate flow rate, and is useful for follow-up monitoring.
- MRI has replaced CT as the best imaging modality and gives both the extent and related anatomy for complex lesions.
- Angiography is reserved for high-flow lesions when suitability for embolization or surgery is being assessed.

Treatment

Treatment is largely conservative:

- Congenital AVMs frequently reduce in size with growth of the child and treatment is rarely easy.
- Adult AVMs only require treatment for complications or occasionally cosmesis.

Interventional radiology

- Percutaneous embolization using wire coils or a foam sclerosing agent under radiological guidance
- Risks include the following:
  - Percutaneous puncture (infection, false aneurysm formation, embolization)
  - Inadvertent embolization of adjacent vessels
  - Tissue necrosis after successful lesion embolization
  - *Postembolization syndrome* may occur with pain at the site of embolization, accompanied by malaise, fever and leukocytosis, and hyperkalemia. This usually settles with symptomatic treatment in 24–48 hr. It is due to tissue necrosis and cytokine release.

Surgery

- Small lesions may be excised completely.
- Obliteration of small, superficial venous malformations can be undertaken by direct puncture and injecting a sclerosing agent such as STD (sodium tetradecyl sulfate).
- Open surgery is mostly confined to high-flow lesions after preoperative embolization.

Carotid disease

Key facts

- A *cerebrovascular accident* (CVA), or stroke, is a sudden onset of irreversible neurological deficit.
- A *transient ischemic attack* (TIA) is a sudden onset of neurological deficit that resolves within 24 hr.
- CVA is the third-most common cause of death in the United States after coronary artery disease (CAD) and cancer.
- CVA has an incidence of 160 per 100,000 population per year.
- Advanced age influences progressive incidence of cerebral infarction.

Pathological features

- Atheromatous plaques form at the bifurcation of the common carotid artery and progress into the external and internal carotid vessels.
- CVA or TIA arises from disease at the origin of the internal carotid artery and may be due to
  - Platelet embolization from the surface of the plaque (usually after an acute rupture or opening of the plaque surface)
  - Embolization of atheromatous material from the plaque.

Clinical features

- Several clinical variants of a classic CVA are recognized:
  - *Stroke in evolution.* Progressive neurological deficit occurs over hours or days. It is indication for emergent endarterectomy.
  - *Completed stroke* is the stable end result of an acute stroke lasting over 24 hr.
  - *Crescendo TIAs* are rapidly recurring TIAs with increasing frequency, suggesting an unstable plaque with ongoing platelet aggregation and small emboli. It is indication for emergent endarterectomy.
- Carotid bruits are detectable in over 10% of patients >60 years of age and do not correlate well with the degree of stenosis or risk of CVA.
- Patients with a significant stenosis may have no audible bruit.

Neurological features

These depend on the territory supplied by the vessel affected by the embolism, the degree of collateral circulation to that territory, and the size and resolution of the embolism.

- *Amaurosis fugax.* Transient monocular visual loss (described as a curtain coming down across the eye) lasts for a few seconds or minutes and involves the central retinal artery.
- *Internal capsular stroke.* Dense hemiplegia usually includes the face and involves striate branches of the middle cerebral artery.
- *Hemianopia.* loss of vision in one-half of the visual field.

Prognosis of patients with TIAs

Some 80% of TIAs are in the carotid territory and the risk of stroke following a TIA is around 18% in the first year, 20% of which may occur in the first month of the TIA. The overall risk is 7 times the risk of stroke for an age-matched population.

Diagnosis and investigation

- Carotid color duplex scan: all patients who have had a TIA or stroke within the last 6 months. There is 95% accuracy for assessment of degree of stenosis.
- MRA/CTA is reserved for those patients in whom duplex is inconclusive or difficult to carry out because of calcified vessels.

Treatment

Medical management

The best medical therapy is an antiplatelet agent (e.g., aspirin, dipyridamole), smoking cessation, optimization of BP and diabetes control, and a statin for lowering of cholesterol.

Surgery: carotid endarterectomy (CEA)

CEA is offered to patients with symptomatic >50% stenosis of the internal carotid artery.

- NASCET (North America Symptomatic Carotid Endarterectomy Trial) has demonstrated a reduction in stroke in the first year following CEA, from 18% with best medical treatment to 3%–5% with surgery and best medical therapy.
- ACAS (Asymptomatic Carotid Artery Stenosis) trial has shown some benefit of CEA to asymptomatic patients with >70% stenosis, but the number needed to prevent one stroke is 22 patients treated.

Technical details

- CEA can be performed under regional block or general anesthesia.
- Use oblique incision anterior to sternocleidomastoid.
- Carotid vessels are controlled after dissection.
- Give IV heparin prior to trial clamp.
- Cerebral circulation is protected in 10% of patients without an intact circle of Willis with a shunt (Pruitt/Javed).
- Shunts should be used if EEG changes are noted or in all patients if no EEG is used.
- Patch closure with Dacron/bovine pericardium is recommended.
- Postoperatively, close monitoring of BP and neurological state is required.

Complications

- Death or major disabling stroke, 1%–2%
- Minor stroke with recovery, 3%–6%
- Myocardial infarction
- Wound hematoma
- Damage to hypoglossal nerve, ansa cervicalis, vagus

The diabetic foot

Foot ulceration is the one of the most common end points of diabetic vascular complications and diabetics are 15 times more likely to undergo major lower-limb amputation than nondiabetics.

Causes and features

Key features of the diabetic foot are
- Ulceration
- Infection
- Sensory neuropathy
- Failure to heal trivial injuries

Ulceration
- Risk factors for ulceration include the following:
  - Previous ulceration
  - Neuropathy (stocking distribution loss and "Charcot's joints")
  - Peripheral arterial disease (more commonly affects the below-knee calf vessels [trifurcation], which are frequently highly calcified, giving rise to falsely elevated ABI readings or incompressible vessels)
  - Altered foot shape
  - Callus, indicating high foot pressures
  - Visual impairment
  - Living alone
  - Renal impairment
- Ulceration is secondary to either large-vessel or small-vessel arterial occlusive disease or neuropathy or a combination of both.
- 45% of diabetic foot ulcerations are purely neuropathic in origin; 10% are purely ischemic; and 45% are of mixed neuroischemic origin.
- Peripheral arterial disease in diabetics

Diagnosis and investigation

Pure neuropathic ulceration
- Warm foot with bounding pulses
- Distended veins
- Evidence of sensory loss leading to unrecognized repeated local trauma
- Normal or high duplex flows

Ischemic or neuroischemic ulceration
- Foot may be cool
- Absent pulses
- Ulcers are commonly on toes, heel, or metatarsal head.
- Secondary infection may be present with minimal pus and mild surrounding cellulitis.
- ABIs may be misleadingly high due to incompressible vessels.
- Duplex ultrasound assessment is required.
- Use angiography for suspected critical ischemia due to stenosis.

Treatment

Prophylactic management

- This is best undertaken in a specialist diabetes foot clinic with multidisciplinary input.
- Conduct regular foot inspection for evidence of pressure or ulceration.
- Always use appropriate wide-fitting footwear.
- Pay attention to nail care with regular visits to a podiatrist.
- Podiatrist debridement of pressure sites or callus is needed if there is adequate vascular supply.
- Keep away from heat and do not walk barefoot.

Established ischemic ulceration

- Treat local or systemic infection.
  - Give broad-spectrum antibiotics (local guidelines).
  - Debride obviously dead tissue.
  - Drain collections of pus.
  - Take plain X-ray for signs of underlying osteomyelitis.
- Consider revascularization if appropriate.
  - Angioplasty
  - Femoral-distal bypass grafts
  - Reconstruction to deal with vascular supply
- Consider amputation for failed medical or surgical treatment.
  - It is often possible to do limited distal amputations.
  - May be progressive if disease spreads

The diabetic surgical patient

- Renal disease requires close monitoring of hydration, BP, and renal function.
- To conduct angiography, metformin needs to be stopped for 48 hr to avoid lactic acidosis.
- Insulin-dependent diabetics starved for any reason require a sliding scale.
- If patient is immobile for any long period, avoid pressure sores with use of foam leg troughs, heel elevation, and prompt attention to any skin breaks.

Amputations

Key facts

- Of all amputations, 90% are for arterial disease (20% of which are in diabetics), 10% are for trauma, and 1% are for pure venous disease.
- Amputation may be a beneficial treatment for pain, to restore mobility, or, occasionally, to save a life in trauma or acute limb ischemia.
- Amputation for arterial disease carries a significant mortality rate and a major morbidity.
- The surgical aim is to achieve a healthy stump for a suitable prosthesis and successful rehabilitation.
- Amputees are at the center of a large team including surgeons, nurses, physiotherapists, prosthetists, occupational therapists, counselors, and the family.

Causes and features

- *Dangerous*: life-saving:
  - Spreading gangrene, e.g., necrotizing fasciitis, gas gangrene
  - Extensive tissue necrosis following burns or trauma
  - Uncontrolled sepsis (diabetic foot) with systemic infection
  - Primary malignant limb tumors not suitable for local excision
- *Dead*: vascular events:
  - Critical limb ischemia with unreconstructable disease
  - Irreversible acute limb ischemia
- *Deformed*: neuropathic or deformed:
  - Failed, complicated orthopedic surgery with severely impaired gait

Level

- The level is chosen according to the following conditions:
  - Lowest level at which tissue is viable for healing
  - Include as many working major joints as possible to improve function.
  - Ideally sited between large joints to allow prosthesis fitting
  - Perform above-knee amputation if patient is non-ambulatory or has flexion contractures at the knee.
- *Above knee*. Most amputations will heal and some patients will achieve walking with a prosthesis.
- *Through knee*. Fewer heal and some patients achieve walking.
- *Below knee*. About two-thirds heal and many more patients achieve walking than those with above-knee amputations.

Types

- *Hip disarticulation* is rarely needed but indicated for trauma or tissue necrosis above the high thigh.
- *Above-knee amputation (AKA)*. Bone is transected at the junction of the upper two-thirds and lower third of femur (12–15 cm above knee joint). AKA is common in end-stage vascular disease.
- *Gritti–Stokes (supracondylar AKA)*. This type is increasingly popular for bilateral amputees as it creates a long stump. It is especially good for wheel chair–dependent patients.
- *Through-knee amputation (TKA)* produces a wide stump, which is difficult for prosthesis fit.

- *Below-knee amputation (BKA)*. Weight bearing on patellar tendon with good prosthetic fit. Good knee function is essential.
  - Posterior flap is the best technique as it produces a better stump for prosthetic fitting.
  - The tibia is transected 8–10 cm distal to the tibial tuberosity and the fibula 2 cm more proximally.
  - Postoperative mobilization is early and temporary limb aids can be used when the wound is sound.
- *Symes (ankle)*. There are few indications for this in vascular patients and it is best avoided other than in trauma or diabetic patients. Prosthetic fitting is difficult and a good BKA is better for walking.
- *Transmetatarsal*. This type is useful in diabetics or when several toes are gangrenous.
- *Ray* is used when digital gangrene extends to the forefoot. It is especially useful for diabetics when infection tracks up the tendon sheath.
- *Digital* amputation is usually done only in the setting of diabetic disease or local trauma.

Treatment
Preoperative care
- Restore hemoglobin levels and correct fluid and electrolyte balance.
- Ensure good diabetes control.
- Cross-match 2 units of blood.
- Give adequate pain relief.
- Obtain ECG and chest X-ray.
- Optimize cardiac function.
- Give prophylactic antibiotics and adjust dosage based on cultures
- Provide counseling if available.

Postoperative care
- Pain control with epidural ± PCA
- Regular physiotherapy to prevent muscle atrophy or contractures, as well as upper-limb exercises
- Early rehabilitation on temporary limb aid
- Own wheelchair to aid early mobilization

Complications
- Infection
- Nonhealing of stump
- Progression of underlying disease and higher level amputation
- Phantom limb pain due to hypersensitivity in divided nerves can be helped with gabapentin, amitryptyline, or carbamazepine.
- For failed mobilization, early regular analgesia and physiotherapy are important.
- Perioperative cardiovascular events are common.

Vasospastic disorders

Many systemic disorders have vasospasm as part of their presentation.

Causes

Rheumatological disease

Vasospasm is often associated with autoimmune disease:

- Systemic sclerosis
- Systemic lupus erythematosus (SLE)
- Rheumatoid arthritis
- Sjögren's syndrome
- Dermatomyositis
- Polymyositis

Neurological disease

- Reflex sympathetic dystrophy
- Post-traumatic vasospasm
- Vibration white finger (due to exposure to handheld vibrating tools, among miners, fitters, builders, platers, etc.)

Drug-induced

α-agonist treatment (ergotamine)

Idiopathic

Raynaud's disease has the following features:

- Male:female ratio is 1:9.
- Affects 20%–30% of young women, with possible familial predisposition
- It is possibly due to deficiency of a potent vasodilator (a calcitonin gene–related peptide) in the digital nerves, which allows action of unopposed cold stress-induced release of the vasoconstrictor endothelin.

Features

Vasospasm of any cause results in Raynaud's phenomenon:

- Intermittent attacks:
  - Initiated with pallor ("white") due to local tissue oligemia
  - Proceeding to cyanosis ("blue") due to venous stasis and deoxygenation
  - Followed by the rubor of hyperemia ("red") due to reactive hyperemia as blood flow is restored

Diagnosis and investigations

Stop all vasoactive treatment 24 hr prior to assessment.

- Digital SBP changes after local cooling to 15 °C (fall >30 mmHg is significant) with measurement of finger Doppler pressures
- Screening: CBC, lytes, urinalysis, thyroid function tests, plasma viscosity, rheumatoid factor, autoantibody screen

Treatment

Medical

- Patient should avoid precipitating factors, e.g., indoor work, electrically heated gloves or socks, and smoking.
- Drug therapy is used If symptoms are severe enough to interfere with work or lifestyle:
  - Calcium channel blockers (e.g., nifedipine, 10 mg/day increasing to 20 mg/day tid) may help, but side effects may limit use.
  - Iloprost (prostacyclin) infusion: weight-related doses are given IV over 48–72 hr according to patient's tolerance of side effects.

Surgical: sympathectomy

This is reserved for patients showing failure to respond to medical therapy or with secondary complications (e.g., digital ulceration).

- *Lumbar.* Open, laparoscopic, or chemical for foot symptoms; effects are mostly short-lived
- *Cervical.* Mostly now endoscopic technique; poor response rate and high relapse rate

Varicose veins

Key facts

- The venous system of the leg is comprised of three groups:
  - *Superficial*: long and short saphenous systems and tributaries
  - *Deep*: between the muscle compartments of the legs
  - *Perforators*: connecting the superficial and deep systems
- Blood passes from the superficial to deep systems via perforators in the calf and also at the saphenofemoral junction (SFJ), saphenopopliteal junction (SPJ), and mid-thigh perforators (MTP), which contain one-way valves.
- Varicose veins are tortuous and dilated segments of veins, associated with valvular incompetence.
- They affect up to 20% of the population.
- Male:female ratio is 9:1.
- There is a familial predisposition.

Causes and features

Classification

- *Spider veins* are intradermal dilated veins; they may be associated with hormonal influences.
- *Flares* are often around the ankle and associated with calf perforator incompetence.
- *Stem veins* are along long or short saphenous systems.
- *Venous malformations*, e.g., congenital (Klippel–Trelaunay syndrome)

Causes

- Primary idiopathic
- Secondary
  - Pelvic masses, e.g., pregnancy, uterine fibroids, ovarian mass, pelvic tumor
  - Pelvic venous abnormalities, e.g., after pelvic surgery or irradiation, previous iliofemoral deep venous thrombosis (DVT)

Clinical features

- *Symptoms* include pain, aching, itching, heaviness, swelling, edema, cramps, being worse at the end of the day, with hot weather, or premenstruation
- *Complications* include eczema, excoriation, phlebitis, lipodermatosclerosis, ulceration, or bleeding.

Diagnosis and investigations

- *General condition*: edema, eczema, ulcers (usually medial calf), lipodermatosclerosis, healed ulceration
- *Standing*: cough impulse, thrill, or saphenovarix at SFJ
- *Tap test*. Tap downward over vein from the SFJ; impulse should be interrupted if valves are competent (frequently unhelpful).
- *Trendelenberg test*. For competence of the SFJ, MTP, and SPJ.
  - With the patient supine, elevate the leg, empty veins, apply tourniquet high in the thigh, and ask patient to stand.
  - Look for venous filling and then release the tourniquet, observing filling of the veins.

- If controlled by the tourniquet and then rapidly fills on release, the incompetent valve is above the level of the tourniquet, i.e., SFJ.
- Then repeat two times with the tourniquet just above the knee and below the knee to test the MTP and SPJ, respectively.
- *Handheld Doppler* (HHD). Listen over the SFJ and SPJ and apply calf compression with the other hand—listen for reflux lasting 1–2 sec. This is the most accurate outpatient method of diagnosis and localization of primary venous reflux disease.
- *Color duplex* is the gold-standard investigation in defining anatomy and incompetence. It is used for recurrent varicose veins and previous DVT, and mismatch between clinical examination and HHD.

Treatment options

Medical

- Microsclerotherapy, laser sclerotherapy, photodynamic therapy
- Foam sclerotherapy
- Compression stockings

Surgical

- Local "stab" avulsions deal with varicosities.
- Saphenofemoral or saphenopopliteal disconnection
- Long saphenous vein stripping (effectively avulses all incompetent thigh perforators). This is never done below the knee because of the risk of saphenous nerve injury.
- Subfascial endoscopic perforator ligation (SEPS) is for calf perforators.

Indications for treatment

- *Cosmetic*—venous flares and spider veins: microsclerotherapy, laser, or photodynamic therapy
- *Varicosities without valvular incompetence*: sclerotherapy, compression stockings, foam sclerotherapy, avulsions
- *Primary varicose veins with valvular incompetence*
  - For SFJ or MTP incompetence: saphenofemoral ligation, long saphenous vein stripping, and stab avulsions
  - For SPJ incompetence: saphenopopliteal ligation and stab avulsions
  - For calf perforator incompetence, there is a controversial role of subfascial endoscopic perforator ligation.

Recurrence can be due to inadequate primary assessment or operation, neovascularization, perforator disease, or disease progression.

Complications of surgery

- Bruising (virtually universal)
- Recurrence (20%)
- Hemorrhage
- Wound infection (most common in groin)
- Saphenous nerve damage with paresthesia (8%)

Experimental treatments

- Endovascular laser therapy (EVLT)
- Endovenous radiofrequency ablation

Deep venous thrombosis

Causes and features

- DVT may develop in association with abnormalities of the vein wall, blood flow, or constituents of blood (Virchow's triad).
- It may be due to vein compression or stasis (immobility, trauma, mass, bed rest, surgery, paralysis, long-distance travel, including airline travel).
- It may be due to inherited hypercoaguability (factor V Leiden, protein C, protein S, or antithrombin insufficiency).
- It may be due to acquired hypercoaguability (surgery, malignancy, polycythemia, smoking, hormone replacement therapy, oral contraceptive pill [OCP], dehydration).
- Severity may vary from isolated asymptomatic tibial or calf thrombosis to severe iliofemoral-segment thrombosis with phlegmasia cerulia dolens (venous gangrene).

Clinical features

- Clinical manifestations may be absent.
- Local features of venous engorgement and stasis:
  - Limb swelling
  - Pain
  - Erythema and warmth to the touch
  - Mild fever and tachycardia resulting from release of inflammatory mediators
  - Homan's sign—calf pain on dorsiflexion of the foot is very unreliable and should *not* be performed.

Complications

- Pulmonary embolism
- Venous gangrene (phlegmasia dolens)

Diagnosis and investigations

- Aim to confirm the presence and extent of thrombosis (to decide on necessity and type of treatment and risk of embolization).
- *Ascending venography* is rarely used now.
- *Duplex scan* is the investigation of choice. It visualizes the anatomy and gives the extent of thrombosis, as it relies on flow of blood and compressibility of vein. Duplex scanning is operator-dependent and has lower sensitivity for calf DVT.
- *VQ scan* is used if there is suspicion or evidence of a pulmonary embolism.
- *CT pulmonary angiography* (CTPA) is the safest, most sensitive, and most specific investigation for suspected pulmonary embolism.

Treatment

- Prophylaxis
- Conservative measures: bed rest, elevation, and good hydration
- *Uncomplicated DVT*: low molecular-weight heparin (LMWH), initially in the hospital; it may be given on an outpatient basis at a dedicated DVT clinic. Subsequent treatment is oral anticoagulation with warfarin for 3–6 months.

- *Complicated DVT*: initially with IV unfractionated heparin (UFH) while converting to oral anticoagulation with warfarin.
- Thrombolysis or surgical thrombectomy are reserved for severe thrombosis with venous gangrene.
- Vena caval filter is percutaneously inserted via the jugular or femoral vein into the infrarenal IVC to catch thromboemboli and prevent PE.
  - This is used for patients with recurrent PEs despite treatment, at risk of major central PE, requiring urgent surgery despite high risk that DVT is present, or other contraindications to anticoagulation.
  - Risks include IVC obstruction, renal vein thrombosis, and complications of insertion.

Chronic venous insufficiency (postphlebitic limb)

This condition is mostly secondary to extensive or recurrent lower-limb DVT.

Clinical features
- Leg or ankle edema
- Varicose eczema, pigmentation, lipodermatosclerosis
- Venous ulceration (medial is more common than lateral)
- Pain relieved by elevation
- Venous claudication (rare)

Assessment
- Many (80%) patients have venous disease alone; others have this mixed with arterial disease.
- History of proven or suspected DVT is common.
- Ulcers are present in many patients—70% are recurrent; 50% are longstanding.

Investigations
- Handheld Doppler pressures to detect arterial disease
- Venous duplex to detect DVT or incompetence and to look for superficial venous disease

Treatment
- Elevation, bed rest, and elevation of foot of bed
- Graduated compression hosiery (when ulcers are healed):
  - Class I: ankle pressure <25 mmHg—prophylaxis
  - Class II: ankle pressure 25–35 mmHg—marked varicose veins and chronic venous insufficiency
  - Class III: ankle pressure 35–45 mmHg—chronic venous insufficiency
  - Class IV: ankle pressure 45–60 mmHg—lymphedema
- Treat stasis ulcers with four-layer compression bandaging (Una boot). There is 75% ulcer healing at 12 weeks.
- Need to confirm ABI >0.7 or Doppler pressures >50 mmHg

Surgery
- Skin grafts (split-skin and pinch grafts)
- Ulcer bed clearance of slough or infection
- Surgery is for superficial venous disease only.
- Its role in mixed superficial and deep venous disease is controversial.
- The patient may need arterial revascularization.

Thrombolysis

Key facts
- Thrombolysis was introduced over 30 years ago.
- Lower doses of thrombolytic agents have reduced the risk of major hemorrhage or stroke.
- It is usually administered as a low-dose intra-arterial infusion or increasingly as an adjunct to surgery intraoperatively.

Agents
- *Urokinase* is expensive, not readily available in the United States.
- *Streptokinase* is cheap but has systemic effects and a 27-min half-life. It has side effects of anaphylaxis, fever, and antibody resistance, thus limiting repeated use. It is widely used for treatment of MI.
- *Recombinant tPA* has powerful clot affinity, lower systemic effects and bleeding complications, and a half-life <6 min. It is most commonly used in the United States.

Indications
- Treatment of acute limb ischemia with viable limb due to *in situ* thrombosis or embolism not suitable for surgery
- Treatment of acute surgical graft complications, e.g., prosthetic graft occlusion <2 weeks and viable limb
- Treatment of residual thromboembolic disease after acute reconstructive surgery
- Thrombosed popliteal artery aneurysm (allows clearance of distal calf vessels)
- It may be suitable to treat venous thrombosis (axillary/femoral), but one needs to balance the risk of hemorrhage and stroke.

Regimen
- Administered via arterial catheter and simultaneous heparin via catheter sheath
- Regular clinical assessment and coagulation checks are needed with clear protocols: half-hour temperature, pulse rate, and BP, as well as foot checks.
- Regular review with angiography (minimum q8hr)
- There is an increased complication rate after 24–36 hr of infusion.

Contraindications
- Increased risk of bleeding (hemorrhagic disorders, peptic ulcer, recent hemorrhagic stroke, recent major surgery, or multiple puncture sites)
- Evidence of muscle necrosis, as this may result in reperfusion syndrome and multiorgan failure
- Urgency such as immediately threatened limb viability

Complications
- *Minor*: allergenic, catheter problems (leak, occlusion), bruising, 15% risk of hemorrhage
- *Major*: 5% risk of major hemorrhage or stroke

Complications in vascular surgery

Complications may occur in the perioperative or early or late postoperative periods. In general, vascular patients are older and have an increased cardiac, cerebral, pulmonary, and renal comorbidity. This is due to the associated risk factors of hypertension, diabetes mellitus, hypercholesterolemia, and smoking.

General
Cardiac
- Atherosclerosis is a systemic disease with a predilection for the cerebral, coronary, peripheral arterial, and renal circulations.
- 40% of patients with peripheral vascular disease (PVD) have at least two of the other circulations affected.
- 20% of patients undergoing noncardiac vascular surgery have evidence of silent myocardial ischemia.
- 70% of the mortality associated with aortic surgery is attributable to perioperative cardiac dysfunction.

Pulmonary
- Worsened by preexisting pulmonary disease, smoking, and obesity
- Ensure adequate analgesia with PCA or epidural and good physiotherapy and early mobilization.

Hemorrhage
- *Perioperative* bleeding is from uncontrolled blood vessels.
- *Postoperative* bleeding is usually due to a breakdown of vascular anastomoses. It is recognized by acute hypotension, shock, abdominal swelling, and pain. Return the patient to the operating room.

Renal failure
- Many vascular patients have preexisting renal impairment due to renovascular disease, drug treatments, or surgery.
- Acute perioperative risks include dehydration, use of IV contrast, and use of NSAIDs or nephrotoxic antibiotics.

Specific
Reperfusion injury
- Due to grossly disordered distal circulation from ischemia during surgery being reperfused into circulation
- Features of acute hemodynamic instability and release of toxins (potassium, myoglobin)
- Injury is prevented by controlled, gradual reperfusion with fluid resuscitation and vasopressor treatment to maintain a good perfusion pressure to the coronary, cerebral, and renal circulations.

Trash foot
- Embolization of debris to the skin or feet after aortoiliac surgery
- Avoided by careful surgical technique and distal vessel clamping first

Swollen limb
- Most swollen limbs are due to reperfusion injury of previously ischemic limbs.
- Consider investigations for DVT if possible.

Lymphocele
- Occurs mostly after groin surgery
- Presents as a fluctuant, non-tender swelling
- Most cases will resolve spontaneously, although larger collections may be aspirated under *strict* aseptic conditions.
- This rarely requires further surgery to oversew the lymphatics.

Gut ischemia
- May follow aortic surgery (ischemic colitis); 2.5% after ruptured AAA surgery, and <1% after elective aortic aneurysm surgery due to loss of gut blood supply
- May present as vague abdominal pain or blood-stained diarrhea
- Sigmoidoscopy usually confirms the diagnosis.
- If there is no evidence of peritonitis, then fluids to rehydrate and close observation are required.
- If there is evidence of peritonitis, an urgent laparotomy is needed with resection of the ischemic bowel.

Impaired sexual function
This is due to damage to the peri-aortic or hypogastric plexus and underlying vascular disease of the blood supply to the pelvis.

Late complications
Graft occlusion
- Early failure after <30 days is due to a technical cause. Occlusion is recognized by acute deterioration in symptoms or acute limb ischemia.
- Late failure is usually due to intimal hyperplasia, continued smoking, or disease progression. It is recognized by progressively worsening symptoms.

False aneurysm
This is usually secondary to infection or occasionally fatigue of graft material (long-term). Further surgery is usually required.

Graft infection
- Mostly from gut bacteria or coagulase-negative staphylococci. MRSA is an increasing problem.
- Infection can be minimized by use of prophylactic antibiotics, meticulous technique, and infection-control policies on vascular wards.
- Once infected, the graft usually has to be removed and alternative extra-anatomic reconstruction is required.
- Infection is recognized by signs of low-grade or chronic sepsis ($\uparrow$ CRP, $\downarrow$ Hb, fever).

Transplantation

Martin Hertl, MD

Basic transplant immunology

The mammalian immune system can be divided into two systems: *innate* and *adaptive*. *Allorecognition* is a function mainly of the adaptive immune response and depends on two main processes. First, alloantigen must be taken up and complexed with surface major histocompatibility complex (MHC) molecules on antigen-presenting cells (APCs) that include B cells, dendritic cells, and Langerhans cells. It is called *direct recognition* when donor APCs within the allograft perform this function and *indirect recognition* when host APCs do this. Second, antigen-specific host T-cell receptors must bind to the peptide fragments of alloantigen complexed with the MHC molecules on APCs (see also Box 16.1).

B- and T-cell diversity

APCs are able to identify, take up, and present alloantigen because of the presence of B-cell receptors (BCRs) specific for each alloantigen. Similarly, T-cell receptors (TCRs) are specific to each alloantigen. The production of a huge number of receptors (approximately 2.5×10^7), each specific to a particular peptide fragment, is possible because of the millions of potential combinations of the thousands of TCR and BCR gene segments.

T-cell activation

When the TCR binds to antigen complexed with MHC molecules, a chain of reactions between intracellular signaling molecules leads to T-cell activation, differentiation, and clonal expansion, resulting in the rapid production of large numbers of cells able to coordinate and effect destruction of tissues bearing the specific alloantigen; this manifests clinically as rejection.

Rejection

There are several types of rejection.
- *Hyperacute rejection* (HAR) is mediated by preformed antibodies that bind to antigens of ABO blood groups, non-self HLA, and xenografts that are similar to antigens found on bacteria and viruses. It results in immediate tissue edema, hemorrhage, and graft thrombosis.
- *Acute rejection* is a function of both the innate and the adaptive immune system, triggered by the recognition of foreign MHC and foreign peptides presented by self-MHC and T cells, and results in tissue destruction over days to many months after transplant.
- *Chronic rejection* is a poorly understood vasculopathy that occurs over years. It is probably a function of the adaptive immune system mediated predominantly through indirect recognition.
- *Cellular rejection* is characterized by cytotoxic T cells destroying a graft. It is usually successfully treated with steroids and an increase in immunosuppression
- *Humoral rejection* is characterized by antibody deposition in the graft, and it is B-cell mediated. Plasmapheresis is used to reduce the amount of circulating antibody, followed by B-cell antibody (Rituxan).

Box 16.1 Glossary of terms in transplant immunology

Adaptive immunity. Learned response to specific non-self antigens

Alloantigen. Antigen from genetically different member of the same species

Allogenicity. Ability of tissue to provoke an immune response when transplanted into a genetically different member of the same species.

Allograft. Transplantation of tissues between nonidentical members of the same species

Allorecognition. Recognition of alloantigen as non-self

Antigen. Cell surface glycoproteins

Antibody. Specific proteins produced by B cells in response to non-self antigen, consisting of two light-chain and two heavy-chain proteins, composing a constant and a variable region. The variable chain region binds with the antigen that triggered the response and the constant region coordinates the cellular response

APC (antigen-presenting cells, dendritic cells). These cells ingest and process antigen, then present it bound to surface MHC to T cells. APCs are most commonly B cells, but other leukocytes can also act as APCs.

Autografts Transplants with the patient's own tissue

B cells. B cells mature in bone marrow. They are APCs that can produce antibodies. In response to antigen they undergo clonal expansion, triggered and coordinated by T helper cells.

Cellular immunity. Adaptive immunity

CD. Cellular differentiation molecule (noted by a number, e.g., CD4)

Clonal expansion. Production of large numbers of identical cells

Costimulatory molecules. Molecule receptors that must be activated, in addition to a main receptor

Direct recognition. Donor APCs present alloantigen to host T cells.

Graft-versus-host-disease. Condition in which immunocompetent donor cells react and destruct recipient tissue

HLA (human leukocyte antigen). Human MHC

Humoral immunity. Innate immunity

Indirect recognition. Host APCs present alloantigen to host T cells.

Innate immunity. Instant response to certain non-self proteins

Isografts. Transplantations between identical individuals (twins)

MHC (major histocompatibility complex). Glycoproteins expressed on the surface of all cells, unique to that individual, coded for by MHC genes on chromosome 6. Alloantigen must be bound to MHC for T cells to recognize it. The two classes of MHC are Class I (HLA molecules A, B, and C), present on all cell membranes, and Class II (HLA molecules DP, DQ, and DR), also known as minor histocompatibility complex, present on only certain cell types. Class II is less allogeneic.

Rejection. Destruction of tissue by host immune response

T cells. T cells mature in the thymus. T cells that bind to thymic tissue (self) are destroyed. T helper cells that are CD4+ coordinate, and cytotoxic T cells (CD8+) effect the response.

Xenograft. Tissue transplanted between species

Immunosuppression and rejection

The goal of immunosuppression is to inhibit the immune response to alloantigen, while preserving the immune response to infection and malignancy. Immunosuppressive drugs (see Box 16.2) are usually dosed higher right after transplant, when the risk of rejection is greatest, and then tapered. A careful balance is maintained between therapeutic and toxic doses of immunosuppression: this is achieved by combining drugs with different mechanisms of action and different side effects.

Acute rejection

Diagnosis

Acute cellular rejection varies in clinical symptomatology depending on the organ transplanted. Clinical features in heart transplantation, for example, include low-grade fever, malaise, reduced exercise tolerance, pericardial rub, supraventricular arrhythmias, low cardiac output, and signs of congestive cardiac failure. Blood tests can reveal a lymphocytosis.

As all patients are on immunosuppression, symptoms may be minimal until rejection is quite advanced, so routine surveillance is undertaken. Hemodynamic measurements with a PA catheter may be helpful, but the gold-standard diagnostic tool is RV endomyocardial biopsy, usually via a right internal jugular percutaneous approach. This is carried out every 7–10 days for a month, tapering to 2- to 6-month intervals. Lymphocyte infiltration and myocyte necrosis is used to grade the severity of cellular rejection. Biopsy-negative cardiac dysfunction raises the possibility of accelerated coronary artery disease or chronic vascular rejection.

Management

- Asymptomatic mild rejection is monitored but not routinely treated. There is danger of a transition to chronic rejection if acute rejections are not completely reversed.
- Myocyte necrosis is a definite indication for increased immunosuppression, but intermediate grades are treated according to clinical context.
- Up to 3 days IV methyprednisolone 500–1000 mg/day for severe acute rejection
- Lower dose (20–60 mg/day po methylprednisolone) on a reducing dosage over several weeks for all other episodes.
- Repeat endomyocardial biopsy after 7–10 days: repeat steroid course if there is no improvement, or give rescue therapy if patient is hemodynamically unstable.
- Rescue protocols include methylprednisolone + thymoglobulin (rarely OKT3).
- Retransplantation might be indicated in certain situations.

Chronic rejection

Chronic rejection manifests as allograft coronary artery disease, detectable in over half of cardiac transplant patients within 5 years of transplantation, and within months in a few patients. Other processes that have been associated with allograft coronary disease include increased donor age, hyperlipidemia, and CMV infection. Ischemia is frequently silent as the heart is denervated. The clinical picture includes ventricular arrhythmias, congestive cardiac failure, and sudden death. Coronary angiography is the gold-standard investigation but may underestimate the extent of disease, as the morphology is diffuse, smooth, intimal proliferation. There is no effective treatment apart from retransplantation. Prophylaxis centers on the same risk reduction strategies used in native ischemic heart disease.

Box 16.2 Immunosuppressive agents

Corticosteroids

Corticosteroids inhibit the immune response at many levels. They decrease production of λ-interferon and interleukins (IL) that would normally cause upregulation of the lymphocyte response, and they reduce macrophage function.

Cyclosporin (CYA)

Cyclosporin is a calcineurine inhibitor: it inhibits the production of IL-2 by T-helper cells, selectively reducing the cytotoxic T-cell response.

Tacrolimus (FK506)

Tacrolimus is also a calcineurin inhibitor with a similar profile.

Mycophenolate mofetil (MMF)

MMF inhibits purine synthesis in lymphocytes, reducing clonal expansion and lymphocyte counts

Azathioprine (AZA)

Azathrioprine causes dose-related bone marrow suppression by suppression of purine synthesis.

Sirolimus (rapamycin)

Sirolimus stops IL-2 triggering clonal expansion of T lymphocytes.

Daclizumub, basiliximab

IL-2 receptor blockers that prevent clonal expansion of T cells

OKT3

OKT3 is a monoclonal antibody produced in mice that binds the CD3 receptor site on cytotoxic T cells, preventing antigen recognition and clonal expansion. Its first dose is associated with severe side effects such as fever, chills, and anaphylactic reaction.

Polyclonal antibodies, e.g., antithymocyte globulin

These are produced by animals (rabbit, horse) after immunization with HLA-antigen: they attach to most circulating lymphocytes, effecting a reduction in cell counts to less than 10% of normal. The side-effect profile is more benign compared to that of OKT3.

Transplant recipients

Indications for transplantation

Cardiac transplantation
- End-stage heart disease with a life expectancy of 12–18 months
- New York Heart Association (NYHA) class III or IV heart failure
- Refractory to medical or surgical therapy
- Patients with ventricular assist devices (VAD)

Lung transplantation
- End-stage lung disease where conventional therapy is not likely to provide acceptable benefits or satisfactorily improve life expectancy

Renal transplantation
All patients with end-stage renal failure should be considered for renal transplant unless there are specific contraindications.

Liver transplantation
- Unacceptable quality of life because of liver disease
- Anticipated remaining length of life is <1 year
- End-stage liver dysfunction as calculated by the MELD score, exception points are given for small HCC (Milan criteria)

Small bowel transplantation (often part of multivisceral)
- Congenital extensive atresia
- Life-threatening complications of TPN in patients with intestinal failure
- Short-gut syndrome after extensive small bowel resection from necrotizing enterocolitis or mechanical complication such as volvulus

Pancreas transplantation
- Type I diabetes mellitus with secondary organ damage (nephropathy, neuropathy, retinopathy, poorly controlled, life-threatening hypoglycemia)

Absolute contraindications to transplantation
- Inability to comply with immunosuppression
- Chronic current systemic infection incompatible with immunosuppression
- Continued abuse of alcohol or other drugs
- Irreversible secondary organ failure not appropriate for combined transplant
- Severe cerebrovascular disease
- Malignancy (except liver transplantation for treatment of HCC or neuroendocrine tumors)
- Other life-threatening medical condition (e.g., AIDS)

Relative contraindications to transplantation
- HIV, hepatitis B/C
- Malignancy except for those treated by transplant
- COPD with FEV_1 <50%, PVR >4 Wood units in heart transplants
- Diabetes with severe target-organ damage (coronary artery disease), but not retinopathy

- Lipid disorders refractory to diet or therapy
- Severe osteoporosis
- Amyloidosis (but possibility of liver after heart transplantation or even combined transplantation)
- Continued smoking

Routine investigations in transplant assessment (varies by organ type)

- A full history and clinical examination
- Chest X-ray with further assessment by CT or ultrasound if indicated
- ECG, transthoracic echocardiogram (TTE), 6-min exercise test, ejection fraction assessment
- Cardiac catheterization and coronary angiography
- Lung function tests
- Urinalyisis, nose swab, and MRSA screen
- Full dental assessment and repair as indicated
- Blood group antibody screen
- FBC, ESR, APTT, PT, INR, fibrinogen, hypercoagulable panel (protein S and C)
- Plasma viscosity
- Urea and electrolytes (U & E), creatinine, creatinine clearance, calcium, phosphate, liver enzymes, cardiac enzymes, fasting blood glucose and lipids, amylase
- Serology for hepatitis B/C, HIV, syphilis, rubella, EBV, herpes varicella and zoster, CMV, toxoplasma.
- Antinuclear factor (ANF) < anti-DNA (by sheep cell agglutination test [SCAT] and LatexAT).
- HLA typing, lymphotoxic antibody screen
- Letter from primary care physician (PCP) confirming previous compliance; interview with social worker, documentation of substance abuse counseling.
- Colonoscopy in patients over age 50 (high rate of stage III and IV colon cancer seen in these patients)

Physiotherapy assessment

Once a patient has been referred, assessment normally takes place in two main stages: an initial, detailed outpatient assessment designed to avoid invasive and costly investigations in a patient who is clearly unsuitable for transplantation, followed in appropriate cases by a 2- to 4-day in patient assessment. The goals of the inpatient assessment are as follows:

- To assess the patient's clinical, psychological, and social suitability
- To ensure that the patient and relatives are fully informed about all aspects of being on the transplant list, the procedure, and aftercare
- To familiarize the patient with the transplant unit and staff
- To optimize the patient's clinical, psychological, and social condition

Accepting a patient onto the transplant list

The results of the above investigations are considered at a multidisciplinary meeting attended by surgeons, anesthetists, organ-specific specialist (nephrologists, cardiologist, pulmonologist, hepatologist, endocrinologist, gastroenterologist), transplant coordinators, and nurses, dieticians, and physiotherapists. The patient is informed of the decision and receives the following:

- A letter stating that he or she is listed for organ transplantation (likewise, a letter has to be sent if the patient is deactivated from the list for medical or other reasons)
- A detailed explanation of the waiting-list procedures (including their responsibility to be available for potential transplant at all times, and the duty to inform the transplant team of any changes in their health, circumstances, medication, and planned holidays)
- A booklet describing this in more detail and explaining what to do when called for surgery, the operation, accommodation for partners, publicity and the media, and wards and departments after surgery

Availability of organs for transplantation

An increasing demand for organ replacement has made transplantation a victim of its own success. The number of potential organ transplant recipients increases every year. There is a national shortage of organ donors despite publicity, donor cards, and the national organ donor registry (UNOS).

Transplant donors

Cadaveric donation

Cadaveric brain-dead beating-heart donors comprise the majority of organ donors (about 8000 in the United States each year). Donation after cardiac death (DCD) donors are accepted more often in recent years, mainly pushed by the organ shortage. The diagnosis is confirmed by CT scan, and a series of clinical tests performed twice by two senior doctors establishes brainstem death. Potential donors undergo a review of their history and clinical examination; ECG; chest X-ray; arterial blood gases; ABO typing; testing for HIV, hepatitis C and B, and CMV; and echocardiography.

Criteria for cadaveric organ donation

- Signed donor card, or consent of next of kin (📖 p. 14)
- No age limit (older donors have been successfully used)
- Hemodynamic stability without high-dose inotropic support
- Absence of septicemia, extracerebral malignancy, HIV
- A shortage of organ supply has resulted in extending the cadaveric donor pool to non-heart-beating donors (DCD)
- Organ-specific criteria include the following:
  - Kidney: age 4–75 years with acceptable renal function
  - Heart: age 1 month–60 years with no known cardiac disease
  - Heart–lung: as above. No pulmonary disease or trauma. PO_2, PCO_2 levels acceptable on less than 50% inspired oxygen
  - Liver: age 1 month–80 years. No known liver disease or drug addiction

Management of cadaveric organ donors

Resuscitation of organ donors requires early recognition and assiduous support. Brain death is associated with a variety of sequelae that include hypothermia, coagulopathy, fall in T_3 and T_4, myocardial depression, and diabetes insipidus.

Therapeutic intervention must be continued up to and throughout the donation procedure. Unnecessary delays should be avoided and the harvested organs must be in optimal condition.

Monitoring

- ECG
- Radial artery line (mean arterial pressure 60–70 mmHg)
- Urine output (more than 1 mL/kg/hr)
- CVP (5–12 cm H_2O PCWP 8–12 mmHg; Swan-Ganz catheterization is recommended in heart donation)
- Temperature (over 35.5°C)

Cardiovascular support

Dopamine may exacerbate any polyuria and cause vasoconstriction with end-organ damage. Dobutamine may exacerbate hypotension. Levophed (norepinephrine) or Neo-Synephrine (phenylephrine) are used for refractory hypotension.

Hormone replacement therapy
- Diabetes insipidus: replace urine loss with 5% dextrose and water via a nasogastric tube.
- Vasopressin via infusion may exacerbate vasoconstriction. Minirin (Desmopressin) is a better antidiuretic. The aim is to achieve an output of 1–3 mL urine/kg/hr.

Respiratory support

Respiratory support requires meticulous asepsis. Oxygen delivery is optimized to achieve a normal $PaCO_2$. High PEEP should be avoided.

Hematological support

Coagulopathies are treated with blood products, and hematocrit is kept at around 30.

Principles of cadaveric organ harvest

The aim is to minimize ischemic times of all organs. Harvest of multiple organs is common: heart and lungs are harvested before abdominal viscera are removed, since they are most vulnerable to ischemia. Respiratory support is continued until the lungs are excised.
- A midline incision from sternal notch to pubis is made.
- 200 IU/kg heparin is given IV just prior to cross-clamping.
- While dissection of abdominal organs is taking place, a median sternotomy is made.
- Organs are carefully examined for evidence of trauma and acquired or congenital disease: the aim is to retain adequate vascular and visceral cuffs to facilitate later anastomosis.

Organ preservation

With current preservation techniques ischemic times as long as 6 hr (heart) to 24 hr (kidney) may be tolerated, but the key to minimizing ischemic injury remains minimizing ischemic time. A variety of storage solutions are used at temperatures of 0°–4°C. Two categories exist: intracellular solutions characterized by high K^+ and low Na^+ such as University of Wisconsin solution (UW solution), and extracellular solutions characterized by low to moderate K^+ and high Na^+ such as Bretschneider (HTK) solution.

Living donors

These are first-degree relatives (parent, child, or sibling) or genetically unrelated individuals (spouse, but also donors that are "emotionally related"). Living donation requires meticulous preparation, ideally by an independent nephrologist and hepatologist or pulmonologist, depending on the organ donated. There were 6700 living donors in the United States in 2006, mostly donating kidneys. "Altruistic" donors are currently accepted mainly as kidney donors.
- All donors undergo blood grouping, tissue typing, and assessment of viral status for hepatitis B and C, HIV, and CMV.

Heart and lung transplantation

Cardiac transplantation

Matching donor to recipient

- **ABO compatibility**. The donor and recipient must be ABO compatible: hyperacute rejection occurs in ABO-incompatible patients.
- **HLA typing**. Although hearts are among the least allogeneic organs, and an HLA mismatch is not a contraindication to transplantation, HLA-A_2 or -A_3 mismatch has been associated with chronic rejection, and some centers choose to avoid this.
- **Size match** is important.

Technique of transplantation

Orthoptopic heart transplantation involves transplanting the donor organ into the space vacated by the recipient heart. There are several techniques of orthoptopic heart transplantation.

- The most commonly used is **the bicaval anastomosis** technique: the donor cavae are attached directly to the recipient cavae.
- In the **original technique** right and left atria of donor and recipient are preserved: anastomosing atria to atria is technically less demanding than bicaval anastomosis.
- In the **total anastomotic technique** each pulmonary vein is individually anastomosed.
- In **heterotopic transplantation**, used in 2.5% of heart transplants, the donor heart is retained and the transplanted heart is anastomosed so that it acts to bypass the left heart. The technique is reserved for severe pulmonary hypertension.

Postoperative care

Monitoring for rejection is done via transvenous endomyocardial biopsy.

Complications

- Infections (nosocomial, opportunistic, or acquired)
  - Bacterial (common nosocomial and opportunistic infections include *Pneumocystis carinii, Mycobacterium* spp)
  - Viral (CMV, HBV, HIV may be transmitted from graft)
  - Fungal (*Candida albicans, Aspergillus*)
  - Most centers put patients on prophylaxis for these infections post-operatively, including TMP/sulfa for pneumocystis pneumonia, clotrimazole for fungal prophylaxis, and acyclovir for viral prevention.
- Rejection (📖 pp. 520, 522) and graft ischemic heart disease
- Hyperlipidemia and diabetes secondary to immunosuppression
- Renal failure (similar risk factors to heart failure, perioperative hypoperfusion, nephrotoxic immunosuppression regimes)
- Hypertension: etiology poorly understood, but most likely due to cyclosporine A (CYA)
- Malignancy: decrease in the T-cell response to Epstein–Barr virus as a result of immunosuppression

Results of cardiac transplantation
- 1-year survival is 87%
- 5-year survival is 72%

Lung and heart–lung transplantation
Matching donor to recipient
- **ABO compatibility**. Donor and recipient must be ABO compatible: hyperacute rejection occurs in ABO-incompatible patients.
- **HLA typing.** Although an HLA mismatch is not a contraindication to transplantation, improved graft survival is associated with matching HLA-B, HLA-A, and HLA-DR loci.
- **Size match** is important.

Technique of transplantation
- **Single-lung transplant** is performed when the remaining native lung will not compromise graft function or present a hazard: emphysema, asthma, and sarcoid require single-lung transplants.
- **Double lung** transplants are performed via a clam-shell incision for cystic fibrosis and bronchiectasis, and have improved survival in cystic fibrosis patients compared to single-lung recipients.
- Because of donor organ shortages **heart–lung transplants** are performed less often with an increase in the use of lung transplants.
- **Domino heart–lung transplants**, where a heart–lung transplant was performed for septic lung disease and the healthy explanted heart then transplanted into a second recipient, is now rarely performed.

Postoperative care
Early postoperative management centers around maintaining a balance between adequate perfusion and gas exchange, while minimizing fluid load, cardiac work, and barotrauma. Cardiovascular management and complications are very similar to those outlined on p. 530.
- Monitoring for rejection is done by transbronchial biopsy and bronchoalveolar lavage.

Complications
- Infections (nosocomial, opportunistic, or acquired)
  - Bacterial (common nosocomial [see p. 530] and opportunistic infections include *Pneumocystis carinii, Mycobacterium* spp.).
  - Viral (CMV, HBV, HIV may be transmitted from graft)
  - Fungal (*Candida albicans, Aspergillus* spp.)
- Vascular stenosis: arterial stenosis results in pulmonary oligemia and venous stenosis in pulmonary edema.
- Tracheal stenosis
- Tracheal ischemia may result in leak and mediastinitis.
- Infection with *Pseudomonas* spp. is common in cystic fibrosis patients. CMV infection is dangerous.

Results of lung transplantation
- 1-year survival is 83%
- 5-year survival is 46%

Kidney and pancreas transplantation

Kidney transplantation
Kidney transplantation is the most common form of organ transplant.

Matching donor to recipient
- **ABO compatibility.** Donor and recipient must be ABO compatible: hyperacute rejection occurs in ABO-incompatible patients. Caveat: recently ABO incompatible transplants are successful with desensitization (plasmapheresis) using living donors.
- **HLA typing.** A favorable match is defined as no more than one mismatch for HLA-A and/or HLA-B and no mismatches for HLA-DR .
- **Children** are given priority.

Technique of transplantation
The kidney is placed non-anatomically into the iliac fossa using an extraperitoneal approach.
- The renal vessels are anastomosed to the external or common iliac vessels. A general rule is to place the first kidney as far distal on the iliac vessels as possible and go more central with subsequent transplants.
- The ureter is anastomosed to the bladder, on the anterior surface of the bladder via a new incision through the bladder wall.
- The ureter is occasionally stented, which will require removal via cystoscopy in 4–6 weeks (it is removed sooner in cases of urinary infection).
- Preoperative native nephrectomy is only occasionally needed for continued or recurrent urinary infection, tuberculosis of the kidney, or massive polycystic kidney disease.

Postoperative care
Early postoperative management centers on maintaining a balance between adequate renal perfusion and blood pressure control.
- Graft function is monitored by urea, creatinine, and creatinine clearance. In cases of increased pain or decreased urine output postoperatively, the transplant kidney is evaluated by renal ultrasound with Doppler evaluation of blood flow into the renal artery and vein, as well as imaging for fluid collections around the kidney. Living donor kidney transplants are expected to have high urine output immediately post-operatively, and low urine output is an urgent complication.
- Oliguria and polyuria are common early after transplantation and are indicative of ischemic injury prior to organ harvest or a prolonged cold ischemic time.
- Biopsy to confirm rejection is done percutaneously, usually with ultrasound guidance.

Complications
- Infection (📖 p. 530)
- Rejection (📖 p. 520)
- Renal vein or artery thrombosis may result in loss of the kidney.
- Ureteric stenosis is treated by ureteroplasty and a stent, or surgery.

- Urinary leak requires urgent surgical repair.
- Lymphocele is managed by percutaneous drainage or by marsupialization into the peritoneum.
- *Note:* in patients with chronic renal failure who may need hemodialysis in the relative near future, as well as patients with kidney transplants, subclavian central venous lines are usually avoided because of the risk of subclavian vein stenosis. Subclavian stenosis precludes dialysis access with an AV fistula or PTFE graft in the future on the side of the stenosis. Internal jugular lines are preferred if central venous access is required. In addition, peripheral IVs are preferentially place below the actecubital fossa for a similar reason, to preserve the veins in the arm for future dialysis access.

Results of kidney transplantation
Cadaveric kidney transplantation
- 1-year survival is 94%
- 5-year survival is 82%

Living donor kidney transplantation
- 1-year survival is 97%
- 5-year survival is 90%

Pancreatic transplantation

Pancreatic transplantation is performed for insulin-dependent diabetes. It is performed either alone (commonly done as pancreas after kidney transplantation [PAK], where the kidney was done previously using a living donor) or in conjunction with kidney transplantation for diabetics in end-stage renal failure. Over 463 PAKs were performed in the United States in 2006, and over 900 as combined kidney–pancreas transplantations.

The transplant operation
The pancreas is harvested as either a segment (tail and body) or as the whole organ with a cuff of duodenum. It is transplanted into an iliac fossa using very similar techniques to those of renal transplantation. The drainage of exocrine function is either to the bladder or to a loop of small intestine by breaching the peritoneum. It is the unwanted exocrine function of the graft that gives rise to significant complications. Bladder-drained exocrine secretions can cause chemical cystitis, the main reason why this technique has largely been abandoned today. Exocrine leakage may occur when it is anastomosed to the intestine, giving rise to peritonitis.

Postoperative monitoring
Immunosuppression is as for kidney transplantation. Bladder-drained graft function may be monitored by assay of urinary amylase. Immunological damage to the pancreas is advanced before changes in blood sugar are recognized; C peptide/insulin levels may be assayed.

Currently, the use of pancreatic islets alone, infused into the portal vein, appears inadequate to render patients insulin-independent.

Insulin is also used sparingly in the immediate postoperative period after pancreas transplant in order to assess the graft function.

Complications
- Infection (📖 p. 530)
- Rejection (📖 p. 520)
- Portal vein thrombosis may result in loss of the pancreas.
- Anastomotic leak resulting in pancreatic fistula

Results of pancreas transplantation
Pancreas transplantation
- 1-year survival is 94%
- 5-year survival is 82%
- 1-year graft survival is 77%
- 5-year graft survival is 53%

Pancreas–kidney transplantation
- 1-year survival is 95%
- 5-year survival is 86%
- 1-year graft survival is 90%
- 5-year graft survival is 76%

Liver transplantation

Approximately 6500 liver transplants are performed each year in the United States, about 300 of them using living donors. The use of "split" livers for size reduction (adult to child) and adult-to-adult living donor liver transplantation has been adopted in recent years.

There is a national shortage of organ donors despite publicity, donor cards, and the national organ donor register. Organs are allocated according to the MELD (Model of End-stage Liver Disease) score, a development of the Child classification, computing bilirubin, INR, and creatinine into a score of 6–40 (see www.unos.org for the exact formula).

Diseases suitable for transplantation

See Table 16.1.
- Chronic HCV disease (hepatitis C virus)
- Alcoholic liver disease—6 months abstinence before consideration
- Primary biliary cirrhosis
- Primary sclerosing cholangitis—excluding complicating cholangiocarcinoma
- Hepatocellular carcinoma in a cirrhotic liver (selected cases)
- Fulminant hepatic failure
- Some cases of patients with neuroendocrine liver metastases

Clinical indications

- Decompensation of chronic liver disease, with an anticipated survival of less than 1 year
- Unacceptable quality of life, due to symptoms of hyperbilirubinemia, including pruritis
- Diuretic-resistant ascites
- Spontaneous bacterial peritonitis
- Hepatorenal failure
- Hepatic encephalopathy

The transplant procedures

Organ retrieval is performed by transplant surgeons. The aorta and the portal vein are both cannulated. The portal vein is perfused with cold UW or HTK solution. Liver preservation is in cold storage in sterile bags. The liver is transplanted within 12 hr of retrieval. The recipient undergoes removal of the native liver, in some centers with placement on venovenous bypass, and placement of the new liver in an orthotopic position, restoring the normal vascular anatomy and an end-to-end choledocho-choledochostomy. Most commonly, immunosuppression is achieved using tacrolimus, MMF, and steroids.

Complications are as for other organs, including rejection, opportunistic infection, and vascular thrombosis. The latter requires immediate retransplantation. Graft survival is 82% at 1 year and about 65% at 5 years, depending on the indication. Patient survival rates are 87% and 72% at 1 and 5 years, respectively.

Table 16.1 Monitoring disease progression using a Child–Pugh score

- Child–Pugh class A, 5–6 points
- Child–Pugh class B, 7–9 points
- Child–Pugh class C, 10–15 points

	1 point	2 points	3 points
Bilirubin (mmol/L)	<34	34–51	>51
Albumin (g/L)	>35	28–35	<28
Prothrombin time (seconds prolonged)	1–3	4–6	>6
Ascites	None	Slight	Moderate
Encephalopathy grade	None	1–2	3–4

Patients in class C should be referred for transplantation.

Intestinal transplantation

Only 170 intestinal transplants were performed in the United States in 2006. Results are still hampered by graft rejection (organ has a lot of lymphatic tissue). Cluster transplantation (with liver, pancreas, stomach, duodenum) has a better long-term outcome, but carries a higher risk of graft vs. host disease (GVHD).

Diseases suitable for transplantation

- Short-bowel syndrome with complications associated with parenteral nutrition
- Irreversible intestinal failure due to
  - Congenital mucosal disorders
  - Chronic pseudo-obstruction of intestine
  - Locally invasive tumors at the base of the intestine

Complications

- Infection (📖 p. 530)
- Rejection (📖 p. 520)
- Anastomotic leaks

Results of intestinal transplantation

Patient survival

- 1-year survival is 80%
- 5-year survival is 50%

Graft survival

- 1-year graft survival is 78%
- 5-year graft survival is 41%

Anesthesia

Jingping Wang, MD, PhD
Warren S. Sandberg, MD, PhD

Preoperative assessment

Introduction

The preoperative assessment is the anesthesiologist's first introduction to a patient and remains a fundamental part of practice. It is important to conduct a thorough history and physical exam, assess and ensure the readiness for surgery, formulate and discuss the anesthetic plan, obtain informed consent, and educate the patient about the expected perio–perative events. The preanesthetic assessment is cost effective, having been shown to reduce cancellations on the day of surgery. It is the first of many interventions aimed at decreasing anesthetic morbidity and mortal-ity. The preoperative interview has also been documented to reduce patient anxiety before surgery and may even decrease postoperative pain and length of hospital stay.

With a healthy patient, preanesthesia assessment and planning is usually straightforward, but this determination is more difficult for elderly patients, those with multiple medical problems, and those contemplating a high-risk surgery. Subspecialty consultation and testing may be needed to better define the extent and impact of intercurrent disease. Such testing may lead to therapy aimed at improving the medical status of the patient to decrease the risk of the surgery.

There are two main goals for the preoperative assessment:
- Evaluation of patient's general health (and optimization if necessary)
- Anticipation of possible complications (and planning to avoid them)

The history should concentrate on symptoms and signs that alert the anesthetist to potential problems during anesthesia as well as those involv-ing the general condition of the patient. The goal is to collect the information needed for planning the optimal anesthetic, and to assess the overall and specific risks of anesthesia.

Basic history

Four components are always required, unless the patient is unable to give a history and emergency prevents obtaining the history from a surrogate.

Allergies

Taking a history of known allergies before prescribing or administering any drug is essential. Be aware of the difference between an allergy and a side effect. For example, opioids frequently cause nausea as a side effect, but many patients report an allergy to the drug class as a consequence.

Medications

Some medications interact with anesthetic agents. Review all prescription medications. Also review over-the-counter, alternative, and illicit drugs as well as tobacco and ethanol use, as these can have serious implications for anesthetic management.

Previous exposure to anesthesia

Review previous anesthetics. Inquire about untoward events, such as
- Adverse reactions to drugs
- Difficult intubation
- Unplanned intraoperative awareness

When such events are discovered in the history, alternative plans may be made to avoid recurrence. A family history of anesthesia problems should also be obtained, as some syndromes, such as plasma cholinesterase deficiency and malignant hyperthermia, are genetically determined.

NPO status

Patients should fast before elective surgery. Obtain a history of the last oral intake of liquids and solids. Depending on the time of last intake, some patients may be considered to have a full stomach, and certain patients are considered to have full stomachs regardless of the time of last oral intake (see section on preoperative fasting, 📖 p. 548). Patients with full stomachs are at risk of regurgitation and pulmonary aspiration during induction of anesthesia, and plans for anesthesia are adjusted to minimize this risk.

Focused medical history and investigation

Medical illnesses may complicate the course of anesthesia and surgery. Concurrent disease guides the anesthesiologist's choice of preoperative testing, consultation, and anesthetic planning.

Cardiovascular system

The history and physical exam should help evaluate the presence of valvular heart disease, congestive heart failure, ischemic heart disease, pacemakers or defibrillators, and hypertension.

Valvular heart disease
- Symptoms of valvular heart disease include dyspnea on exertion, paroxysmal nocturnal dyspnea, palpitations, dizziness, fainting, and angina.
- In general, all diastolic murmurs, loud systolic murmurs, and those accompanied by a thrill are abnormal and indicate underlying structural heart disease.
- With a thorough history and clinical examination, the cardiovascular reserve and degree of stenosis, regurgitation, and mobility of the valves can be estimated.
- The most accurate method of diagnosing the cause of a cardiac murmur is echocardiography. A transthoracic echocardiogram (TTE) should be obtained in patients with murmurs concerning for aortic and mitral stenosis.
- Patients with valvular heart disease or prosthetic valves have a greater risk of developing endocarditis. Prophylactic antibiotic coverage is warranted for most procedures in these patients.

Congestive heart failure (CHF)
- Signs of left ventricular failure include tachycardia, gallop rhythm, fine basal inspiratory crepitations, evidence of an enlarged heart, and displaced apex beat.
- Right heart failure produces a raised jugular venous pressure wave, hepatic enlargement, and peripheral edema.

- Perioperative mortality appears to be more dependent on the patient's condition at the time of surgery than on the myocardial depressant effects of anesthesia. CHF should be aggressively and adequately treated before major elective surgery.
- Therapy is aimed at reducing ventricular filling pressures in addition to improving cardiac output. Medications proven to reduce morbidity and mortality include ACE inhibitors, beta-blockers, and spironolactone. Digoxin and diuretics reduce morbidity without reducing mortality.

Ischemic heart disease

- Ischemic heart disease may be silent but is indicated by a history of angina or myocardial infarction. Precipitating factors such as anemia or valvular heart disease should be sought. Angina associated with dyspnea indicates left ventricular dysfunction.
- A recent history of myocardial infarction increases the risk of perioperative myocardial reinfarction, and elective surgery should be deferred.
- Patients with risk factors for coronary artery disease (CAD) should be risk stratified using the most recent guidelines of the American Heart Association,[1] and additional indicated testing and risk analysis should be performed prior to elective surgery.

Pacemakers or defibrillators

- Patients with cardiac pacemakers or defibrillators should be identified during the history.
- Potential pacemaker interference is a consideration if using electrocautery, particularly with demand-type pacemakers.
- Implanted defibrillators can interpret monopolar electrocautery as a cardiac dysrhythmia and deliver unwarranted therapy.
- Simple electrodessication of small lesions located distant to the pacemaker poses negligible risk.
- The patient's cardiologist should be notified in advance if the defibrillator requires inactivation.

Hypertension

- Hypertension is a risk factor for the development of CAD and a major cause of CHF, renal failure, and cerebrovascular disease.
- Patients with hypertension are at a higher risk for labile blood pressure and for hypertensive emergencies during surgery and immediately following extubation. In the perioperative period, poorly controlled hypertension is associated with an increased incidence of myocardial ischemia, MI, left ventricular dysfunction, dysrhythmia, and stroke.
- Patients should continue taking antihypertensive medications throughout the perioperative period.
- In the perioperative environment, IV esmolol, labetalol, or nitroprusside may be used for acute hypertensive episodes, whereas calcium channel blockers or ACE inhibitors may be used in less acute situations.
- Preoperative anxiolytics or sedation and adequate postoperative pain control are important for alleviating unwanted stress and anxiety, which contribute to undesirable elevations in blood pressure.

1 http://circ.ahajournals.org/cgi/content/full/116/17/e418

Pulmonary system

Postoperative pulmonary complications contribute significantly to perioperative morbidity and mortality. Pulmonary complications occur much more often than cardiac complications in patients undergoing elective surgery on the thorax and upper abdomen. Their frequency varies from 5% to 70%. Postoperative pulmonary complications prolong hospital stay by an average of 1–2 weeks.

Smoking

- Current smokers have a 2-fold increased risk of postoperative complications, even in the absence of COPD. The likely mechanism is that abrupt absence of the irritant effect of cigarette smoke in the postoperative period inhibits coughing and leads to retention of secretions and small airway obstruction.
- The risk is highest in patients who have smoked within the last 2 months. Patients who quit smoking for more than 6 months have a risk similar to those who do not smoke.
- The beneficial effects of smoking cessation, including improvement in ciliary and small airway function and a decrease in sputum production, occur gradually over several weeks.
- Counseling, nicotine replacement therapies, bupropion (Zyban), and varenicline (Chantix) improve the quit rate and should be used aggressively.

Chronic obstructive pulmonary disease (COPD)

- Patients with severe COPD (forced expiratory volume in 1 sec [FEV_1] <40% predicted) are 6 times more likely to have a major postoperative complication. The benefits of elective surgery must be weighed against this potential risk.
- A careful preoperative evaluation of patients with COPD should include identification of high-risk patients and aggressive treatment. Elective surgery should be deferred in patients who are symptomatic, have poor exercise capacity, or have acute exacerbation until their condition has been optimized.
- Bronchodilators, smoking cessation, antibiotics, and chest physical therapy may help significantly reduce COPD-related pulmonary complications.

Asthma

- Inadequate preoperative control of asthma may increase the risk of postoperative complications.
- Optimal asthma control is defined as the absence of symptoms and an FEV_1 of >80% of predicted or personal best.
- Perioperative systemic corticosteroids are recommended for persistent symptoms if the peak flow rate and FEV_1 are <80% predicted or previous best.

Sleep apnea

- Patients with sleep apnea are at increased risk of worsened sleep-disordered breathing, airway obstruction, severe hypoxemia, and hypercapnia in the postoperative period. The diagnosis should be confirmed and the severity assessed preoperatively with a formal polysomnographic sleep study.

- Individuals with sleep apnea who are also obese may present difficulties with endotracheal intubation or early postoperative upper-airway obstruction, requiring reintubation or other therapies. The intraoperative and postoperative use of sedatives and narcotics should be minimized.
- Postoperative nasal continuous positive airway pressure (CPAP) therapy is beneficial. Further, patients with sleep apnea often benefit from regional anesthesia rather than general anesthesia.

Endocrine system
Thyroid
- Hypo- and hyperthyroidism should be controlled prior to elective surgery.

Diabetes mellitus
- Diabetic patients have poor wound healing and an increased propensity for infections. This becomes critical when areas of microvascularization, such as the digits, are the proposed sites of surgery. Also, peripheral neuropathy and the high prevalence of microangiopathy in the skin make wound healing in acral sites more difficult in this population.
- Diabetic gastroparesis is common, so diabetic patients are considered to have full stomachs.
- Ideally, the patient's blood glucose level should be fairly controlled, and the insulin doses should be adjusted as needed.
- As a rule of thumb, insulin-dependent patients require one-half of their non-fasting insulin doses while fasting.

Laboratory testing
Routine preoperative lab testing in asymptomatic healthy patients is not cost effective and does not benefit the patient. Five percent of healthy people have abnormal test results and these have very low predictive values. Patients undergoing minimally invasive surgery after a careful medical history have little potential to benefit from more laboratory testing. Instead, such testing may result in further unnecessary workup and delays in surgery. Lab tests should be ordered on the basis of information obtained from the history and physical exam, the age of the patient, and the complexity of the surgical procedure.

Recommendations for the use of preoperative ECG testing in healthy asymptomatic patients are based on the two factors that increase a patient's cardiovascular risk: increasing age and male gender. Most institutions recommend preoperative ECGs for male patients >40–45 years of age and female patients >50 years of age. Additional risk factors for cardiac disease identified during the history that would warrant a preoperative ECG include hypertension, hypercholesterolemia, cigarette use, diabetes, obesity, positive family history for coronary artery disease, pulmonary disease, CNS disease, a history of radiation therapy, and ETOH (ethyl alcohol) use.

Preoperative screening chest X-rays have a very low yield for finding new abnormalities in surgical patients under 70 years of age and should not be used unless there is some feature of the history that increases the yield. Even in elderly patients, the yield of new abnormalities is low, and changes in management based on X-ray findings are rare.

Examinations specific to anesthesia management

Dentition

The teeth are vulnerable to damage during airway instrumentation. The presence of damaged, loose, or unhealthy teeth should be noted and the risk of further damage discussed with the patient.

Airway assessment

During the physical examination, particular attention is paid to the airway, due to the lethal consequences of failed airway management. Various scoring systems have been created using orofacial measurements to predict difficult intubation. The most widely used is the Mallampati classification (see Box 17.1), which identifies patients in whom the pharynx is not well visualized through the open mouth (see Fig. 17.1). High Mallampati scores predict difficult intubation with reasonable sensitivity.

Evaluation of the oropharynx is accomplished by sitting the patient erect, and, while looking eye-to-eye, asking the patient to open their mouth and stick out their tongue (without vocalizing). Performing the exam with the patient in craniocervical extension, with the examiner still eye-to-eye, improves the positive predictive value. Classification is according to the scale in Box 17.1 and comparison to Figure 17.1.

Box 17.1 Mallampati classification

Class I: Entire uvula and tonsillar pillars visible
Class II: Tip of uvula and pillars hidden by tongue
Class III: Only soft palate visible
Class IV: Only hard palate visible

Assess cervical range of motion, mouth opening, and thyromental distance, all of which will impact the actual intubation prior to surgery. Limited range of motion, poor mouth opening, a high Mallampati score, and a thyromental distance of less than three finger-breadths independently predict difficult intubation, and multiple "positives" among these further increase the likelihood of difficulty.

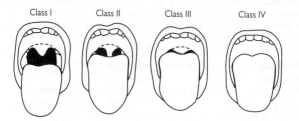

Fig. 17.1 Illustration of Mallampati classes. Reproduced with permission from Allman K, Wilson I (2006). *Oxford Handbook of Anesthesia*. Oxford: Oxford University Press.

- Summarizing, predictors of difficult airway management in the general population include the following:
  - High Mallampati score
  - Small or receding jaw
  - Prominent maxillary teeth
  - Short neck
  - Limited neck extension
  - Poor dentition
- Unique factors complicating airway management include the following:
  - Tumors of the face, mouth, neck, or throat
  - Oral or pharyngeal infection
  - Facial trauma
  - Interdental fixation
  - Hard cervical collar
  - Halo traction

The American Society of Anesthesiologists (ASA) publishes an algorithm for the assessment and management of the difficult airway.[2] Systematic use of this guideline has probably reduced anesthesia morbidity and mortality.

Completing the preoperative assessment

A written plan for anesthesia is required. This should include assignment of an ASA physical status classification, preoperative management of medical diseases bearing on the anesthetic, preoperative medication management, and documentation of informed consent.

2 http://www.asahq.org/publicationsAndServices/Difficult%20Airway.pdf

ASA physical status classification

The ASA has established patient physical status classifications I–VI (see Box 17.2). These reflect the overall medical status of the patient prior to surgery and have good interobserver reproducibility, even when assigned by non-experts.

Box 17.2 ASA physical status classification

Class I A normal healthy patient

Class II A patient with mild systemic disease

Class III A patient with severe systemic disease that limits activity, but is not incapacitating

Class IV A patient with incapacitating systemic disease that is a constant threat to life

Class V A moribund patient not expected to survive 24 hr with or without surgery

Class VI A brain-dead organ donor

E is added to above if operation is an emergency surgical procedure

---

Medication management

Routinely used medications have many potential interactions with anesthetics, but few situations prohibit concurrent administration. The half-life of routinely used medications and adjustment of the dose according to the perioperative schedule must be considered. Many medications must be continued through the perioperative period, with the last dose taken with a sip of water up to 2 hr prior to the procedure, and resumed during recovery. Other drugs must be stopped, replaced, or transiently administered by another route. For example, beta-blockers have potential adverse effects when discontinued abruptly and should be given parenterally in the perioperative period. Switching to an alternative formulation of the same drug may involve a change in dose due to differing bioavailability of the active drug. Additional monitoring of the patient or plasma drug concentrations may be required when different treatments or formulations are used perioperatively.

The components of perioperative medication management are as follows:

• Accurate documentation of preoperative medication
• Establish and document decisions for stopping or changing medications prior to surgery.
• When applicable, monitor appropriate chemistry study results to determine dosages and minimize the occurrence of adverse effects.
• Appropriate management of pain
• Administration of adjunctive medications
• Use of appropriate formulations and alternative products when needed
• Review of discharge medications to ensure discontinuation of surgery-specific drugs (e.g., anticoagulants, analgesics) to avoid polypharmacy and drug errors

Preoperative fasting

Minimizing gastric volume reduces the risk of regurgitation and aspiration during anesthesia; see the 1999 American Society of Anesthesiologists (ASA) Practice Guidelines for Preoperative Fasting and Table 17.1. These are intended for healthy patients at low risk of pulmonary aspiration undergoing elective procedures (not for women in labor) and are applicable to general anesthesia, monitored anesthesia care (MAC), conscious sedation, and regional anesthesia. The guidelines may need to be modified for patients with conditions that might affect gastric emptying or gastric fluid volume. Patients beyond the first trimester of pregnancy and up to 6 weeks postpartum are considered "full stomach" and should be npo of both solids and liquids for a period of 8 hr. Following the guidelines does not guarantee complete gastric emptying.

Ambulatory children and adults may drink clear liquids up to 2 hr preoperatively and still be considered at no increased risk for pulmonary aspiration during general anesthesia if they do not have conditions often associated with increased volume of gastric contents. If more than 2 hr have passed after drinking clear fluids, endogenous gastric secretion is the principal determinant of the pH and volume of stomach contents in the typical ambulatory patient. A longer fluid fast does NOT further reduce aspiration risk. "Clear" liquids are defined as non-coagulating, non-emulsion, or non-particulate-containing fluids.

Examples of clear liquids include water, fruit juices without pulp, carbonated beverages, clear tea, and black coffee. Because nonhuman milk is similar to solids in gastric emptying time, the amount ingested must be considered in determining appropriate fasting period. A light meal typically consists of toast and clear liquids. Meals that include fried or fatty foods or meat may prolong gastric emptying time. Both amount and type of foods ingested must be considered in determining appropriate fasting period.

Table 17.1 Fasting recommendations to reduce risk of pulmonary aspiration[3]

Ingested material	Minimum fasting period (hr)
Clear liquids	2
Breast milk	4
Infant formula	6
Nonhuman milk	6
Light meal	6
Solids	8

3 http://www.asahq.org/publicationsAndServices/NPO.pdf

Informed consent

The most important goal of informed consent is that the patient has an opportunity to be an informed participant in their health-care decisions. Complete informed consent includes a discussion of the following elements: (1) the nature of the decision and procedure; (2) reasonable alternatives to the proposed intervention; (3) the relevant risks, benefits, and uncertainties related to each alternative; (4) assessment of patient understanding; and (5) the acceptance of the intervention by the patient.

For consent to be valid, the patient must be competent to make the decision at hand and the consent must be voluntary. The informed-consent process should be seen as an invitation for the patient to participate in their health-care decisions. The discussion should be carried on in layperson's terms and the patient's understanding should be assessed along the way.

Intraoperative management

Overall goals in the operating room

Maintaining patient safety in the operating room is a major concern. Circumventing preventable complications is essential. Traditionally, nursing and anesthesia staff have managed most safety issues in the operating room, but modern practice involves all members of the team, including the surgeon or proceduralist.

Key aspects of patient safety in the operating room include following the universal protocol for patient identification and establishing the procedure to be performed, thoughtful patient positioning, ocular protection, proper handling of electrocautery, fire prevention, minimization of electrical hazards, attention to sterile technique when inserting and accessing catheters, and airway management.

Along with patient safety in the OR, staff safety is a major concern. An uncluttered, adequately lit environment is essential. Exposure to body fluids should be minimized by appropriate use of barriers, eye protection, gloves and "safety" devices for vascular access.

Finally, anesthesiologists share control of many variables affecting outcomes from surgery. For example, infection prophylaxis by timely administration of preoperative antibiotics, maintenance of normothermia and, in some situations, providing hyperoxia, is largely within the anesthesiologist's purview. There are developing lines of evidence suggesting that control of pain, inflammation, and cardiovascular stress on the day of surgery all improve long-term outcomes.

Patient identification and verification of procedure

On the day of surgery, the anesthesiologist shares responsibility to ensure that the correct procedure is performed on the correct patient. Check the following:
- Patient name
- Date of birth
- Medical record number
- Procedure to be performed
  - Site
  - Laterality
  - Approach

These should be checked with the patient while the rest of the team (nurses, surgeon or proceduralist) is present. Be very alert to possible inconsistencies.

Monitoring

Purpose and standards for monitoring

Physiologic monitoring during anesthesia is intended to optimize patient care, and has been credited with the steady reduction in morbidity and mortality. The ASA promulgates standards for intraoperative monitoring,[4] but simply meeting the standard cannot guarantee any specific patient

4 http://www.asahq.org/publicationsAndServices/standards/02.pdf

outcome. The standards apply to all general anesthetics, regional anesthetics, and monitored anesthesia care. The ASA standard monitors include the following:

- Standard I
  - Qualified anesthesia personnel shall be present in the room throughout the conduct of all general anesthetics, regional anesthetics, and monitored anesthesia care.
- Standard II
  - During all anesthetics, the patient's oxygenation, ventilation, circulation, and temperature shall be continually evaluated.
  - Oxygenation: There will be appropriate monitors to ensure adequate oxygen concentration in the inspired gas and the blood during all anesthetics.
  - Ventilation: to ensure adequate ventilation of the patient during all anesthetics
  - Circulation: to ensure the adequacy of the patient's circulatory function during all anesthetics
  - Body temperature: to aid in the maintenance of appropriate body temperature during all anesthetics

In practice, the minimum monitor set will be the following:
- An oxygen analyzer for the inspired fresh gas
- Capnography
- Pulse oximetry
- Noninvasive or invasive blood pressure
- Electrocardiography
- Temperature (available)

Invasive monitoring

Invasive monitoring includes arterial, central venous and pulmonary artery catheterization, and Foley catheterization.

Arterial catheterization (see Fig. 17.2)
- *Indications*: An arterial catheter is indicated when there may be wide swings in blood pressure where such swings may be deleterious, such as in patients with cardiac or cerebrovascular disease. It is also indicated when frequent blood gas analysis will be necessary, for example, in a patient with severe, chronic pulmonary disease.
- *Contraindications*: Local infection, preexisting ischemia of the extremity, and Raynaud's phenomenon.

Central venous catheterization
- *Indications*: Cases with major fluid shifts, either acutely or over several hours of surgery. This is also indicated for aspiration of air emboli, insertion of transvenous pacing wires, and administration of potent inotropes and vasoconstrictors (such as dopamine, norepinephrine, and epinephrine).
- *Contraindications* include local infection at the insertion site or placement of the line in the surgical field. Coagulopathies are not an absolute contraindication to central venous catheterization.

Pulmonary artery catheters (see Fig. 17.3)
- *Indications*: The pulmonary artery catheter is indicated for patients who are undergoing major surgery with major fluid shifts who have severe LV dysfunction (and/or cardiac failure), pulmonary hypertension, or cor pulmonale. However, routine use even in these patients is being questioned because it is unclear that the benefits outweigh the risks.
- *Contraindications*: (1) mechanical heart valves (absolute); (2) hypercoagulable states; (3) recently inserted transvenous pacemaker, bifascicular heart block, coagulopathy, frequent dysrhythmias, history of pulmonary stenosis (all relative contraindications).

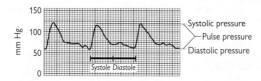

Fig. 17.2 Illustration of arterial catheter waveform.

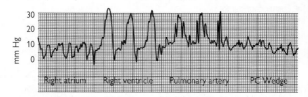

Fig. 17.3 Pulmonary artery waveform and pressures.

Foley catheterization
- *Indications*: Urine output is a very sensitive indicator of renal perfusion, which in turn reflects intravascular volume. If the case involves significant fluid shifts, is going to be long, or is to be performed in a patient with borderline renal function, a Foley catheter is indicated.

General anesthesia

The type of anesthesia used is based on several factors, including the patient's physical condition, the type of surgery to be performed, previous anesthesia history, reactions to medications, the patient's and surgeon's preferences, and information provided during the preoperative interview. General anesthesia (GA) is given to patients when the surgical area cannot be adequately anesthetized with a local or regional nerve block, or when patient or procedural factors argue for unconsciousness. Attributes of general anesthesia include the following:

Advantages
- After induction, it makes no psychological demand of the patient.
- GA allows complete stillness for prolonged periods of time.
- It facilitates complete control of the airway, breathing, and circulation.
- It permits simultaneous surgery on widely separated areas of the body.
- It can be used in cases of hypersensitivity to local anesthetic agents.
- It can be administered without moving the patient from the supine position.
- It can be adapted easily to procedures of unpredictable duration or extent.
- It usually can be administered rapidly.

Disadvantages
- GA requires anesthesia personnel.
- It requires complex and costly machinery.
- It is usually associated with some degree of physiological trespass.
- It carries the risk of major complications including death, brain damage, myocardial infarction, pulmonary aspiration, blindness, and stroke.
- Roughly 0.2% of general anesthetics are complicated by unintended intraoperative awareness.
- It is commonly associated with less serious complications such as nausea or vomiting, sore throat, headache, shivering, and delayed return to normal mental functioning.
- It is uniquely associated with malignant hyperthermia, a rare, inherited muscular condition in which exposure to some (but not all) general anesthetic agents results in acute and potentially lethal temperature rise, hypercarbia, metabolic acidosis, and hyperkalemia.

Complications
A given patient's risk for complications as a direct result of GA is small but depends largely on his or her medical comorbidities. Death attributable to anesthesia is thought to occur at rates of less than 1:10,000, but these are average figures incorporating both elective and emergency patients with all types of physical conditions. Minor complications occur at predicable rates, even in previously healthy patients.

The frequency of problems during the first 24 hr following ambulatory surgery is as follows:

- Bleeding, vomiting, nausea: less than 5%, although nausea and vomiting rates can be much higher
- Fever: 5%–15%
- Dizziness, headache, drowsiness, hoarseness: more than 15%
- Sore throat: 25%
- Incision pain: 30%

Four phases of general anesthesia

Premedication and sedation

This phase is usually conducted in a preoperative holding area. The goal is to have the patient arrive in the operating room in a calm, relaxed frame of mind, while causing minimal interference with breathing and cardiovascular status.

- The most commonly used premedicants are short-acting benzodiazepines. Midazolam syrup is often given to children to facilitate calm separation from their parents prior to anesthesia.
- In anticipation of surgical pain, NSAIDs or acetaminophen can be administered preemptively.
- Antacids, metoclopromide, and/or H2 blockers may be administered to patients with gastroesophageal reflux.
- An unresolved debate is whether to administer preoperative and intraoperative beta-blockers to those with risk factors for coronary disease to prevent myocardial infarction.

Induction

The transition from the unanesthetized to anesthetized state is called *induction* of anesthesia. Induction of general anesthesia is achieved by IV injection of induction agents (drugs that work rapidly, such as thiopental and propofol), or by the slower inhalation of anesthetic vapors from a face mask, or a combination of both. Rarely, induction is achieved by intramuscular injection.

Adult patients and most children are induced with IV drugs, this being a rapid and minimally unpleasant experience for the patient. In addition to the induction drug, most patients receive an injection of opioid analgesic. This helps preempt undesirable responses to endotracheal intubation and skin incision. Opioids potentiate the ability of induction agents to induce anesthesia.

The next step of the induction process is the securing of the airway. This may be a simple matter of manually holding the patient's jaw such that their natural breathing is unimpeded by the tongue or may demand the insertion of a prosthetic airway device such as a laryngeal mask airway or endotracheal tube. A variety of factors are considered when making this decision. The major issue is whether the patient requires an endotracheal tube. Indications for endotracheal intubation under general anesthesia include the following:

- Potential for airway contamination (full stomach, gastroesophageal [GE] reflux, GI or pharyngeal bleeding)
- Surgical need for skeletal muscle paralysis

- Predictable difficulty with endotracheal intubation or where anesthetist's access to the airway during the case will be difficult (lateral or prone position)
- Surgery of the mouth or face
- Prolonged procedure is anticipated

If airway control is anticipated to be difficult, the airway may be secured using specialized techniques *prior* to induction.

Surgery through the muscular walls of the thorax and abdomen is usually facilitated by muscle relaxation with an intermediate or long-acting muscle relaxant. This paralyzes muscles indiscriminately, including the muscles of breathing. Therefore, the patient's lungs must be ventilated using positive pressure, usually via an endotracheal tube.

Maintenance
The patient must be kept anesthetized with a maintenance agent. Some induction drugs can be used for maintenance, but anesthesia is most commonly maintained by the delivery of anesthetic gases (more properly termed *vapors*) into the patient's lungs. These may be inhaled as the patient breathes on his or her own or be delivered under pressure by each mechanical breath of a ventilator.

As the procedure progresses, the level of anesthesia is altered to give the minimum amount necessary to ensure adequate anesthetic depth. Excessive anesthetic depth is associated with decreased heart rate and blood pressure, and, if carried to extremes, can jeopardize perfusion of vital organs or be fatal.

Traditionally, depth of anesthesia has been a matter of clinical judgment, but several continuous monitors of neurologic function give the anesthetist a simplified output corresponding to anesthetic depth.

As the surgical procedure draws to a close, the patient's emergence from anesthesia is planned. Experience and close communication with the surgeon enable the anesthesiologist to predict when the incision will be closed and application of dressings, casts, etc., will be complete. In advance of that time, anesthetics are decreased or even switched off entirely to allow time for metabolism, redistribution, or excretion.

Emergence
The patient's neuromuscular blockade must be reassessed and residual muscle paralysis is reversed using specific drugs. Adequate long-acting opioid analgesic is administered to keep the patient comfortable in the recovery room. If a ventilator has been used, the patient is restored to breathing on their own and, as anesthetic drugs dissipate, the patient emerges to consciousness. Once the patient is reversed, awake, suctioned, and extubated, care must be taken in transferring the patient to the gurney and oxygen must be readily available for transportation to the recovery room or post-anesthesia care unit (PACU).

Monitored anesthesia care and IV sedation

IV sedation and monitored anesthesia care are used as adjuncts to regional anesthesia to potentiate the regional block and allow the patient to tolerate the procedure. IV sedation causes minimal CNS depression and may be administered by a nurse under direction of the proceduralist.

Basic physiologic monitoring is required. Drugs commonly used for IV sedation include the following:

- Midazolam in doses (cumulative) of 0.5–2.0 mg
- Opioids, such as fentanyl (25–250 µg, cumulative dose), meperidine (25–150 mg, cumulative dose)
- Supplemental oxygen should be provided.
- IV sedation should only be used where some member of the team is trained to secure and maintain the airway, or where such assistance is readily available.

Monitored anesthesia care achieves significant CNS depression, but the airway and spontaneous ventilation are maintained and the patient is able to respond to verbal commands.

- Drugs used for monitored anesthesia care include those listed for IV sedation above, and potentially include all of the induction and maintenance agents used for general anesthesia

Meticulous attention to monitoring is required to guard against airway obstruction, oxygen desaturation, and pulmonary aspiration. Consequently, monitored anesthesia care is performed only by qualified anesthesia personnel.

Regional anesthesia

The benefits of regional anesthesia may include minimal impact on the sensorium while providing excellent immobility and loss of sensation. Regional anesthesia decreases the incidence of aspiration, nausea, early postoperative pain, and postanesthesia disorientation. Regional anesthesia is divided into neuraxial (chiefly spinal and epidural anesthesia) and peripheral techniques. Neuraxial techniques are suitable for surgery of the trunk and lower extremities, while peripheral techniques are suited primarily to extremity surgery.

The two most common neuraxial techniques are single-shot spinal anesthesia and continuous epidural anesthesia via a catheter. Compared with spinal anesthesia, epidural anesthesia takes more time to perform, has a slower onset of action, and may not produce as profound a block; however, the duration of an epidural block can readily be extended intraoperatively or postoperatively if necessary by reinjecting the catheter. Neuraxial regional techniques require assiduous aseptic technique to avoid potentially devastating infection and should not be performed in coagulopathic patients for fear of an epidural hematoma.

In regional anesthesia local anesthetic drugs are used that block neuronal sodium channels. Opioids are useful adjuvents in neuraxial techniques. Care should be exercised in choosing a local anesthetic for neuraxial blockade:

- Spinal lidocaine may be associated with a transient radicular irritation.
- Bupivacaine and tetracaine may be associated with prolonged motor block.
- Neuraxial opioids may produce pruritus, urinary retention, nausea and vomiting, and respiratory depression.

Various dosing regimens have been proposed to minimize these side effects.

Epidural anesthesia

Epidural anesthesia is a neuraxial block technique with many applications. Both single injection and catheter techniques can be used, although catheter techniques predominate. Epidural techniques may be used as a sole anesthetic, as an analgesic adjuvant to general anesthesia, and for postoperative analgesia in procedures involving the lower limbs, perineum, pelvis, abdomen, and thorax.

The advantage of epidural over spinal anesthesia is the ability to maintain continuous anesthesia after placement of an epidural catheter, thus making it suitable for procedures of long duration. The catheter may be used into the postoperative period for analgesia, using lower concentrations of local anesthetic drugs or in combination with different agents. Postoperative epidural analgesia facilitates early ambulation and return of bowel function after abdominal surgery.

Epidural anesthesia has a low but real incidence of major complications, including epidural hematoma or abscess. Either can cause permanent neurologic damage, including paralysis if not diagnosed promptly and evacuated. Back pain is an unreliable symptom of epidural abscess or hematoma. Declining motor strength or sensation in the face of a stable epidural infusion rate should prompt consultation with an anesthesiologist to evaluate if there is a problem.

Absolute contraindications to epidural anesthesia

- Patient refusal
- Coagulopathy or therapeutic anticoagulation. If bleeding occurs into the epidural space, a hematoma may form and compress the spinal cord. Patients with a low platelet count or receiving anticoagulant drugs such as heparin or warfarin are at risk
- Skin infection at the injection site poses an unacceptable risk of neuraxial infection.
- Raised intracranial pressure

Relative contraindications

- Uncooperative patients
- Preexisting neurological disorders
- Hypovolemia
- Fixed cardiac output states
- Anatomical abnormalities of vertebral column

Spinal anesthesia

Spinal anesthesia is induced by injecting small amounts of local anesthetic into the cerebrospinal fluid (CSF) in the subarachnoid space. The injection is usually made in the lumbar spine below the level at which the spinal cord ends (L2). Spinal anesthesia is easy to perform and has the potential to provide excellent operating conditions. If the anesthetist has an adequate knowledge of the relevant anatomy, physiology, and pharmacology, profound anesthesia can easily and safely be obtained to the mutual satisfaction of the patient, surgeon, and anesthetist.

Spinal anesthesia is best reserved for operations below the umbilicus, e.g., hernia repairs, gynecological and urological operations, and any operation on the perineum or genitalia. Spinal anesthesia is particularly suitable for older patients and those with systemic disease such as chronic respiratory disease and hepatic, renal, and endocrine disorders such as diabetes. Many patients with mild cardiac disease benefit from the vasodilation that accompanies spinal anesthesia, except those with stenotic valvular disease or uncontrolled hypertension.

Advantages of spinal anesthesia
- The costs associated with spinal anesthesia are minimal.
- The majority of patients are very happy with the technique and appreciate the rapid recovery and absence of side effects.
- Spinal anesthesia produces few adverse effects on the respiratory system as long as unduly high blocks are avoided.
- There is a reduced risk of airway obstruction or the aspiration of gastric contents.
- Spinal anesthesia provides excellent muscle relaxation for lower abdominal and lower limb surgery.
- Blood loss during the operation is less than when the same operation is done under general anesthesia.

Disadvantages of spinal anesthesia
- Hypotension may occur with higher blocks, so the anesthetist must know how to manage this situation with the necessary resuscitation drugs and equipment immediately at hand.
- Some patients are not psychologically suited to be awake, even if sedated, during an operation. They should be identified during the preoperative assessment. Likewise, some surgeons find it very stressful to operate on conscious patients.
- Even if a long-acting local anesthetic is used, a spinal is not suitable for surgery lasting longer than approximately 4 hr. Patients find lying on an operating table for long periods uncomfortable. If an operation unexpectedly lasts longer than this, it may be necessary to convert to a general anesthetic or supplement the anesthetic with IV ketamine or with a propofol infusion if that drug is available.
- There is a theoretical risk of introducing infection into the sub-arachnoid space and causing meningitis. This should never happen if equipment is sterilized properly and an aseptic technique is used.
- A postural headache may occur postoperatively.

Contraindications to spinal anesthesia
- Patient refusal
- Inadequate resuscitation drugs and equipment. No regional anesthetic technique should be attempted if drugs and equipment for resuscitation are not immediately at hand.
- Clotting disorders and therapeutic anticoagulation—see contraindications to epidural anesthesia above.
- Hypovolemia from whatever cause, e.g., bleeding, dehydration due to vomiting, diarrhea or bowel obstruction. Patients must be adequately rehydrated or resuscitated before spinal anesthesia or they will become very hypotensive
- Infection at or near the site of lumbar puncture

- Neurological disease
- Elevated intracranial pressure
- Transient neuropathies—long-acting agents are less problematic

Peripheral regional anesthesia

Peripheral nerve blocks are achieved by injecting anesthetic solution around a major nerve or plexus to produce anesthesia in the distribution of that nerve. The blocks are particularly advantageous when infiltration anesthesia may cause unacceptable distortion of the surgical site or require an amount of anesthetic that exceeds the maximum recommended dose. Regional blocks allow a smaller amount of anesthetic to be used, thereby reducing the risk of systemic toxicity. Regional blocks also allow anesthesia of larger surface areas with less distortion of the surgical site.

- Regional blocks require complete knowledge of the anatomic landmarks and the location of the nerve to be blocked, keeping in mind individual variation.
- Peripheral nerves are located using specially designed nerve stimulators or with ultrasound visualization.
- If local anesthetic is injected intravascularly, cardiotoxicity (malignant ventricular dysrhythmias and cardiovascular collapse) will likely occur. Hence, aspiration should always be performed before the anesthetic is injected to verify that the needle tip does not lie within a blood vessel.
- The length and type of needle are determined by the estimated distance from the injection site to the nerve targeted for the block.

Numerous peripheral regional-anesthesia techniques have been developed, practically creating a subspecialty of anesthesia. Description of the individual techniques is beyond the scope of this chapter.

Early postoperative management

In the recovery room, the anesthetic plan is continued until discharge. Concerns that are directly the responsibility of the anesthesiologist in the immediate postoperative period include nausea and vomiting, hemodynamic stability, and pain management. Shorter-acting narcotics and NSAIDs are administered for pain relief, and any of several agents may be given for control of nausea and vomiting. Other concerns include continuing awareness of the patient's airway and level of consciousness, as well as follow-up of intraoperative procedures such as central-line placement and postoperative X-rays to rule out pneumothorax. Recovery of normal muscle strength and sensation (including proprioception of the lower extremities, autonomic function, and ability to void) should be demonstrated after spinal or epidural anesthesia.

Postoperative nausea and vomiting (PONV)

PONV is one of the most common side effects associated with surgical procedures. The medical complications of PONV include possible wound disruption, esophageal tears, gastric herniation, muscular fatigue, dehydration, and electrolyte imbalance. There is also a risk of pulmonary aspiration of vomitus. PONV may cause anxiety about undergoing future surgery. The cost implications of PONV can be major because of delayed recovery and discharge, as well as increased medical resource utilization.

PONV risk factors

Large multifactorial trials have identified four major risk factors for PONV:

- Female gender
- Nonsmoker
- History of PONV or motion sickness
- Planned postoperative use of opioid analgesics

Each of these risk factors, if present, increases PONV likelihood to the same degree. Presence of three or more risk factors virtually assures PONV and warrants chemoprophylaxis.

Detailed analysis of risk factors for PONV divides them into patient risk factors, procedural risk factors, anesthetic risk factors, and postoperative risk factors, many of which map onto the major factors listed above.

Patient risk factors

- *Gender*. The prevalence of PONV is three times higher in women than in men. This gender difference is not evident in prepubertal children or in the elderly, indicating that there may be hormonal involvement.
- *Age*. Children are two times more likely to develop PONV than adults. PONV is rare in very young children, increases up to the age of 5, and is highest in children between the ages of 6 and 16 years
- *Obesity*. Fat-soluble anesthetics may accumulate in adipose tissue and continue to be released for an extended period, resulting in prolonged side effects, including PONV.

- *Migraine*. Patients with a history of migraine are more likely to experience PONV.
- *Preoperative fasting status*. Adequate preoperative fasting reduces the risk of PONV, whereas excessive starvation appears to increase the risk. In emergency surgery where there has not been an adequate fast, PONV risk is increased.
- *History of PONV or motion sickness*. Such patients may have a lower threshold to nausea and vomiting than the rest of the population. Anxiety from a previous experience of PONV may add to the risk.
- *Gastroparesis*. Patients with delayed gastric emptying secondary to an underlying disease may be at increased risk of PONV.

Procedural risk factors
The following surgical-procedure categories increase the incidence of PONV:
- Gynecological
- Abdominal, especially gastrointestinal
- Laparoscopic
- Ear, nose, and throat
- Ophthalmic

Anesthetic agents
- Preoperative use of opioid analgesics
- Nitrous oxide
- Inhalation agents
- Greater depth of anesthesia

Use of propofol as a maintenance agent is PROTECTIVE.

Postoperative risk factors that can influence the risk of PONV
- *Pain*. Relief of pain is often associated with the relief of nausea, even though the use of opioid analgesics may exacerbate the risk because of their known emetic potential. However, some patients may be willing to tolerate a degree of pain provided they are free of nausea and vomiting
- *Use of opioids*. The use of opioids may exacerbate the risk of PONV because of their known emetic potential.
- *Early ambulation*. Early or sudden movement can increase the risk of PONV, especially if patients have received opioids.
- *Dizziness*. PONV is increased in patients who experience dizziness.
- *Hypotension*. Postoperative hypotension is common and can trigger PONV.
- *Premature oral intake*. It is generally considered wise to restrict oral intake, and then to recommend small sips of water to minimize the risk of PONV.

Pharmacologic treatment of PONV (see Table 17.2)
No single drug or class of drug is fully effective in controlling PONV, presumably because none block all pathways in the vomiting center. Because of the multireceptor origin of PONV, combination therapy is widely employed and more effective than monotherapy.

Table 17.2 Agents for PONV prophylaxis and rescue

Agent	Dose	Comments and side effects
Propofol	10 mg IV, repeated dose	Intuitive hesitance to use induction agent in PACU for PONV
Ondansetron and other 5-HT3 antagonists	1.0–4.0 mg IV (ondansetron)	Effective; can cause headache, constipation, transiently increased LFTs
Dexamethasone	4.0–8.0 mg IV	Theoretical risks of adrenocortical suppression, delayed wound healing, fluid retention, electrolyte disturbances, psychosis, osteoporosis; all minimal with one-time exposure
Butyrophenones: droperidol and haloperidol	0.5–1.0 mg IV (haloperidol)	Sedation, restlessness, dysphoria, acute dystonic reactions, dysrhythmia
Metoclopramide	10–20 mg IV	Avoid in bowel obstruction; can cause extrapyramidal reactions
Scopolamine	0.1–0.6 mg SC, IM, IV	Muscarinic side effects, somnolence
Dimenhydrinate	25–50 mg IV	Drowsiness, dizziness

Postanesthetic Discharge Scoring System (PADSS)

Postanesthetic management of the patient includes periodic assessment of respiratory and cardiovascular function, neuromuscular function, mental status, temperature, pain, nausea and vomiting, wound drainage, bleeding, and urine output.

- PADSS is a structured scale (Table 17.3) used to evaluate patients' readiness for discharge within a framework that is consistent across institutions.
- The total possible score is 10; patients scoring ≥9 are considered fit for discharge home.
- Clinical judgment always supersedes these guidelines if the patient's condition is not satisfactory in a given area. Whenever doubt exists about diagnosis or patient safety, discharge should be delayed.

Table 17.3 PADSS axes for evaluation

Category	Score	Explanation
Vital signs	2	Within 20% of preoperative value
	1	Within 20% to 40% of preoperative value
	0	Within 40% of preoperative value
Activity, mental status	2	Oriented and steady gait
	1	Oriented or steady gait
	0	Neither
Pain, nausea, vomiting	2	Minimal
	1	Moderate
	0	Severe
Surgical bleeding	2	Minimal
	1	Moderate
	0	Severe
Intake/output	2	Oral fluid intake and voiding
	1	Oral fluid intake or voiding
	0	Neither

Pain management

Nonopioid analgesics

The most commonly used analgesic agents are drugs such as aspirin and the nonsteroidal anti-inflammatory drugs (NSAIDs). These are the main analgesic treatment for mild to moderate pain.

NSAIDs have both analgesic and anti-inflammatory actions. Their mechanism of action is predominantly by inhibition of prostaglandin synthesis by the enzyme cyclo-oxygenase, which catalyses the conversion of arachadonic acid to the various prostaglandins that are the chief mediators of inflammation. NSAIDs are more useful for superficial pain arising from the skin, buccal mucosa, joint surfaces, and bone. They may be usefully combined with opioids due to their different modes of action.

Analogs of gamma-aminobutyric acid, such as gabapentin have also proven useful as nonopioid analgesics.

Opioids

Opioids act at CNS receptors. Initially, three distinct receptor groups were described (mu, kappa, and sigma) on the basis of their binding characteristics. Various opioids have differing affinities for these receptors and are described by their receptor affinities as either full or partial agonists. Major side effects include nausea, vomiting, constipation, and respiratory depression. Tolerance may occur with repeated dosage but this is highly unlikely to become apparent during the first week of continuous treatment. Opioids are antitussives.

- **Codeine** is a weak opioid analgesic derived from opium alkaloids (as is morphine). Codeine is metabolized to morphine, which is the active compound. In contrast to morphine, codeine has predictable absorption when given orally. Codeine is effective against mild to moderate pain in most patients, although many African Americans lack the enzyme required for metabolism to morphine. In these patients, codeine is inefficacious.
- **Morphine, hydromorphone**, and **oxycodone** have intermediate half-lives and are useful for moderate to severe pain. All are metabolized in the liver and clearance is reduced in patients with liver disease, in the elderly, and in the debilitated. Morphine and hydromorphone are most frequently administered parenterally. Rapid IV injection of morphine doses releases histamine, causing flushing, bronchospasm, and hypotension. Equianalgesic doses of hydromorphone are free of this side effect. Oxycodone is administered orally, where its predictable absorption and bioavailability are assets.
- **Methadone** is well absorbed orally. It is slowly metabolized in the liver and has a very long half-life. The resultant prolonged duration of action makes it more suitable for use in chronic pain rather than acute postoperative pain. However, intravenous methadone has been used successfully for acute pain management.
- **Fentanyl** is used chiefly for intraoperative analgesia because of its relatively short duration of action. It has similar actions and side effects to those of morphine and is metabolized in the liver. Postoperatively it has been used intrathecally or epidurally.
- **Meperidine** produces effects similar to those of morphine but is a unique chemical entity. Consequently, its actions differ somewhat from those of other opioids, including reduced antitussive and anti-diarrheal actions, predictable increases in heart rate, and more euphoria. Currently it is used for preanesthesia sedation and for relief of moderate to severe pain, particularly in obstetrics and postoperative situations.

Opioid overdoses produce respiratory depression and hypotension. The specific antidote naloxone is indicated for coma or very slow respiration.

Patient-controlled analgesia (PCA)

Patients control their own IV analgesia (within limits) and so titrate the dose to their own end-point of pain relief using a button trigger for a small microprocessor-controlled pump. The limits include

- Size of the bolus dose
- The minimum time period between doses (the lock-out period)
- The maximum cumulative dose allowed over 1 hr

In theory, the plasma level of the analgesic will be relatively constant and high plasma opioid levels from large boluses will be eliminated. Almost every opioid drug has been used for PCA. The ideal drug should have rapid onset, moderate duration of action (to prevent the need for frequent demands), and a high margin of safety between effectiveness and troublesome side effects.

Successful and safe PCA requires that the patient understand how the device works, and this should be explained in detail before the operation.

Despite the apparent inherent safety of the PCA design, patient injury does sometimes occur. One potential mechanism is "PCA-by-proxy," wherein doses are administered by individuals other than the patient. Opioid-induced sedation prevents patients from accidental overdose, but only if they are the only person triggering doses.

Neuraxial analgesia

As described above, epidural catheters have many advantages as postoperative analgesics. Low concentrations of local anesthetic combined with low-dose epidural opioid provide effective analgesia for most trunk and lower-extremity procedures when given as a continuous infusion. Patients have excellent mobility, minimal sedation, and quick return of bowel function.

Opioids may be administered by the intrathecal route as well. Intrathecal and epidural opioids have been used following a wide variety of surgical procedures and other acutely painful conditions. Intrathecal opioids are easy to administer either to provide surgical anesthesia or as an additional technique when general anesthesia is given.

Neuraxial routes of analgesia are not free of side effects. These include nausea, vomiting, pruritis (which is much more common with morphine than with other drugs), and urinary retention. Of most concern, however, as with any opioid, is the possibility of respiratory depression.

Ambulatory surgery

Appropriate operations for the ambulatory setting have minimal physiologic trespass, low anesthetic complexity, and uncomplicated recovery. The design of the ambulatory facility may impose limitations on types of operations or patients that can be accommodated. Such limitations may be secondary to availability of equipment, recovery room nursing expertise and access to consultants, and availability of ICU or hospital beds.

Traditionally, ASA PS 1 or 2 patients were considered ideal ambulatory patients. However, a subset of ASA class 3 and 4 patients is suitable for ambulatory surgery, although such patients also face increased risk for prolonged recovery or unplanned hospital admission.

Many currently used anesthetics, opioids, and muscle relaxants have rapid recovery profiles. Titration of anesthetics to indices of CNS activity (e.g., the bispectral index or similar monitors) may result in decreased drug dosages, faster recovery from anesthesia, and fewer complications. Use of a supraglottic airway, such as the laryngeal mask airway (LMA), rather than an endotracheal tube, is ideal in the outpatient setting because lower doses of induction agent are required to blunt the hypertension and tachycardia associated with its insertion. However, supraglottic airways do not protect against aspiration.

Commonly used drugs in anesthesia

Inhaled anesthetics

Isoflurane
- Pros: Inexpensive; excellent renal, hepatic, coronary, and cerebral blood flow preservation
- Cons: Slow onset and offset; pungent and irritating so cannot be used for inhalation induction

Sevoflurane
- Pros: Nonirritating so can be used for inhalation induction; extremely rapid onset and offset
- Cons: Expensive; must be used at flows >2 L/min to minimize risk from "Compound A" exposure; theoretical potential for renal toxicity from inorganic fluoride metabolites

Desflurane
- Pros: Extremely rapid onset and offset
- Cons: Expensive; stimulates catecholamine release; requires special active-temperature-controlled vaporizer because of high vapor pressure; irritating so cannot be used for inhalation induction

Nitrous oxide
- Pros: Decreases volatile anesthetic requirement, very inexpensive, less myocardial depression than volatile agents
- Cons: Diffuses into gas-filled spaces (bowel, pneumothorax, middle ear, gas bubbles used during retinal surgery) faster than nitrogen diffuses out, causing distension, decreases FiO_2, increases pulmonary vascular resistance, supports combustion

IV anesthetics

There are four major IV anesthetics in wide use. Only one, propofol, is truly suitable for maintenance of anesthesia. Allergy to IV anesthetics is extremely rare. However, propofol is supplied in a lipid emulsion containing egg lecithin. True anaphylaxis to eggs indicates that the patient is likely allergic to the propofol vehicle.

Thiopental
- Pros: Excellent brain protection: stops seizures and raises the seizure threshold; inexpensive
- Cons: Myocardial depression, vasodilation, histamine release, laryngospasm; bronchspasm; can precipitate porphyria crisis in susceptible patients

Propofol
- Pros: Antiemetic; quick recovery if used as solo anesthetic agent
- Cons: Pain on injection; relatively expensive; supports bacterial growth; myocardial depression; vasodilation

Etomidate
- Pros: Excellent cardiovascular stability—least myocardial depressant effect of IV anesthetics
- Cons: Pain on injection; adrenal suppression (? significance if used only for induction); myoclonus; most emetogenic of the IV agents

Ketamine
- Pros: Works IV, PO, PR, IM—good choice in uncooperative patient without IV; indirect sympathomimetic → provides cardiovascular stability with adequate adrenal reserve; often preserves airway reflexes
- Cons: Dissociative anesthesia with postoperative dysphoria and hallucinations; increases ICP/IOP and $CMRO_2$; sympathetic nervous system stimulation bad for patients with ischemic coronary disease; increases airway secretions

Local anesthetics
- **Esters**: Metabolized by plasma esterases—one metabolite is PABA, which can cause allergic reactions. Patients with "allergy to novacaine" usually do well with amides for this reason. All have only one *i* in their name, e.g., procaine, tetracaine
- **Amides**: Metabolized by hepatic enzymes. All have at least two *i*'s in their name, e.g., lidocaine, bupivacaine. Allergy to this class of drugs is very rare
- Some **local anesthetics** are used for infiltration anesthesia. During such use, one must avoid accidentally giving a toxic dose (see Table 17.4).
  - Cardiotoxicity consists of ventricular dysrhythmias and profound vasodilation, causing cardiovascular collapse.
  - Central nervous system toxicity consists of sedation, disorientation, seizures, and loss of consciousness.
- Addition of epinephrine to the anesthetic solution delays systemic absorption, effectively raising the dose that may be administered without causing toxicity.

Table 17.4 Maximum recommended doses of local anesthetics for infiltration

Drug	Max dose without epinephrine (mg/kg)	Max dose with epinephrine (mg/kg)
Lidocaine	4.5	7
Mepivacaine	7	
Bupivacaine	2	3
Tetracaine	3	

Skeletal muscle paralyzing agents

Depolarizing

Succinylcholine activates the skeletal muscle acetylcholine receptor and passively diffuses off the membrane, while circulating drug is metabolized by plasma esterases. These agents are associated with increased ICP/IOP, muscle fasciculations, and postoperative muscle aches; triggers MH; and increases serum potassium, especially in patients with burns, crush injury, spinal cord injury, muscular dystrophy, or disuse syndromes. They are rapid and short acting.

Nondepolarizing

There are many different kinds, all ending in -*onium* or -*urium*. Each has different site of metabolism, onset, and duration, making choice depend on the specific patient and case. Some examples are as follows:

- **Pancuronium.** Slow onset, long duration, tachycardia due to vagolytic effect
- **Cisatracurium.** Slow onset, intermediate duration, Hoffman (nonenzymatic) elimination, so attractive choice in liver or renal disease
- **Rocuronium.** Fastest onset of nondepolarizers, making it useful for rapid sequence induction, intermediate duration

Reversal agents

Antiparalytic drugs

All currently available drugs are acetylcholinesterase inhibitors, thereby allowing more acetylcholine to be available to overcome the neuromuscular blocker effect at the nicotinic receptor, but also causing muscarinic stimulation (leading to bradycardia and asystole without coadministered anticholiergic).

- **Neostigmine.** Shares duration of action with glycopyrrolate
- **Edrophonium.** Shares duration of action with atropine
- **Physostigmine.** Crosses the blood–brain barrier, therefore useful for atropine overdose
- **Sugammadex** (investigational). Not a cholinesterase inhibitor. It works by specifically and tightly chelating steroidal non-depolarizing neuromuscular blocking drugs, completely removing the paralyzing agent from the neuromuscular junction.

Narcotic antagonists

- **Flumazenil.** Useful for reversal of benzodiazepine effect
- **Naloxone.** Useful for reversal of opioid effect.
  - Use multiple small doses of 0.04 mg, each separated by approximately 3 min. With this approach, unwanted sedation and respiratory depression can be reversed without reversing analgesia.

Anticholinergics

These are given with cholinesterase inhibitor reversal agents to block the muscarinic effects of cholinergic stimulation; they are also excellent for treating bradycardia and excess secretions.

- **Atropine.** Used in conjunction with edrophonium, crosses the blood–brain barrier, causing drowsiness; may be used as premedication for children to avert bradycardia with intubation
- **Glycopyrrolate.** Used in conjunction with neostigmine, does not cross the blood–brain barrier

Orthopedic surgery

Joshua Alpert, MD
Peter Asnis, MD

Examination of a joint

Develop an ordered system when evaluating a joint.[1]

Ask

- History: What is the mechanism of injury (how did it happen)? Is it acute (<6 weeks) or chronic (>6 weeks), traumatic or atraumatic.
- Is there a recent history of an infection, or a systemic illness?
- Is there a specific area of tenderness?
- Is the patient able to bear weight through the joint?
- Is the pain worse with active or passive range of motion (ROM)?

Look

- Compare both sides.
- Skin: Evaluate for redness, warmth, bruising, masses, scars, foreign objects, and drainage.
- Is there any swelling? If so, is it an effusion, synovitis, or bony deformity?
- Look for muscle wasting around the joint and in the whole limb.

Feel

- Examine the unaffected or least painful side first and explain this to the patient. Then examine the affected side.
- Is the skin normal, hot, cold, or moist?
- Is there any local tenderness? Look at the patient's face—does the patient appear to be in pain?
- Is there an effusion (transilluminates, fluid shifts with compression), synovitis (nonmovable fluid feel), hemarthrosis (doughy feel), or bony swelling?
- Always examine the joint above and below (e.g., shoulder and wrist exam for complaints of elbow pain).

Move

- Ask the patient to move the joint through a full range of motion.
- Look for pain (patient's face) or limitation of motion.
- Is the limitation mechanical (blocked) or restrictive (resisted by the patient because of pain)?
- Compare active to passive ROM.
- Examine and compare the contralateral joint.
- Evaluate the ability of the patient to bear weight (i.e., walk or stand) on the affected extremity.
- Listen and feel for any clicking, catching, or locking during ROM testing.
- Assess the patient's neurovascular status: muscle motor grading, sensory exam, reflexes, pulses, and capillary refill.

Special tests—shoulder

- Impingement test: resisted pain with forward flexion
- Rotator cuff (supraspinatus) testing: Weakness with forearm abduction to 90° and forward flexion to 30° is indicative of rotator cuff pathology.

- Lift-off test: Place the dorsum of the patient's hand against their back. If they are unable to lift it off the back they have a subscapularis injury.
- Anterior apprehension test: Abduction and external rotation causes patient fear of dislocation, which indicates anterior instability.

Special tests—knee

- ACL testing (Lachman): With the knee flexed at 30°, pull the tibia forward while stabilizing the femur. Laxity and lack of an end point are consistent with an ACL tear.
- PCL testing (Posterior Drawer Test): With the knee flexed at 90°, place thumbs over the anterior tibia at the joint line, and use posterior-directed force. Laxity is consistent with PCL tear.
- Meniscus: Signs of meniscus tear include swelling, joint line tenderness, pain with hyperflexion, pain with hyperextension, and difficulty squatting.
- Medial collateral ligament testing: With the knee flexed to 30° (off edge of table), place valgus stress (laterally directed force on tibia) and evaluate for laxity.
- Lateral collateral ligament testing: With the knee flexed to 30° (off edge of table), place varus stress (medially directed force on tibia) and evaluate for laxity.

Signs or symptoms of joint (intra-articular) infection

The following signs are consistent with an intra-articular infection, which usually indicates a medical emergency:
- Pain out of proportion to exam (i.e., extreme pain with any range of motion of the joint)
- Pain with passive motion (when examiner moves knee)
- Redness, warmth, swelling around joint
- Systemic signs: fever, chills, general malaise
- Abnormal lab values: elevated WBC, ESR, CRP
- To definitively diagnose a septic joint, aspirate the joint and send the fluid for Gram stain, culture, cell count, and crystals.
- If there is any concern about an infected (septic) joint, have a low threshold to aspirate.

1 Myers A, Sickles T (1998). Preparticipation sports examination [review]. *Prim Care* **25**(1):225–236.

Examination of the limbs and trunk

Develop your own system that you feel comfortable with. Always compare the opposite extremity. Make allowances for the dominant side.

Muscles and joints

- Look for deformity, asymmetry, and twitching (fasciculation).
- Move each joint through its full range.
- Learn to recognize flaccidity (floppy), increased tone (rigidity), and spasm. Are there alterations in any of the above through the whole range of movement?
- Is the rigidity through whole movement or only initially (spasticity)?
- Are there involuntary movements such as twitches or tremors? If so, do these movements change with movement or relaxation of the limb?
- Always examine the joint above and below the area being evaluated.

Motor (muscle) strength testing

Grade 0   No movement
Grade 1   Flicker of movement only
Grade 2   Movement with gravity eliminated
Grade 3   Movement against gravity
Grade 4   Movement against resistance
Grade 5   Normal power

Test all muscle groups within their relevant myotomes according to the patient's history.

Coordination

- Ask the patient to touch their nose with their index finger with eyes open and then shut with both fingers. Alternatively, ask the patient to put their right heel on to their left knee and run it down the shin and vice versa. Note whether these movements are smooth or jerky.
- Romberg's test: Stand with feet together and eyes shut. A positive result will cause the patient to become unstable or fall; be prepared!

Reflexes

- Biceps C5
- Brachioradialis C6
- Triceps C67
- Abdominal, T8–T12
- Knee jerk L4
- Ankle jerk S1/2
- Plantar response. Normal flexor, abnormal extensor (Babinski's sign)
- Clonus at ankle (normal 2 beats or less)

Grading
0 Absent
1 Hypoactive
2 Normal
3 Hyperactive, no clonus
4 Hyperactive ,with clonus

Sensation

Explain what you are about to do clearly to the patient and test them with their eyes closed. Compare symmetrical sides of the body at the same time. Map out the abnormalities.

- Pinprick, light touch, and temperature are tested in a dermatomal pattern.
- Vibration sense is tested with a 128 MHz low-pitched tuning fork on a bony prominence. Start distal and, if abnormal, move from proximal side.
- Proprioception (joint position sense) is tested by moving the metatarsophalangeal joint of the hallux up and down; the patient confirms the correct movement.
- Know the dermatomal pattern of sensory nerves.

Fracture healing

Fracture healing occurs as either primary or secondary bone union.
- *Primary bone union* occurs when bone edges are anatomically aligned perfectly (e.g., in fractures treated operatively with rigid internal fixation).
- *Secondary bone union* occurs via callus formation when the bone edges are close to each other but not perfectly aligned (e.g., those fractures treated with splinting, casting, or external fixators).

Secondary bone union

Immediate response
- After a fracture occurs, bleeding begins and a hematoma will form between the bone ends and extend into the surrounding soft tissues.
- The size of the hematoma will depend on the blood supply to the bone and the violence of the injury.
- The hematoma can continue to expand during the first 36 hr.

Inflammatory response
- Injury to tissue and platelet activation cause an inflammatory cascade recruiting various cytokines.
- This attracts various cells such as macrophages into the hematoma to encourage the process of removing any dead and devitalized tissue, together with proliferation of osteoblasts and fibroblasts to help in the next phase.

Repair response
- Fibroblasts and chondroblasts organize the hematoma into collagen and granulation tissue.
- Osteoblasts proliferate and begin forming primary callus, which can be external (bridging), medullary (internal), or periosteal.
- The amount of callus is dependent upon local factors such as the type of fracture, proximity of the bone ends, amount of hematoma, and amount of movement present at the fracture site.
- New blood vessels migrate into the callus, causing calcification and subsequent ossification into woven bone.

Remodeling response
- Further consolidation of the woven bone occurs and lamellar bone is laid down.
- Finally, remodeling occurs, in which swelling around the fracture site decreases and trabeculae can be radiographically seen crossing the fracture site.
- Remodeling is most marked in children and follows the mechanical forces applied to the bone in a physiological environment.

Primary bone union

- This occurs when bone is held rigidly with the use of compression of the fracture with a *lag screw* and/or a *plate device*. The bone ends are placed anatomically together and compressed tight.
- The inflammatory response is much reduced and the bones heal by direct union end-to-end.
- This is achieved by osteoclasts acting as "cutting cones" passing directly across the fracture site. The channel produced by them is filled in with new bone.
- No callus is formed and union takes much longer to achieve, with the strength of the construct during the healing process being borne by the mechanical plate device.

Factors adversely affecting fracture healing

- Severe local trauma, bone loss, soft tissue interposition
- Large displacement of bone ends
- Inadequate immobilization
- Infection
- Disturbances of ossification, e.g., metabolic bone disease, osteoporosis, and local pathological tumor
- Poor nutrition, smoking, drugs (especially NSAIDs)
- Site of fracture—e.g., common sites for poor union include intracapsular neck of femur, distal third of tibia, scaphoid and talar fractures
- Increasing age

How long do fractures take to unite?

Perkins rules

- Fractures of cancellous (metaphyseal) bone (e.g., those around joints) will take 6 weeks to unite.
- Fractures of cortical (diaphyseal) bone (e.g., shafts of long bones) will take 12 weeks to unite.
- Fractures of the tibia (because of poor blood supply) will take 24 weeks to unite.
- Time to union for children equals the age of the child in years + 1, e.g., a tibial fracture in a 2-year-old child will unite in 3 weeks. Use common sense when applying the rule to fractures of cancellous bone in older children.

Delayed union

Union fails to occur in 1.5 times the normal time for a fracture union.

Non-union

Union fails to occur within 2 times the normal time for a fracture union. However, expect open fractures to normally take 2 times the normal Perkins rule.

Non-union can be broadly divided into the following categories:
- Hypertrophic: normally due to excess mobility, i.e., good healing potential
- Atrophic: normally due to poor blood supply, i.e., poor healing potential

Reduction and fixation of fractures

Remember that a fracture is a soft tissue injury with a broken bone at the bottom of it. Thus the principles of management are to treat the soft tissues with respect while reducing and maintaining a reduction of the fracture.

Modern fracture reduction and treatment were pioneered by the AO Group and centers around four key principles[1]:

- Fracture reduction and fixation to restore anatomical relationships
- Stability by fixation or splinting, as the personality of the fracture and the injury dictates
- Preservation of the blood supply to the soft tissue and bone by careful handling and gentle reduction techniques
- Early and safe mobilization of the part and patient

Fracture reduction can be achieved by closed[2] (manipulation) or open (direct) methods. Maintenance of the reduction may also be achieved via closed methods, which can be nonsurgical (plaster or brace) or surgical (intramedullary nail, external fixation, "K" wires), or via open methods such as rigid internal fixation with plates and screws.

Splinting or casting

- Splinting: plaster material around a portion of the extremity allowing for swelling. This is not as rigid as a cast, and is done in acute settings.
- Cast: plaster or fiberglass material circumferentially around the fractured area. A cast is more rigid, and rarely done in an acute setting.
- Typically involves splinting of joints either side of a long-bone fracture
- Simplest and cheapest to apply
- No incision, low risk of surgical complications such as infection

Cast bracing

- Stabilization of a fracture across a joint with plaster but the joint itself is left free of plaster and a brace is applied
- Has the advantage of allowing early movement of the joint without the use of weight bearing, e.g., for tibial shaft fractures

Internal fixation

Indications

- Rehabilitation is facilitated more quickly with internal fixation after anatomical reduction.
- Intra-articular fractures: to prevent or reduce the incidence of osteoarthritis
- Neurovascular damage. Fracture stability must be achieved before the delicate repair of vessels or nerves takes place.
- Polytrauma. Multiple injuries are better managed by fixation to facilitate nursing care and to allow early mobilization.
- Elderly patients tolerate immobilization and prolonged bed rest poorly.
- Fractures of long bones (e.g., forearm, femur, tibia). Failure of conservative therapy (loss of acceptable alignment)
- Pathological fractures

Methods of internal fixation
- Compression plates and screws, K wires, intramedullary nails, tension band wiring

Complications
- Infection, which increases with the length of incision and exposure required
- Neurovascular injury
- Implant failure, and subsequent fracture through a bony defect (stress riser) if the implant is removed

External fixation

Indications
- Initial stabilizing device for any fracture for which "damage control" surgery may be appropriate to get the patient initially stable until further surgery can be planned.
- Open (compound) fractures, especially of the tibia
- Life-saving splinting procedure in pelvic fractures

Methods
External fixators allow the soft tissue envelope around the fracture to be addressed by grafts or flaps if required. This method requires good nursing or community care and patient compliance for pin site care.

Complications
These include pin site infection and possible osteomyelitis from transosseous pins.

Internal and external fixation—locking plates

- A plate with screws with threads on the shaft and head so that the screw head itself is physically screwed into the plate and locks tight, preventing movement and a backing out of the screw
- The locking plate gives angular stability and is much stronger than a normal plate.
- Advantages are
  - A strong fixation in osteoporotic fractures
  - They can be placed percutaneously (avoiding stripping of soft tissue and blood supply from a fracture site).

1 Ruedi TP, Murphy WM (2000). *AO Principles of Fracture Management.* New York: Thieme Medical Publishers.
2 McRae R, Esser M (2002). *Practical Fracture Treatment*, 4th ed. Edinburgh: Churchill Livingstone.

The skeletal radiograph

A plain X-ray is an important part of the overall orthopedic assessment. However, X-rays do not substitute for an accurate history and physical examination.

Evaluation

Systematically review every X-ray in a similar fashion.[1,2]

- Know the patient's history prior to reading the X-ray. It will help you focus your attention to the proper areas.
- When evaluating images, confirm the proper date on the X-ray, as well as the patient's name and age, and the side being imaged.
- Always take a minimum of two views at 90° to each other. It is very easy to miss a fracture or dislocation with only one view.
- Examine the film on a viewing box with a bright spotlight or on a digital computer with appropriate resolution.
- When describing the lesion, think of side, anatomical site, nature, displacement, and soft tissue components.
- Keep it simple.
  - A—adequate views and alignment
  - B—bones
  - C—cartilage (soft tissues)
- Look for cortical or medullary changes, periosteal reactions, deformity, soft-tissue swelling, and cortical breach (definition of a fracture).
- Supplement plain radiological findings with advanced imaging studies such as CT scan (better to evaluate bone), MRI (better for soft tissues), ultrasound, bone scan, or spectrometry scan, as indicated.

Radiological features

Osteoporosis

- This is the most common form of bone disease.
- It is characterized by low bone mass and deterioration of the microarchitecture of bone tissue with a consequent increase in bone fragility and susceptibility to low trauma fractures.
- It affects middle-aged and elderly women, predisposing them to fractures of the distal radius, femoral neck, and vertebral bodies.
- Localized osteoporosis follows disease, e.g., after joint fusion.
- The cortices are thin with reduced medullary trabeculae—i.e., the bone is essentially normal; there is just too little of it.

Osteomalacia

There is reduced mineralization of osteoid.

- The trabeculae are blurred.
- Symmetrical transverse or oblique cortical defects appear (Looser's zones, pseudofractures).
- In children, changes are most marked at the metaphysis (rickets).

Diffuse increase in density

Think of neoplasia, fluorosis, sarcoidosis, and bone dysplasia (osteopetrosis).

Abnormalities of bone modeling

Developmental disorders, e.g., osteochondrodysplasia, are often present from birth. Look for abnormalities of the eyes, heart, and ears. Thorough assessment by a biochemical and genetic specialist is required.

Local abnormalities may occur in congenital disorders, e.g., endro-chondromatosis (Ollier's disease), fibrous dysplasia, and neurofibromatosis, or in acquired disorders, e.g., Paget's disease.

Solitary lesions

Always think of sepsis, primary bone tumors, or secondary metastasis. Location and age are important—e.g., an epiphyseal lesion in a child may be a chondroblastoma and a subarticular lesion in a young adult may be a giant cell tumor. The older the patient the more likely it is a metastasis.

Describing a fracture

- List details, including date of radiograph, and describe the type of view (AP of right ankle, lateral of C-spine).
- Be systematic. Comment on the whole radiograph, starting with foreign bodies and including monitoring equipment and evidence of surgery such as prostheses and surgical clips. Go on to describe soft tissues and any extra bones visible (e.g., upper cervical spine on a skull radiograph).
- Which bone is involved? It is useful to compare with a skeleton if available.
- Is it a fracture? Structures that may be mistaken for fractures include suture lines between bones, vascular channels, and physes in immature skeletons. Anatomic structures are more likely to be symmetrical, if not midline.
- Is the fracture visible in multiple views?
- Is it displaced? In which direction is the displacement? Are there more than two fragments (comminuted or multifragmentary)? Is there an associated joint dislocation?
- Is it an open fracture (compound)? Radiographic clues include air or foreign material in the soft tissues overlying the fracture or, more ominously, in the cranial cavity. Look for asymmetrical fluid levels in the sinuses suggestive of bleeding from a fracture.
- A ring structure (e.g., the bony pelvis) rarely fractures in only one place—look for further fractures when one is found.

1 Raby N, Berman L, de Lacy G (2005). *Accident and Emergency Radiology: A Survival Guide*, 2nd ed. London: Saunders.
2 Nicholson DA, Driscoll P (1995). *ABC of Emergency Radiology*. London: BMJ Books.

Fractures of the phalanges and metacarpals

Terminology and anatomy
- *Metacarpal bone*: bone between carpal bones and phalanges (finger)
- *Proximal phalanx (P1)*: between metacarpal and middle phalanx
- *Middle phalanx (P2)*: between P1 and distal phalanx (P3)
- *Distal phalanx (P3)*: fingertip

Metacarpal fractures
The cause of these fractures is usually a direct blow (i.e., punching a wall). The "Friday night" or "Boxer's" fracture most commonly affects the small finger.

Fracture types
Metacarpal fractures are transverse, oblique, spiral, or comminuted. The majority are fractures of the metacarpal neck. Angulations of the shaft are less well tolerated and are associated with a higher rate of rotational deformity.

Treatment
Isolated fractures with no rotational deformity present can be "buddy-strapped" to an adjacent finger, or placed in a splint and immobilized. If malrotated, unstable, or severely angulated, these fractures require either closed reduction and percutaneous K-wire fixation or open fixation with mini-fragment screws.

Multiple fractures are usually better treated with fixation methods if the adjacent metacarpal is involved. Less deformity is acceptable at the second and third metacarpals.

Proximal and middle phalanx fractures
These fractures are caused by a direct blow or twisting injuries.

Treatment
If the fracture is stable, use buddy taping and immobilization. If it is unstable, rotated, or severely angulated or involves the joint, consider closed reduction and K-wire fixation or open reduction and fixation with mini-fragment screws.

Fracture of distal phalanges
These fractures are usually caused by a crush injury that can be comminuted, open, and associated with nail bed injuries.

Types
- Longitudinal, comminuted, transverse

Treatment
Use a splint x4 weeks, closed reduction, and percutaneous pin if the fracture is unstable. If there is an open fracture or associated nail bed injury, treat with irrigation and debridement, simple nail bed repair if needed, and primary suture or Steri-strip® with pressure dressing. Inspect the wound at 48 hr. Antibiotics may be required.

Mallet finger (avulsion of extensor digitorum longus)

The cause is a direct blow causing flexion of the distal phalanx, i.e., catching injury.

Fracture type

Injury is avulsion of the extensor tendon from the terminal phalanx either with or without a piece of bone.

Treatment

Keep finger hyperextended in a mallet finger splint 24 hr/day for 6 weeks; the splint can then be worn only at night for 2 weeks. If the bone fragment is large and does not reduce in the splint, then percutaneous pinning or open fixation is required.

Thumb

Thumb fracture is caused by a blow to the tip of the thumb, or forced opposition of the thumb.

Fracture types

The fracture type depends on location of the fracture: distal phalanx, proximal phalanx, metacarpal shaft, metacarpal base, or carpometacarpal joint fracture with or without associated dislocation.

Treatment

Reduce under traction; apply plaster splint with the distal phalanx free for 4 weeks. Up to 30° of angulation can be accepted.

Basal fracture dislocation (Bennett's and Rolando fractures)

This is an intra-articular fracture of the base of the thumb metacarpal that is unstable and frequently presents with joint subluxation. *Bennett's fracture* is an avulsion type leaving a volar lip fragment behind; A *Rolando fracture* is more comminuted, generally in a T or Y pattern.

The treatment of choice is closed reduction and percutaneous K-wire fixation from the thumb metacarpal base to either carpus or index metacarpal. Open reduction and fixation with mini-fragment screws may also be a fixation method.

Thumb carpal metacarpal dislocation

Reduce under ring block and immobilize in plaster splint.

Immobilization for hand injuries (intrinsic plus position)

To prevent stiffness, the metacarpal-phalangeal joint should be immobilized in 90° of flexion and the proximal interphalangeal joints in extension with the wrist extended at 30°.

Wrist injuries

Scaphoid fractures

These fractures[1] are caused by a fall onto the outstretched hand with forced dorsiflexion.

Examination

- Generally occurs in young patients (<50 years of age)
- Evaluate for anatomical snuffbox tenderness (between dorsal first and third extensor tendon compartments).
- Tenderness also with exam on the volar surface of the scaphoid
- Wrist movement, particularly pronation followed by ulna deviation, may be painful.
- Pain on compression of the thumb longitudinally or on gripping may be present (scaphoid compression test).

Investigation (radiographs)

Order "scaphoid series" films:

- PA wrist in neutral and ulnar deviation
- Lateral wrist in neutral
- PA in 45° pronation and supination
- There is a false negative rate of <5%.
- If X-rays are negative but suspicion persists, splint the wrist and repeat films in 2 weeks. Bone scan or MRI is obtained for diagnosis if there is continued suspicion at 2 weeks.
- Obtain a CT scan to assess if a nondisplaced fracture is truly nondisplaced.

Treatment

- Cast in neutral position (RCTs show that the thumb does not need to be included[2]). Cast for 8 weeks, although the fracture may take 12 weeks to unite.
- Displacement of >1 mm requires open reduction and internal fixation with a compression screw.

Complications

- Non-union occurs with proximal fractures due to blood supply running from distal to proximal in the bone. If not united at 12 weeks, proceed to open reduction and internal fixation (compression screw (Herbert, Acutrack, AO cannulated). The patient may need bone grafting.
- Avascular necrosis occurs with proximal and displaced fractures (see above). Treatment is by internal fixation and bone grafting, which may need to be a "vascularized" graft.
- Degenerative changes may occur after non- or malunion, and is treated by limited wrist fusion (four-corner fusion, scaphoidectomy, and radial styloidectomy).

---

1 Ring D, Jupiter JB, Herndon JH (2000). Acute fractures of the scaphoid, *J Am Acad Orthop Surg* 8:225-231.

2 Clay NR, Dias JJ, Costigan PS, et al. 1991. Need the thumb be immobilized in scaphoid fractures? A randomised prospective trial. *J Bone Joint Surg Br* **73** (5):828–832.

Other carpal fractures

- The most common one is a hook of *hamate fracture*. The hamate is fractured by a direct blow to the palm of the hand or repeated direct contact (e.g., motorcyclists, golfers, racquet sports).
- Treatment is usually excision but internal fixation may be attempted if the fragment is large.

Ligamentous injuries of the wrist

- Such injuries are common. They are difficult to diagnose and thus easily missed.
- If left untreated they can cause long-term disability.

The proximal row of carpal bones forms an intercalated segment—i.e., they are connected and work together as a unit. Injury may occur to the ligaments connecting the bones.

Scapholunate ligament

Injury to this ligament is common in isolation or in association with fractures (especially distal radius) and shows a "Terry Thomas" sign, i.e., increase in the space between scaphoid and lunate on a clenched-fist PA view.

Acute ruptures may be repaired but chronic injuries may require reconstruction or fusion.

Lunotriquetral ligament

Injury to this ligament is less common. Acute repair may be successful but chronic injuries require lunotriquetral fusion.

Carpal dislocations

Complete ligamentous injury may allow the carpus to dislocate.

- This occurs with either the lunate remaining in place, a *perilunate dislocation*, or the carpus staying in place and the lunate moving, a *lunate dislocation*.
- On rarer occasions the scapholunate ligament remains intact and the scaphoid fractures result in a *transcaphoid perilunate dislocation*.

Treatment

Severe injury requires reduction, which is best done open, as it allows formal repair of the disrupted ligaments as well as stabilization of the carpus. If the scaphoid is fractured it should be internally fixed as well.

Carpometacarpal fracture dislocation

- Usually as the result as a punch injury; affects little or ring fingers
- Commonly missed with poor history and examination
- Indicated by tenderness at the carpometacarpal base
- Diagnosed with a *true* lateral (not the standard lateral oblique) X-ray (shows subluxation or dislocation at the carpometacarpal joint)

Treatment

For an unstable injury, reduce with traction and local pressure, then stabilize the joint with K-wire fixation for 4 weeks.

Triangular fibrocartilage complex (TFCC) injury

The TFCC = triangular fibrocartilage and the ulna small ligaments of the hand. An acute tear is usually peripheral and the result of trauma including a fracture to the ulna styloid. It will present with ulna-based wrist pain in ulna deviation with or without rotation.

Treatment

If TFCC injury is associated with a large ulna styloid fracture, this can be internally fixed with a tension band wire technique. Arthroscopic debridement or repair of the tear has been attempted but is technically demanding.

Fractures of the distal radius and ulna

- These fractures are usually caused by a fall onto the outstretched hand.
- They comprise nearly 1 in 6 of all fractures treated.
- Scaphoid and ligamentous wrist injuries may also be present.

Classification

- There are many classification systems: the AO system,[1] the Frykman system,[2] and the Fernandez system.[3] Others use a "4-part" system to classify fractures based on a fracture involving the radial styloid, volar or dorsal lunate facet, and scaphoid facet.[4]
- Adult fractures of the distal radius and ulna are very common and may still be called by historical eponymous terms (Colles, Smith's). It is better to stick to describing the fracture by anatomical methods, e.g., dorsally displaced fracture of the distal radius with shortening and ulna deviation.
- In children the fracture usually involves the epiphyseal region; these fractures are classified by the Salter–Harris system.[5] Salter–Harris type II is the most common injury of the distal radius.
- In adults the injury is usually just proximal to the joint and may include fracture to the ulna styloid, and possible TFCC injury (📖 p. 584).
- The fracture may involve the articular surface of the radiocarpal or the distal radioulnar joint (DRUJ).
- Intra-articular fractures carry a worse prognosis because of the risk of wrist osteoarthritis.

X-rays

- For all patients, get PA, lateral, and oblique views of the wrist. AP and lateral X-rays of the forearm and elbow should be obtained as well to evaluate for associated injury.
- All children should have contralateral X-rays of the wrist and elbow for comparison.

Treatment

Children

- Fractures are generally treated by closed reduction (manipulation) and application of a well-molded plaster splint or cast.[6] Try to minimize the number of closed-reduction attempts in children.
- Operative indications are radius and ulna "both-bone" fractures, severe displacement, open fractures, or if the fracture reduction is lost in plaster after manipulation.
- Operative treatment consists of internal fixation with percutaneous K wires or, more rarely, open reduction and internal fixation with plates and screws.

Adults

A fracture is deemed stable when
- Radial inclination <12° on PA X-ray
- Radial shortening <5 mm on PA X-ray
- Dorsal tilt <15° on lateral X-ray
- <2 mm articular step-off on any view[4]

Fractures with dorsal displacement (Colles fractures)
- Undisplaced + stable. Below-elbow plaster immobilization for 6 weeks
- Displaced + stable. Closed reduction and plaster immobilization for 6 weeks
- Displaced + unstable. Closed reduction and either percutaneous K-wire fixation or external fixation. Open reduction and internal fixation with plates and screws can also be used for complex articular fractures.
- Dorsal comminution is a common problem and must be taken into account in the method chosen.
- Bone structural substitutes, e.g., Biobon, lack RCT data to back up their use and considerable expense.

Fractures with volar displacement (Smith's fracture)
These are unstable and are usually treated by a volar buttress plate (which supports a fracture like a shelf, propping up or supporting the distal fragment).

Intra-articular fractures with volar displacement (Barton's fracture)
Internal fixation is mandatory, as this is a highly unstable fracture.

Ulnar styloid fractures
These fractures can usually be ignored unless the fragment is large, in which case it may represent a TFCC injury (📖 p. 584), treated by internal fixation.

1 http://www.trauma.org/ortho/aoclass.html
2 Frykman G (1967). Fracture of the distal radius including sequelae—shoulder–hand–finger syndrome, disturbance in the distal radio-ulna joint and impairment of nerve function. A clinical and experimental study. *Acta Orthop Scand Suppl* **108**:3.
3 Fernandez DL (1993). Fractures of the distal radius. Operative treatment [review]. *Instr Course Lect.* **42**:73–88.
4 Ilyas AM, Jupiter J (2007). Distal radius fractures—classification of treatment and indications for surgery [review]. *Orthop Clin North Am* **38**:167–173.
5 Salter RB, Harris WR (1963). Injuries involving the epiphyseal plate. *J Bone Joint Surg Am* **45**:587–632.
6 http://www.eradius.com/

Fractures of the radius and ulna shaft

Causes
- The most common mechanism is a fall onto the outstretched hand.
- They may also be due to a direct-blow injury (e.g., the arm is raised to protect the head, leading to an isolated transverse ulnar fracture, the "nightstick fracture")
- All displaced "both-bone" forearm fractures require surgery.

X-rays
- All patients require AP and lateral X-rays of the wrist, forearm, and elbow.

Fracture types
Children
- Usually transverse fractures of the radius and ulna
- May be angulated only, with one boney cortex still intact ("greenstick fracture")
- May sustain a fracture dislocation as in adults

Adults
- Usually either a transverse or oblique fracture of the radius and ulna, which are often displaced
- Remember, the forearm is a "force parallelogram" and that a fracture of only one bone will usually result in a dislocation of the other bone at the proximal or distal joints. These fracture dislocations are characterized as follows:
  - *Monteggia fracture*: proximal ulna fracture with dislocation of the proximal radial head
  - *Galeazzi fracture*: distal radial fracture with dislocation of the DRUJ
  - *Essex-Lopresti fracture*: fracture of the radial head and associated DRUJ dislocation

Treatment
Children
- Greenstick fractures. Closed reduction and cast immobilization from wrist to above the elbow
  - In-line traction is always the key to any initial reduction and often all that is required to reduce and realign the fracture.
  - Use minimal force. If the periosteal hinge is broken during reduction, the fracture may displace completely and become unstable.
- Displaced fractures are often unstable and can be treated by open reduction and internal fixation with plates and screws, or by flexible intramedullary nail fixation.
- Fracture dislocations. Closed manipulation and cast immobilization (failed reduction may require open reduction)

Adults
- It is usually impossible to achieve or maintain a closed reduction for adult forearm shaft fractures, so these are usually treated with open reduction and compression plate fixation.
- Nightstick fractures of the ulna: Accept <10° angulation and >50% bony opposition. It can be treated with splinting or casting, then early-protected motion with an elbow cast-brace is indicated. If the fracture is displaced more than 50% or angled more than 10°, then open reduction and compression plate fixation should be used.
- Fracture dislocations are treated with open reduction and internal fixation to accurately reduce and hold the associated dislocations.

Complications
- Malunion or non-union. Close follow-up of closed, manipulated fractures is required. An X-ray at 1 and 2 weeks is mandatory to watch for slip of position. Malunion can present with functional problems with forearm rotation.
- Non-union is normally treated by open reduction, debridement of the non-union site, and compression plate fixation with or without bone grafting.
- It is not usually necessary to remove hardware from the radius and ulna unless they cause significant problems after the fracture has healed. Radial-plate removal has been associated with a significant risk of neurovascular complications. Children treated with intramedullary fixation of both bone forearm fractures have the IM rods removed after the fracture has healed.

Fractures and dislocations around the elbow in children

These are the second most common injury in children (8% of childhood fractures).[1]

- The cause is usually a fall onto the outstretched hand.
- Ossification centers in a child are important for diagnosis
- Capitellum, 2 years old; radial head, 4 years old; medial epicondyle, 6 years old; trochlea, 8 years old; olecranon, 9 years old; lateral epicondyle, 11 years old

Salter–Harris injuries of the elbow occur through the lateral condyle and radial neck.

X-rays

- Reading a pediatric elbow X-ray is difficult and should be done systematically.
- Always obtain AP and lateral views of BOTH elbows, as well as AP and lateral views of the forearm and wrist to assess for associated injuries.
- The anterior humeral line should bisect the capitellum on the lateral view.
- A posterior fat pad indicates an intracapsular fracture.

Supracondylar fractures
Types
Peak incidence is at 5–7 years of age.

There are two mechanisms of injury: *extension type* and *flexion type*. Classification has been classically associated with the modified *Gartland* system.[2] Grade I is nondisplaced; in grade II angulation is present but the posterior cortex is in contact; grade III is complete displacement.

Treatment

> Displaced supracondylar fractures are an orthopedic emergency, especially if complicated by an absent distal pulse. Do not delay treatment.

- Type 1 (non-displaced) fractures are treated with immobilization in a long arm cast.
- Most type II and all type III fractures are urgently reduced under sedation or general anesthesia by straight-arm traction (up to 5 min may be required).
- Use manipulation to correct rotation, varus/valgus tilt, and, finally, any extension deformity.
- Try to flex the elbow up past 90° with the forearm pronated (this may be difficult because of anterior soft-tissue swelling—the reduction technique itself can cause loss of pulse in the flexed position).
- Internal fixation with two crossed condylar K wires, one medial (beware of ulnar nerve) and one lateral, is used to fix the fracture. Alternatively, two lateral pins can be placed.

Complications

Vascular

- Injury to the brachial artery is rare and the pulse usually returns after fracture reduction.
- True loss of the radial pulse may be due to the following:
  - Vascular spasm, typified by good capillary refill after reduction but slow return of the pulse. Failure of pulse return may be due to other injuries and requires a vascular surgical opinion.
  - Partial injury (endothelial flap), treated by direct repair
  - Complete transection or disruption may be treated by direct repair or, more often, interposition vein graft.
- Contracture. Untreated vascular injury will result in fibrosis and contracture of the forearm (Volkman's ischemic contracture). This is a devastating and debilitating condition and should be avoidable with early (<12 hr) exploration and/or repair or vascular damage.
- Neurological injury
  - Most common: anterior interosseous (branch of medial nerve)
  - Median nerve and, rarely, ulnar nerve
  - Radial nerve
- Malunion. Incorrectly reduced fractures will not remodel and can lead to cubitus valgus and a "gunstock deformity."

Lateral condyle fractures

Types

These fractures are classified according to Milch, depending on how much of the intra-articular surface is involved.

Treatment

- Displaced fracture: open reduction and internal fixation with either two cannulated screws, or two parallel K wires
- The fragment is always considerably larger than expected from the X-ray because the condyle is not fully ossified.
- If not reduced and fixed, the fragment will displace because of the pull of the wrist extensors, arising from the lateral epicondyle. This will lead to a cubitus valgus deformity and can present in later life with an ulna nerve palsy, as it has been chronically stretched around the displaced condyle ("tardy" ulnar nerve palsy).

Other, less common pediatric elbow fractures

- Capitellum fractures
- Olecranon fractures
- Medial condylar and epicondylar fractures
- Distal humerus physis fractures
- Conoid process fractures
- Nursemaid's elbow = radial head subluxation

---

1 Goodwin RC, Kuivila TE (2002). Pediatric elbow and forearm fractures requiring surgical treatment. *Hand Clinic* **18**(1):135–148.
2 Wilkins KE (1997). Supracondylar fractures: what's new? *J Paediatr Orthop B* **6**(2):110–116.

Fractures around the elbow in adults

Olecranon fractures

These fractures are usually caused by a direct blow, such as a fall onto the point of the elbow, but may occur as a fall onto the outstretched hand where the triceps avulses the olecranon process.

Types

Colton[1] types:
- Undisplaced (displacement <2 mm) or displaced (>2 mm)
- Type A (avulsion), B (transverse), C (comminuted), or D (fracture dislocation)

Treatment

- Undisplaced: place in broad arm sling, avoiding flexion beyond 90°
- Displaced: open reduction and internal fixation with tension band-wire technique
- Comminuted: plate and screws

Radial head fractures

These fractures[2] are caused by a fall onto the outstretched hand.

Types

Mason classification:
- Type 1, undisplaced
- Type 2, marginal fracture with significant displacement
- Type 3, comminuted fractures

Treatment

- Type 1: early mobilization ± aspiration of the joint acutely for excellent early pain relief
- Type 2: If no mechanical block, as for type 1. If there is a mechanical block, treat by open reduction and internal fixation with compression screw and/or miniplate.
- Type 3: open reduction and internal fixation vs. excision if no ligamental disruption or dislocation, vs. excision and radial head replacement if there is ligamental disruption or dislocation

Humeral condyle fractures

These fracture are usually due to impaction injury (the olecranon is driven into the humerus via a direct fall and the condyle usually splits into a T- or Y-shaped pattern).

Types

- Supracondylar
- Isolated medial or lateral condyle fracture
- Intercondylar fracture (most common): The fracture line extends from the articular surface to the supracondylar region in a T- or Y-shaped pattern.

Treatment

All of these are intra-articular fractures and therefore must be treated by open anatomical reduction, rigid internal fixation, and early mobilization.

- Use a posterior approach with either a triceps splint or, more commonly, an osteotomy of the olecranon to visualize the whole elbow joint.
- Fixation by compression plate (if bone quality is poor, locking plate) and screws

These fractures may be difficult to treat if they are heavily comminuted and the bone quality is poor.

- They may be treated by no surgical procedure but early mobilization to try to maintain as much function as possible ("bag of bones" technique).
- Non-union is not uncommon following these fractures and sometimes salvage surgery in the form of elbow replacement may be considered.
- In the elderly, primary elbow replacement is sometimes used if the fracture cannot be fixed.

Capitellar fractures

Radiographs

On the lateral view, the capitellum is out of line with the radial head, having been sheared off. There may be an associated radial head fracture.

Treatment

If the fragment is small, excise it. If not, then this is an intra-articular fracture and must be treated with open reduction via a lateral (Kocher) approach, rigid internal fixation with compression screw, and early mobilization.

Complications of elbow fractures

- Joint stiffness and reduction of function
- Degenerative joint disease (osteoarthritis)
- Heterotopic ossification
- Neurovascular injury and its sequelae

1 Colton CL (1973). Fractures of the olecranon in adults: classification and management. *Injury* **5**:21–29.

2 Tejwani NC, Mehta H (2007). Fractures of the radial head and neck: current concepts in management. *J Am Acad Orthop Surg* **15**(7):380–387.

Dislocations and fracture dislocations of the elbow

The elbow is the second most common major joint after the shoulder to dislocate.[1]

Causes

- **Posterior**. Fall onto an outstretched hand with the elbow in extension. Most common; may be posterior, posteromedial, or posterolateral
- **Anterior**. Fall onto a flexed elbow or as a direct blow from behind (e.g., side-swipe injury when driving a car with the elbow resting out the window)
- **Divergent**. Radius and ulna separated proximally (rare)

Associated fractures (complex injury)

- Radial head, medial epicondyle, and olecranon
- Coronoid: caused by avulsion of brachialis origin with hyperextension injury
  - Type 1: avulsion of the tip alone (can be ignored)
  - Type 2: <50% of the process
  - Type 3: >50% of the process is associated with a very high re-dislocation rate as the complex is very unstable. This fracture should be openly reduced and internally fixed with a screw.
- The worst combination for highly unstable injuries is the *"terrible triad"* of radial head, coronoid, and medial collateral ligament injury.

Treatment

- Reduction is usually achieved by gentle traction and a gradual increase in flexion while pushing the olecranon back over the distal humerus.
- Place the arm in a posterior splint acutely followed by a hinged elbow brace, as the injury is usually stable.
- If the joint re-dislocates during reduction, then fully pronate the forearm and repeat. If necessary, place arm in a backslab or hinged brace with an extension block at the point of instability.
- Complex fracture dislocations require open reduction and internal fixation to help stability and allow early mobilization. This may include radial head prosthetic replacement and medial or lateral ligament repair.

Complications

- Vascular: similar range of injuries as in childhood injuries (📖 p. 590). Always check the radial pulse before and after reduction.
- Neurological: injury to median/ulnar nerves
- Myositis ossificans. Excess calcification of brachialis. *Rest*; then move.
- Stiffness. Early motion at 1 week is useful in preventing this.

---

1 Ring D, Jupiter JB (1998). Fracture-dislocation of the elbow [current concepts review]. *J Bone Joint Surg Am.* **80** (4):566–580.

Fractures around the shoulder

Clavicle

Clavicle fractures are caused by a fall onto the outstretched hand or the point of the shoulder, and account for 4% of all fractures.

Types

- Injury occurs in the middle (75%), lateral (20%), or medial (5%) third.
- Lateral injury can be associated with coracoid fractures or tearing of the coracoclavicular ligament.

Treatment

- Most clavicle fractures[1] can be treated conservatively with a sling to take the weight of the arm.
- Absolute operative indications are skin tenting, skin necrosis, and neurovascular injury. Open fractures require open reduction and internal fixation with a plate and screws.
- Relative operative indications are polytrauma patients who may need the extremity for weight bearing, "floating shoulder," and some highly displaced and shortened fractures.
- Distal-third (lateral) fractures associated with acromioclavicular disruption may also need open reduction and fixation with a specialized "Hook" plate.

Complications

- *Malunion*: rarely causes any functional deficit.
- *Non-union*: A minimum of 12 weeks post-injury, symptomatic patients may be treated with open reduction and internal fixation with bone grafting.
- *Acute complications*: neurovascular injury (including brachial plexus injury), neurovascular compression (costoclavicular syndrome), pneumothorax from bony penetration of the pleura

Scapula

Scapula fractures are caused by direct trauma, usually a high-velocity injury. Always have a high clinical suspicion of other possible injuries such as rib fracture, pulmonary contusion, and pneumo- or hemothorax.

Treatment

- *Simple* (no involvement of the glenoid [glenohumeral joint]): adequate analgesia (this is a very painful injury and may require admission) and early mobilization
- *Complex* (involving the glenoid): may need open reduction and internal fixation after further imaging such as CT or MRI scanning

Proximal humerus

This injury is usually due to indirect force from a fall onto the outstretched hand.

Types

Proximal humerus fractures are classified by the number of fracture fragments, i.e., two-, three-, or four-part, and whether associated with dislocation of the joint (a fragment must be 1 cm displaced and 45° angulated to qualify as a part). This is best known is the Neer[2] classification.

Treatment

- *Undisplaced or impacted*: sling with early pendulum mobilization
- *Displaced* fractures usually require open reduction and internal fixation by a "locking" plate, proximal humeral intramedullary nails or cannulated screws, and K wires with or without tension band wiring.
- *Comminuted*: Severely comminuted fractures (4-part), especially those including fracture dislocations, have a high rate of avascular necrosis, which is usually treated with hemiarthroplasty and soft tissue reconstruction of the rotator cuff to the prosthesis.

Complications

Non- and malunion, avascular necrosis of the humeral head, and osteoarthritis of the shoulder joint are most common. High-velocity injuries may also cause neurovascular injuries, particularly of the brachial plexus.

Humeral shaft

Fractures of this type are caused by indirect and direct trauma.

Types

Specify by location proximal, middle, distal third. Fractures may be transverse, oblique (direct injury), spiral (rotational injury), or comminuted.

Treatment

- *Conservative*:[3] if <25° of angulation, <3 cm of shortening (no functional or cosmetic deficit). Either by hanging cast (U-slab of plaster around the elbow to the humerus with a sling to support the wrist) or a functional humeral brace. Union usually takes up to 12 weeks.
- *Surgical*. Normally reserved for polytrauma, ipsilateral forearm fractures, open or pathological fractures, spiral fracture of the distal third with associated radial nerve palsy (Holstein–Lewis fracture), or associated vascular injuries requiring intervention. Fixation is usually through a screw and plate or occasionally an intramedullary nail.

Complications

- Always examine for radial nerve palsy; most are transient neurapraxias.
- Malunion and non-union

Pediatric humeral fractures

- These usually occur at the surgical neck or through and around the proximal humeral epiphysis.
- They may be indicative of a nonaccidental injury.
- Most require no treatment apart from collar and cuff with mobilization as for adults. Remodeling potential is good in this area.

1 Denard PL, Koval KJ, Cantu RV, Weinstein JN (2005). Management of midshaft clavicle fractures in adults. *Aam J Orthoped* **34**(11):527–536.

2 Neer CS (1970). Displaced proximal humeral fractures. I. Classification and evaluation. *J Bone Joint Surg Am* **52-A**:1077–1089.

3 Sarmiento A, Zagorski JB, Zych GA, Latta LL, Capps CA (2000). Functional bracing for the treatment of fractures of the humeral diaphysis. *J Bone Joint Surg Am* **82-A**:478–486.

Dislocations of the shoulder region

Sternoclavicular joint

- *Cause*: fall onto an outstretched hand
- *Types*: usually dislocates anteriorly; posterior dislocation is rare. The deformity is at the medial clavicle.
- *Complications*: Tracheal compression may occur with posterior dislocation.

Treatment

- Anterior dislocation is treated symptomatically with a sling, analgesia, and early mobilization.
- Posterior dislocation with tracheal compression requires closed reduction, or open reduction if this fails (with cardiothoracic surgical help).

Acromioclavicular joint

- *Causes*. Fall onto the outstretched hand or the point of the shoulder. Common to contact sports such as rugby, football, and ice hockey
- *Classification*. Rockwood[1] classification has six types, with increasing numbers relating to increasing severity of ligamentous disruption and displacement

Treatment

- Broad arm sling and early mobilization when pain allows. Persistent pain or functional limitation is treated by reconstruction.
- Conservative vs. surgical treatment depends on the grade of injury.
- Acute repair may be indicated in a professional-level athlete.

Anterior dislocation of the glenohumeral joint

This injury is caused by forceful abduction and external rotation of the glenohumeral joint.[2,3]

Pathology

- In the young patient the anterior glenoid labrum may be torn from the bone (with or without a rim fracture). This is called a Bankart lesion.
- Elderly patients may also sustain a rotator cuff tear.

Features

- The shoulder looks "square," as the deltoid is flat and a sulcus can be visible where the humeral head may be.
- The patient supports the arm, which is abducted and very painful.
- X-rays (AP, axillary lateral, and scapular Y lateral views) show the humeral head anterior and inferior to the glenoid. Used to exclude a fracture of the humerus or glenoid.

Treatment

- Reduced urgently
- The patient should be safely sedated and relaxed with IV medications.
  - The simplest, extremely reliable method is gentle, continued straight-line traction with the arm abducted about 10°–20° from the trunk. This may take 10–15 min, but patience is the key, not force.
  - Countertraction can be placed across the truck with a broad sheet.

Types of shoulder dislocation

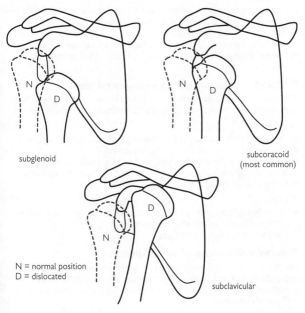

subglenoid

subcoracoid
(most common)

N = normal position
D = dislocated

subclavicular

Fig. 18.1 Types of shoulder dislocation.

- An alternative technique is to have the patient lying prone on the table in a quiet, relaxed environment with the arm hanging freely down and weighted (e.g., 3 L bag of saline or 10 pounds of weights) (Stimpson's technique).
- If there is an associated humeral neck fracture the reduction should be done under general anesthesia (GA) with flouroscopy.
- Place the arm in a sling. Repeat the X-ray (axillary lateral view is key!) to confirm reduction and that there has been no iatrogenic fracture.
- Always document neurological status (axillary nerve) before and after reduction.

Posterior dislocation of the glenohumeral joint

This type of injury is rare and due to forced internal rotation or a direct blow to the anterior shoulder (e.g., after an epileptic fit or electric shock).

Features

- The arm is held internally rotated and no external rotation is possible.
- The humeral head should be palpable posteriorly.
- AP X-rays may show the humeral head as a light bulb shape (internally rotated), but this is not diagnostic of posterior dislocation.
- Axillary lateral X-ray shows the dislocation.

Treatment

- Use in-line traction method (as above) but consider general anesthesia if this is difficult—avoid excessive force.
- The patient may be very unstable.

Recurrent dislocation of the shoulder

Recurrent dislocation is usually due to a Bankart lesion or capsular redundancy (stretched and floppy). It is common in young patients after their first dislocation. [(100 − age at first dislocation) = % recurrence rate; >40 years, recurrence <10%).]

Treatment—surgery

- Labral repair, fixation of the anterior Bankart lesion
- May be done open or arthroscopically
- Capsular laxity is treated by capsular shift, an overlapping "pants-over-vest" procedure to improve proprioceptive joint sensation.

1 Rockwood CA Jr, Green DP (Eds.) (1996). *Rockwood and Green's Fractures in Adults*, 4th ed. Philadelphia: Lippincott-Raven, pp. 1247–1251.
2 Robinson CM, Dobson RJ (2004). Anterior instability of the shoulder after trauma [review]. *J Bone Joint Surg Br* **86-B**:469.
3 Levine WN, Rieger K, McCluskey GM 3rd (2005). Arthroscopic treatment of anterior shoulder instability. *Instr Course Lect* **54**:87–96.

Fractures of the ribs and sternum

Causes
- Single rib fractures occur as a result of direct injury such as a fall.
- Fractures of the lower ribs may occur with coughing.
- Sternal fractures occur with direct injury, e.g., contact with the steering wheel or by restraint by a seat belt.
- High-velocity road traffic accident (RTA) or large crush injuries can result in a flail chest, i.e., multiple rib fractures, each fractured at two sites.

Treatment
- Single rib fracture: symptomatic with analgesia
- Multiple ribs fracture: If ≥3 ribs are involved, the patient should be admitted for observation overnight, but treat symptoms with analgesia and chest physiotherapy.
- Sternal fracture: Symptomatic treatment but observe for associated injuries (see Complications)
- Flail chest or extensive multiple rib fractures is a potentially life-threatening injury and may present with severe respiratory distress.
  - Flail segments move paradoxically, preventing adequate ventilation.
  - Multiple fractures restrict respiratory effort, severely impairing ventilation
  - Treat with high-flow O_2 and analgesia. CPAP and even IPPV (📖 p. 126) may be required.

Complications
The incidence of complications[1] rises dramatically if the injury involves
- More than 3 ribs
- First, second, or third ribs
- Sternum
- Scapula

They are all indicators of high energy transfer injury.

Cardiac tamponade (📖 p. 416)
- Bleeding into the pericardial cavity causes severe hemodynamic shock and may be the cause of a cardiac arrest at presentation.
- Diagnosis is by high clinical suspicion, muffled heart sounds, raised JVP, and no signs of a tension pneumothorax.
- Treat by immediate pericardiocentesis with transfer to cardiothoracic unit for repair of the defect.

Pneumothorax (📖 p. 416)
- Usually due to direct pleural injury by bone fragments during injury
- Often associated with hemothorax
- Signs are respiratory distress, absent breath sounds, hyperresonant percussion note (pneumothorax), or shock.

- Tension pneumothorax is life threatening and requires immediate decompression via a 16G needle placed into the second anterior intercostal space, followed by definitive chest drain placement.
- If in any doubt, always treat first on clinical grounds rather than waiting for X-rays.

1 American College of Surgeons (1997). *Advanced Trauma Life Support (ATLS) Student Manual*, 6th ed, Chicago: American College of Surgeons, pp. 125–141.

Fractures of the pelvis

Causes
- Age <60 years: usually from a motor vehicle accident (MVA) or high energy falls
- Age >60 years: usually injury from a fall at home

The force required to fracture the pelvis in the young is considerable and as a result the mortality can be as high as 20%. It is the main cause of death in multiple-trauma patients.

Types
- The pelvis is a ring made of both bones and ligaments (e.g., sacroiliac).
- An isolated break at any part is stable (the ring will not separate).
- Two breaks in the ring make it unstable (allow the two halves to separate).
- The most commonly used classification is that of Young and Burgess[1] (descriptive):
  - Lateral compression (impact from side)
  - AP compression (impact from the front or rear)
  - Vertical shear (usually a fall from height)
  - Combined mechanical (mixture of all of the above)

Treatment
Single ring fracture (stable)
- Check for an occult sacroiliac ligament injury (local bruising and tenderness with pain on stressing the joint); this makes the injury unstable there.
- Fractures of both superior and inferior pubic rami on the same side are a single break in terms of ring stability.
- Isolated fractures of the ilium, ischium, or pubis are normally treated with bed rest, analgesia, and early mobilization as soon as the pain allows.
- Fractures that extend to the acetabulum (joint) and are displaced are usually treated with open reduction and internal fixation with screws and plates to restore congruency of the joint to reduce the risk of future osteoarthritis.

Multiple-ring fractures (unstable)

Unstable fractures are associated with massive hemorrhage within the pelvis. This is mostly because the pelvic ring is grossly displaced during the injury and tearing of the extensive posterior presacral venous plexus occurs. A patient's entire blood volume can be lost; hence the 20% mortality rate.

Establish hemodynamic control

- Hypotension is very common, but so are associated multiple injuries.
- Establish at least two large-bore IV infusions and commence resuscitation with warmed crystalloid 1000 mL and be prepared to repeat.
- Send blood for urgent cross-match of 4 units. Uncross-matched blood is occasionally necessary as part of resuscitation.
- Continued bleeding must be controlled by preventing the broken pelvic ring from expanding and thus compressing the soft tissues within. This may be achieved by the following means:
  - Binding a bed sheet tightly around the pelvis and internally rotating the hips. This is very effective as an emergency procedure.
  - Application of an external pelvic fixator is a more definitive solution but should be done in the operating room.
- Laparotomy is contraindicated unless there are life-threatening intra-abdominal injuries that must be treated, since this effectively decompresses the pelvis again superiorly.
- Urethral injury occurs, especially with anterior compression bony injuries. If there is blood at the urethral meatus, perineal bruising, hematuria, or a high-riding prostate on rectal examination, then catheterization should only be performed by an experienced urologist (very often suprapubically). Investigation for injury is with a retrograde urethrogram or IV urogram once the patient is stable.
- Definitive treatment is usually by continuation of external fixation or, more commonly, by open reduction and internal fixation with plates and screws.

Complications

- Hemorrhage, shock, and death from exsanguinations
- Open fractures carry a 50% mortality rate and need to be treated aggressively by both orthopedic and general surgical teams.
- Urogenital injury
- Pelvic venous thromboembolism (due to disruption of the venous intima)
- Paralytic ileus
- Malunion may lead to difficulty with pregnancy.
- Osteoarthritis

1 Burgess A, Young JWR, et al. (1990). Pelvic ring disruptions: effective classification system and treatment protocols. *J Trauma* **30**(7):848–856.

Hip fractures

Hip fractures include femoral neck,[1] intertrochanteric, and subtrochanteric fractures.

Causes

- These are the most common fractures in the elderly, with an exponential increase in incidence with age.[2]
- They are usually associated with osteoporosis and caused by a fall. Insufficiency stress fractures also occur.
- Fractures in the young are usually a result of major trauma.

Classification

Hip fractures should be described anatomically and then by bony features (displacement, fragments).
- *Femoral neck = intracapsular* fractures. They occur just below the head (subcapital) or in the neck (transcervical).
- *Trochanteric area = extracapsular* fractures. They occur either in the trochanteric region at its junction with the femoral neck (basal), between trochanters (intertrochanteric), or ≤5 cm below the lesser trochanter (subtrochanteric).
- Classify the fracture as *displaced* or *non-displaced*.

Features

- Among the elderly, the inability to bear weight is a common presenting feature.
- If the fracture is displaced (common) the leg will be shortened, adducted, and externally rotated. Straight-leg raise and hip movements are globally inhibited by pain.
- X-rays: AP pelvis, AP hip, lateral hip
  - Displaced fractures are usually obvious.
  - Non-displaced fractures may be difficult to visualize. If a patient cannot bear weight or do a straight-leg raise despite analgesia, they may have a hip fracture.
  - A bone scan (highly sensitive, poor specificity) or MRI (gold standard) is diagnostic for occult hip fracture.

Treatment

Femoral neck, intracapsular

- *Non-displaced* fractures are treated by internal fixation with cannulated screws.
- *Displaced* fractures are treated by urgent open reduction internal fixation (ORIF) in young patients. In the elderly they can be treated with ORIF, hemiarthroplasty, or total hip arthroplasty (depending on whether there is preexisting arthritis).[3]

Trochanteric area, extracapsular

- *Non-displaced*: Open fixation with the use of a DHS or intramedullary hip screw (IMHS; or gamma nail).
- *Displaced*: ORIF with dynamic hip screw (DHS), or IMHS

In children or young patients, whatever the displacement of fracture, internal fixation is employed. In the very active elderly patient, total hip arthroplasty has been proposed if there is preexisting arthritis.

Complications

- Overall mortality in the elderly is 20% at 90 days. Here the fracture is more a marker of generally poor condition than an injury leading to acute surgical perioperative complications.
- Avascular necrosis of the femoral head occurs much more frequently with intracapsular than with extracapsular fractures (the blood supply of the femoral head flows mostly up via the femoral neck).
- Dislocation of arthroplasty
- Non-union
- Infection
- Lower-limb thromboembolic disease

1 Koval KJ, Zuckerman JD (1994). Hip fractures: I. Overview and evaluation and treatment of femoral-neck fractures. *J Am Acad Orthop* Surg **2**:141–149.
2 Parker MJ, Pryor GA, Thorngren KG (1997). *Handbook of Hip Fracture Surgery*. Oxford: Butterworth-Heinemann.
3 Parker MJ, Khan RJ, et al. (2002). Hemiarthroplasty versus internal fixation for displaced intra-capsular hip fractures in the elderly. A randomised trial of 455 patients. *J Bone Joint Surg Br* **84-B**:1150–1155.

Femoral shaft fractures

Causes

- The most common cause is a high-energy MVA in young adults.
- They are also caused by falls from height.
- Commonly these fractures are part of polytrauma.

Classification

- The AO system can be used but is complex.
- Anatomical description is the simplest:
  - Location (proximal 1/3, mid 1/3, distal 1/3, etc.)
  - Configuration (transverse, oblique, spiral, segmental, comminuted)
  - Number of fragments

Associated injuries

- Polytrauma is common: look for head, chest, and abdominal injuries.
- Ipsilateral femoral neck fracture (up to 5%)
- Knee joint injuries: both bony or ligamentous (e.g., ACL rupture)
- Soft-tissue injury to skin, muscle, neurovascular structures
- Sciatic nerve traction injury (uncommon)

Treatment

Resuscitation

- Establish large-bore IV access and give 1000 mL crystalloid—initial hemodynamic compensation is common in the young and may hide a large blood loss into tissues around a long-bone fracture.
- Send blood for type and cross for 2 units PRBC.
- Reduce and splint the leg, if possible.
- If open, copiously irrigate the wound. Place a sterile dressing over the wound. Start IV antibiotics and update tetanus if indicated.

Children[1,2]

- <2 years: hip spica cast or inpatient traction if unable to obtain reduction
- 2–6 years: hip spica cast
- >6 years: IM flexible nail, external fixation, ORIF
- In older children, operative internal fixation is becoming much more common because of the advantages of early mobilization and discharge from hospital. Options are a flexible intramedullary nail ("elastic" nail) or ORIF with a plate and screw.

Adults

Most adult patients are treated operatively to allow early mobilization.[3]

Intramedullary nail

- Closed reduction and fixation with a nail (reamed or not). The nail is locked both proximally and distally to stop fracture ends from rotating.
- A reconstruction nail must be used if there is an associated fracture of the femoral neck to allow passage of a lag screw up the femoral neck into the head.

Plate fixation

This procedure is technically demanding and not as strong as nail fixation because of the forces acting on the plate. A wide exposure is required, which increases infection risk; it is seldom used.

External fixation

- This is most useful for immediate treatment of fractures associated with polytrauma (damage-control surgery) and where there is extensive soft tissue damage.
- The fixator can be changed for an intramedullary nail when the patient's condition allows.

Complications

- Fat embolus (1%) and possible ARDS
- Infection: 5% after open; 1% after closed nailing
- Non-union
- Thromboembolic disease
- Malunion, rotation being the most symptomatic
- Pressure sores, bronchopneumonia, UTI on conservatively treated patients

1 Metaizeau JP (2004). Stable elastic intramedullary nailing for fractures of the femur in children [operative technique]. *J Bone Joint Surg Br* **86-B**:954–957.
2 Flynn JM, Schwend RM (2004). Management of pediatric femoral shaft fractures *J Am Acad Orthop Surg* **12**:347–359.
3 Wolinsky P, et al. (2001) Controversies in intramedullary nailing of femoral shaft fractures [instructional course lecture]. *J Bone Joint Surg Am* **83-A**:1404–1415.

Fractures of the tibial shaft

- This is the most common long bone fracture.
- It is caused by MVAs and sports injuries (e.g., football and skiing).
- The tibia is subcutaneous in its medial border and has poor soft tissue coverage. This means that it commonly presents as an open fracture.
- The blood supply is poor and the time to union is quite long, resulting in the risk of infection, non-union, and malunion.

Classification

- The AO system can be used but is complex.
- Anatomical description is the simplest:
  - Location (proximal, middle, distal third, etc.)
  - Pattern (transverse, oblique, spiral, segmental, comminuted)
  - Number of fragments
- Open injuries are normally classified additionally by the Gustilo–Anderson system.[1]

Treatment

There is no one method of treatment[2,3] that is appropriate for all fractures. The best rule is to judge each fracture and associated soft tissue injury on an individual basis and treat appropriately.

Splinting

- Used for non-displaced fractures and low-energy displaced fractures in children that can be closed reduced
- Long leg splint acutely, then cast, with the knee flexed 20° and the ankle in neutral position
- Non-weight bearing, on crutches with X-rays weekly for the first 4 weeks to check alignment.
- Start weight bearing at 8 weeks in a weight-bearing contact Sarmiento cast.
- Union takes approximately 14–16 weeks.
- *Advantages.* simple and avoids all operative risks.
- *Disadvantages.* takes a long time; requires good follow-up and patient compliance. Stiffness at the knee and ankle is common and unstable injuries are very difficult to manipulate and control in plaster alone.

Locking plate fixation

- Mostly used for fractures near the joint surface
- Plates used in the shaft have a high rate of infection and non-union caused by the large soft tissue exposure required.
- *Advantages.* simple, quick, rapid mobilization and avoids the need for plaster.
- *Disadvantages.* risk of infection, non-union, and implant failure

Intramedullary nailing

- Currently this is the treatment of choice in most centers but requires increased operating time and experience.
- It may be used in open fractures, especially where soft tissue flaps are required, since it gives relatively unlimited access to the tibia.
- This is best for mid-shaft fractures. It is poor at controlling proximal and distal fractures within 5–10 cm of the knee and ankle joints.
- *Advantages*: early mobilization, quicker rehabilitation than closed methods, soft tissue undisturbed by technique, easy access for flaps
- *Disadvantages*: chance of chronic anterior knee pain (site of nail insertion—not recommended for kneeling profession, (e.g.,carpenters).

External fixation

- This technique is often used in open fractures as it produces the least disturbance of soft tissue. The fracture can be placed in an extremely rigid configuration to allow stability. Rigidity can then be reduced sequentially in outpatients.
- Circular external fixators (Ilizarov) can be used for difficult fractures around the knee or ankle.
- *Advantages*: technically simple; allows early mobilization; avoids further soft tissue damage
- *Disadvantages*. Pin-site infections are common but usually easily treated. External fixation requires good nursing backup and patient compliance. Pin sites need to be planned carefully with the plastic team if flaps are used, so as not to compromise soft-tissue cover.

Other complications

Compartment syndrome

This syndrome[4] is an orthopedic emergency. Immediate fasciotomy is required if the compartment pressures are measured and meet specific criteria. The most consistent and reliable clinical signs are pain out of proportion to the exam, and pain with passive stretch. Paraesthesia, pallor, and pulseless (P's of acute ischemia) are late signs and usually the limb is unsalvageable by the time these appear.

1 Gustilo RB, Anderson JT. (1976). Prevention of infection in the treatment of one thousand and twenty-five open fractures of long bones: retrospective and prospective analyses. *J Bone Joint Surg Am* **58-A**:453–458.

2 Schmidt AH, et al. (2003). Treatment of closed tibial fractures [instructional course lecture]. *J Bone Joint Surg Am* **85-A**:352–368.

3 Bhandari M, et al. (2001). Treatment of open fractures of the shaft of the tibia [review]. *J Bone Joint Surg B* **83-B**:62–68.

4 Elliott KG, Johnstone AJ (2003). Diagnosing acute compartment syndrome [review]. *J Bone Joint Surg Br* **85-B**, 62–68.

Fractures of the ankle

- Fractures of the ankle[1] are the most common fracture of the lower limb.
- They are normally caused by a combination of rotation and abduction or adduction forces (e.g., football tackle, skiing injury).
- Like the pelvis, the ankle should be thought of as a ring, and stability is conferred by the following:
  - The bones (medial and lateral malleoli, talus)
  - The ligamentous supports (lateral tibiofibular ligaments, medial deltoid ligament, and central syndesmosis)
- Remember that a fracture of the proximal fibula (at the knee) is associated with an ankle fracture or dislocation until proven otherwise.

Classification

- AO/Danis Weber system:
  - Type A: below the syndesmosis
  - Type B: at the syndesmosis
  - Type C: above the syndesmosis
- A distal tibial fracture involving the articular surface is known as a Pilon fracture.

Features

- Often there is obvious deformity. Isolated tenderness and inability to weight bear due to pain are highly suspicious.
- Examine for medial and lateral bony tenderness as the medial injury may be ligamentous only. Also examine the proximal fibula.
- X-rays are AP, mortise (15° internally rotated), and lateral views.

Treatment

Stable injuries

- Lateral malleolus fracture with no displacement in the mortise and no medial tenderness can be treated in a weight-bearing splint or CAM boot.

Unstable injuries

- Displaced medial malleolar fractures, bimalleolar fractures, and fractures of the posterior cortex >25% all require open reduction and internal fixation.
- Treat by open reduction and internal fixation with plates and screws.
- Minimal talar displacement (≤2 mm) in the mortise may be acceptable in the elderly or patients with multiple comorbidities and treated by splinting or casting.

Syndesmosis disruption

- Treat with 1–2 cortical screws placed 2–5 cm above the joint if syndesomotic disruption[2] and the fibular fracture is >4.5 cm from joint. Screws are generally removed at 12 weeks.

Displaced fracture or dislocation

- Reduce the fracture immediately in the ER and apply a below-knee posterior mold splint. Always take post-reduction X-rays.
- A displaced fracture or dislocation is an orthopedic emergency and is usually clinically obvious. Displacement is often more than expected due to soft tissue swelling.

Complications

- Wound breakdown
- Nonunion
- Infection: superficial or deep
- Post-traumatic arthritis

1 Vander Griend R, Michelson JD, Bone LB (1996). Fractures of the ankle and the distal part of the tibia [instructional course lecture]. *J Bone Joint Surg Am* **78-A**:1772–1783.
2 Zalavras C, Thordarson D (2007). Ankle syndesmotic injury. *J Am Acad Orthop Surg* **15**:330–339.

Fractures of the tarsal bones and foot

Talus

Cause
- Usually a fall from height or an MVA
- Sometimes seen in private pilots with injury from the rudder bar—"aviators' fracture"

Classification
- By anatomical site, i.e., head, neck, body, or lateral process
- Talar neck fractures are given Hawkins classification types I–IV (indicating increasing levels of displacement with increasing grade).

Treatment
The foot is commonly very swollen and possibly deformed. Take care to assess that adequate circulation is present.
- *Non-displaced*: strict non-weight bearing in below-knee cast for 6 weeks
- *Displaced*: ORIF with lag screws—treat as an emergency if the skin is compromised.

Complications
- Avascular necrosis. The rate increases with displacement (10% in type I to 90% in type III).
- Osteoarthritis of the joint(s) may occur in patients without avascular necrosis. If the patient is symptomatic, salvage surgery by arthrodesis (fusion) of the affected joint may be useful.

Calcaneus
- Calcaneus fracture[1] is caused by a fall from height. Injury is often bilateral.
- Remember to look for commonly associated injuries, i.e., spinal fracture.
- Gross swelling can cause compartment syndrome acutely.

Classification
- Extra- or intra-articular
- Intra-articular fractures involve the subtalar joint and are classified according to their CT appearance by the Sanders system.

Treatment
- *Extra-articular or non-displaced intra-articular fractures*. Conservative treatment includes elevation, ice, bed rest, and observation of soft tissues overnight. Treat non-weight-bearing injury with a removable splint to stop equinus at the ankle. Early subtalar passive mobilization should be initiated.
- *Displaced intra-articular fractures* are usually treated with ORIF with a specialized lateral calcaneal plate.
  - *Advantages*: Anatomical reduction improves heel shape, prevents lateral impingement, and may reduce post-traumatic arthritis, although this remains unproven.
  - *Disadvantages*: High incidence of wound breakdown

Complications

Broad heel, skin necrosis if grossly swollen, and malunion into varus or valgus. Persistent heel pain and post-traumatic arthritis are common.

Lisfranc injury

Fracture dislocation at the tarso-metatarsal joint (named after Lisfranc, who described it in cavalrymen whose feet got trapped in their stirrups).[2] Lisfranc's ligament runs from the base of second metatarsal to medial cuneiform.

Causes and features

- Foot being trapped under the brake or clutch pedal in a MVA. This is a common injury in football players.
- The base of the second metatarsal is damaged. This is the keystone for the forefoot, so injuries here are highly unstable and forefoot dislocation occurs.
- Consider the injury in all patients with forefoot pain and swelling. It may occur as a ligamentous injury alone (with a worse prognosis).

Treatment

Treatment is with ORIF vs. primary arthodesis with transfixion of the tarsometatarsal joints with screws.

Complications

- Foot compartment syndrome in acute injuries
- Metatarsalgia, post-traumatic arthritis in untreated injuries

Metatarsal and phalanges

Causes and features

- Crushing or twisting injuries (e.g., the foot being run over)
- Fifth metatarsal fracture occurs after an inversion injury and can be mistaken for an ankle fracture if not examined correctly.
- Always be suspicious of compartment syndrome in severe crush injuries.
- Always obtain X-rays.

Treatment

- Conservative with mobilization as pain allows. Use plaster only if mobilization is too painful.
- Phalangeal fractures—simple strapping
- Operative fixation is for multiple metatarsal fractures if the first or fifth rays are broken as well as the middle rays.
- Non-union of the fifth metatarsal sometimes requires ORIF with bone grafting if problematic (rare).

1 Sanders R. (2000). Displaced intra-articular fractures of the calcaneus [current concepts review]. *J Bone Joint Surg Am* **82-A**:225–250.
2 Lattermann C, Goldstin JL, Wukich JK, Lee S, Bach BR Jr (2007). Practical management of Lisfranc injuries in athletes. *Clin J Sports Med* **17**(4):311–315.

Injuries and the spinal radiograph

If a patient complains of central pain in the spinal column after trauma, always obtain radiographs.[1,2] This should not delay resuscitation, as a spinal fracture can be immobilized and life-threatening problems corrected first.

Spinal injuries can be associated with other injuries and the patient may not be able to communicate this to you because they are

- unconscious;
- intubated;
- shocked; or
- anesthetized distal to a cord lesion.

Common injuries associated with spinal trauma are the following:

- Bilateral calcaneal fractures: thoracolumbar fractures
- Facial fractures: cervical fracture or dislocation
- Severe head injury: cervical injuries, especially C1/C2
- Sternal dislocation: thoracic spine fracture
- Ankylosing spondylitis: cervical and thoracic fractures
- Cervical fracture: 10% rate of fracture at another level

X-ray interpretation

- Develop a mental picture of the normal spinal radiograph. If you feel that the X-ray just doesn't look right, then it probably isn't! Always check the lateral masses of cervical vertebrae, which are symmetrical.
- Try to develop a system and use this for every fracture you see, even when you know it will be normal. This practice gets you into the habit.
- *C-spine*: Obtain AP and lateral views. All views should visualize C1–T1. Get a swimmer's view or open-mouth views to better visualize C1, C2. Oblique views are better to assess for facet dislocation. Pay close attention to the relationship of C1 and C2. The lateral masses of C1 should never overlap the lateral margin of C2 on a centered AP open-mouth view; ≥3 mm space between the front of the odontoid peg and back of the anterior arch of C1 is abnormal and may indicate instability
- Check the paraspinal soft tissues—a retropharyngeal space of >3 mm indicates a hematoma and is highly suspicious of fracture. The paravertebral pleura should run parallel to the aorta; if not, suspect a hematoma.
- If you are unable to visualize to T1 or unable to adequately assess the C-spine, have a low threshold to obtain a CT scan.
- Obtain an MRI if there is concern about facet dislocation and neurologic compromise to rule out a herniated disc.
- *Lumbar spine*: Obtain AP, lateral, and oblique views of the lumbosacral spine.
- Beware of empty vertebrae; this may imply damage to the spinous process.
- Check the transverse processes; they become displaced when fractured.
- Check pedicles on the AP view as separation indicates displacement.

- If there is an obvious spinal injury, ensure that the associated soft tissue, e.g., thoracic viscera, retroperitoneal structures, and spinal cord injury, are excluded and that the patient is stable before requesting further radiological investigation, e.g., CT scanning.
- If in any doubt, consult senior colleagues immediately for a further opinion.
- The thoracolumbar spine is the most common area for vertebral column injuries.

Structure of the spine

The spine has three structural columns:
- *Anterior*: anterior half of the vertebral body
- *Middle*: posterior half of the vertebral body to the posterior longitudinal ligaments
- *Posterior*: facet joints and their intervertebral ligaments, spinous processes and their interspinous ligaments

Signs that imply spinal instability[3]

- With increasing column involvement there is increasing instability, i.e., one-column injury usually stable, three-column injury highly unstable.
- Neurologic compromise along with two-column disruption (Denis Classification) is associated with instability
- Associated kyphosis.
- Complete vertebral dislocation or translocation.
- Fractures in a previously fused spine, especially ankylosing spondylitis.
- Signs of movement: malalignment, avulsion fractures, and evidence of paravertebral swelling.

1 Raby N, Berman L, de Lacy G (2005). *Accident and Emergency Radiology: A Survival Guide*, 2nd ed. London: Saunders.
2 Nicholson DA, Driscoll P (1995). *ABC of Emergency Radiology*. London: BMJ Books.
3 Wood KB, Khanna G, Vaccaro AR, Arnold PM, Harris MB, Mehbod AA (2005). Assessment of two thoracolumbar fracture classification systems as used by multiple surgeons. *J Bone Joint Surg Am* **87**(7):1423–1429.

Spinal injuries

Any patient with major trauma arriving in the ER should be assumed to have a cervical injury[1] unless proven otherwise. Remember that the A in the primary survey of ATLS resuscitation stands for *airway with cervical spine control*—i.e., it is top priority.[2]

- Cervical spine is the most common area to have a major spinal injury.
- Other areas of concern are at transition zones, e.g., C7/T1, T12/L1, and L5/S1 junctions.
- The main reason for delay in diagnosis of spinal injuries is failure to have a high clinical index of suspicion in all major-trauma patients.

Structure of the spine

With increasing column involvement there is increasing instability—i.e., one-column injury is usually stable, three-column injury is highly unstable.

Neurological assessment

Full accurate and detailed neurological assessment includes Glasgow Coma Scale (GCS), cranial nerve function, power, sensation (three modalities), reflexes, tone, and proprioception, to be performed as part of the secondary survey and documented with date and time.

Principles of treatment

- Establish if the injury is stable or unstable.
- Unstable injuries may have no neurologic injury but are at high risk for compromise if handled incorrectly.
- Correct, initial immobilization of the cervical spine involves a correctly sized semi-rigid collar and proper positioning on the spine board.

Stable injury

Treat with pain relief, bed rest, and mobilization when pain allows.

Unstable injury

- Reduce dislocations.
- Maintain reduction and avoid mobilization until patient is stabilized. Traction or internal fixation may be required.

Cervical injury

Stabilize the injury with a hard collar and spine board. Do not permit flexion or rotation. Assign a competent person (ATLS trained) to do this. Longitudinal traction with the head in neutral position has been recommended. Inform the anesthesia team of injury in case of need for airway management.

Thoracolumbar injury

- Transport patient prone or supine according to need. The patient should be transported on a long spinal board, but removed as soon as possible once in a spinal bed to prevent skin pressure problems. The patient must be "log rolled" as appropriate.

- Use of corticosteroids in acute spinal cord injury is controversial.[3] They must be used early (<24 hr) in consultation with the regional spinal-injuries unit.
- Specialized care is needed. Major spinal injuries should be treated in specialist regional spinal-injury centers.

Spinal shock

- Defined as the immediate loss of all power, sensation, and reflexes below the level of injury due to neurogenic loss of autonomic tone
- Characteristically the spinal reflexes are lost, e.g., bulbocavernous.
- If this is a transient phenomenon, recovery is usually within 24–48 hr.
- No return of function by 48 hr suggests that the prognosis for recovery is poor and the cord lesion is referred to as "complete."
- Clinically the patient has a low blood pressure and low heart rate.
- Cardiovascular shock, e.g., hypotension, delayed capillary return, in a spinal-injured patient should always be assumed to be hypovolemic.
- The patient will have low blood pressure and bradycardia, which should be treated aggressively with fluid resuscitation and investigation of hypovolemic causes.

"Incomplete" spinal cord syndromes

If there is preservation of some modalities of cord function distal to the injury level, the cord lesion is referred to as "incomplete." Several recognized patterns exist.

Central cord syndrome

- Extension injury: usually age >50 years
- Tetraplegia with upper limbs > in lower limbs is common.
- Recovery is no better than 75%.

Anterior cord syndrome

- Flexion injury
- There is dense motor or sensory loss but proprioception and vibration sense (posterior column) are spared.
- Poor prognosis with only 10% recovery

Brown–Sequard syndrome

- Penetrating trauma
- Hemisection of the cord, giving ipsilateral motor, vibration, and proprioceptive loss and contralateral loss of pain and temperature
- Variable recovery

Posterior cord syndrome

- Proprioception and vibration sense are lost but motor power is intact (rare).

1 Delamarter RB, Coyle J (1999). Acute management of spinal cord injury. *J Am Acad Orthop Surg* 7:166–175.

2 Skinner D, Driscoll P (1999), *ABC of Major Trauma*, 3rd ed. London: BMJ Books.

3 Bracken MB, et al. (1997). Administration of methylprednisolone for 24 or 48 hours or tirilazad mesylate for 48 hours in the treatment of acute spinal cord injury. Results of the Third National Acute Spinal Cord Injury Randomized Controlled Trial. National Acute Spinal Cord Injury Study. *JAMA* 277(20):1597–1604.

Acute hematogenous osteomyelitis

This is a disease of growing bones.[1] It is common in infants and children but rare in adults unless they are immunocompromised or diabetic.

Etiology

- Infants: *Staphylococcus aureus, Streptococcus*, and *Escherichia coli*
- Children: *S. aureus, Streptococcus, Haemophilus influenzae* B
- Adults: *S. aureus*
- Sickle-cell patients: *Salmonella* spp.
- Rare causes: *Brucella*, TB, spirochetes, and fungi

Pathological features

The organisms settle near the metaphysis at the growing end of a long bone. The following stages typically occur.

- *Inflammation.* Acute inflammation with venous congestion
- *Suppuration.* After 2–3 days, pus forms in the medulla and forces its way out to the periosteum.
- *Necrosis.* After 7 days, the blood supply is compromised and infective thrombosis leads to necrosis and formation of a pocket of dead tissue (sequestrum).
- *Repair.* At around 10–14 days new bone is formed from the subperiosteal layer that was stripped with the swelling (involucrum).
- *Discharge.* Involucrum can develop defects (cloacae), allowing discharge of pus and sequestrum to aid in resolution. This can also be achieved by surgical release and debridement.

Clinical features

- Usually a child with a preceding history of trauma or infection (skin or respiratory)
- Fever, pain, and malaise develop after a few days.
- The child may be limping or refusing to weight bear.
- On examination there may be localized swelling or redness.
- Infants may present with a failure to thrive, drowsiness, or irritability.
- Neonates may present with life-threatening septicemia in which obvious inflammation of a long bone develops, or a more benign form in which the symptoms are slow to develop but bone changes are extensive and often multiple.

Investigation

- Plain X-rays may be normal for the first 10 days. Do not be reassured!
- ^{99}Technetium bone scan is usually positive in the first 24–48 hr and is effective in confirming diagnosis early.
- ^{67}Gallium bone scan and ^{111}indium-labeled white cell scans are more specific but generally not available in most units.
- MRI is very sensitive but not specific and is difficult for children.
- CT scanning can define the extent of bone sequestration and cavitation.

1 Lazzarini L, Mader JT, Calhoun JH (2004). Osteomyelitis in long bones [current concepts review]. *J Bone Joint Surg Am* **86-A**:2305–2318.

X-ray features
- Soft tissue swelling is an early sign; look for displacement of fat planes.
- Patchy lucencies develop in the metaphysis at around 10 days.
- Periosteal new bone may be seen.
- Involucrum formation is only apparent at around 3 weeks.
- Sequestrum appears radiodense compared to the surrounding bone, which is osteopenic.
- Normal bone density occurs with healing.

Laboratory tests results
- WBC ↑, normally with an elevated neutrophil count
- ESR ↑
- CRP ↑
- Blood cultures are positive in 50% of cases (use to inform and adjust antibiotic therapy).
- Evaluate LFTs and glucose level.

Treatment
- Pain relief by bed rest, immobilization, and analgesics
- Give IV antibiotics according to local guidelines (after blood cultures and aspiration cultures are taken), e.g., Ancef IV then orally for up to 6 weeks, dose-adjusted according to age; clindamycin if the patient is penicillin-allergic; vancomycin for MRSA; ampicillin for *Hemophilus*.
- Surgical drainage of mature subperiosteal abscess with debridement of all necrotic tissue, obliteration of dead spaces, adequate soft-tissue coverage, and restoration of an effective blood supply

Complications
- Disseminated systemic infection, e.g., septicemia, cerebral abscess
- Chronic osteomyelitis
- Septic arthritis
- Deformity due to epiphyseal involvement

Chronic osteomyelitis

Causes
- Most common following contaminated trauma and open fractures
- Occasionally follows acute hematogenous osteomyelitis
- Can occur after joint replacement surgery
- Also presents as a primary chronic infection of bone

Secondary to acute osteomyelitis

Features
- Sinus formation due to sequestra or resistant bacteria
- Prevented by adequate treatment of the initial acute attack

Treatment
- Conservative (simple dressings) treatment may be appropriate (in the elderly). Recurrent attacks with spontaneous recovery may occur and surgery should be reserved for cases where an abscess forms.
- A chronic abscess may require incision and drainage, debridement of all necrotic tissue, and obliteration of dead spaces. This may involve plastic surgery to achieve soft-tissue coverage and restoration of an effective blood supply.
- Closed-suction drainage or irrigation systems (i.e., wound vacs) can be effective, especially if irrigation fluid contains antibiotics. The disadvantage is that early blockage of the system can occur.
- Antibiotic (gentamicin or vancomycin) impregnated beads deliver high local levels and may be beneficial in areas of poor blood supply.
- Unresolving cases may require amputation.

Secondary to trauma (open fractures)
- Prevention is by an early, aggressive approach to open fractures with debridement and lavage of contaminated tissue.
    - Excise all dead tissue widely and remove all devitalized bone fragments, i.e., with no soft tissue connections.
    - Copious lavage is necessary, as "the solution to pollution is dilution" (≥10 L is common).
    - Skeletal stabilization is mandatory.
    - Give IV antibiotics, e.g., IV cefuroxime 9 metronidazole, if anaerobes are involved.
- Treat established, chronic infection as above with removal of internal foreign bodies, e.g., metalwork, and possible application of external fixation.

Secondary to joint replacement surgery
- This is rare (≤1%) but is often a disaster for the elective patient.
- Prevention is better than cure. Dedicated laminar flow rooms, sterile technique, and prophylactic IV antibiotics are mandatory.
- Most patients will require surgical intervention.
    - In acute situations, initial joint irrigation, debridement, polyethelene liner exchange, and tissue sampling can be attempted if the prosthesis is still solid and not "loose."

- If grossly infected, the prosthesis must be removed, the surfaces debrided, and an antibiotic cement spacer placed on the raw bone ends to allow the soft tissue envelope to settle.
- Once inflammatory markers have settled (CRP is the best) and the clinical infection has resolved, a second-stage reimplantation of the prosthesis is performed.
- In instances of chronic, recurrent infection, the implant is removed and the infection is eradicated as described previously, but no prosthesis is reimplanted.

Chronic osteomyelitis as an initial presentation

Brodie's abscess
- This is an isolated, well-contained, chronic abscess.
- *Treatment* is with operative drainage with excision of the abscess wall and antibiotics.

Tuberculosis
- Usually associated with other systemic features of the disease
- May present acutely
- Muscle atrophy develops and spontaneous discharge of a "cold" abscess may lead to sinus formation and destruction of bone.
- Spinal TB may cause vertebral collapse, leading to acute-neurology "Pott's paraplegia."

Syphilitic osteomyelitis
- Associated with advanced, tertiary disease in adults. This type features diffuse periostitis (with sabre tibia) or localized gummata with sequestra, sinus formation, and pathological fractures. X-rays show periosteal thickening with "punched-out" areas in sclerotic bone.
- Infants with congenital disease have epiphysitis and metaphysitis. X-rays show areas of sclerosis near the growth plate that are separated by areas of rarefication.

Mycotic (fungal) osteomyelitis
- This typically occurs in immunocompromised patients.
- Bone granulomas, necrosis, and suppuration present without worsening acute illness.
- It usually occurs as spread from primary lung infections such as coccidiomycosis, cryptococcosis, blastomycosis, and histoplasmosis.
- *Treatment* is with amphotericin B and/or surgical excision.

Peripheral nerve injuries

Pathological features

Neuropraxia

- There is stretching or compression of the nerve. The nerve remains anatomically intact.
- Focal demyelination occurs at the site of injury, which is repaired by Schwann cells.
- Recovery is usually complete, occurring in days or weeks. There is no axonal degeneration.

Axontemesis

- The axon is divided but the covering connective-tissue component remains intact, i.e., the nerve cylinder remains. This is usually a traction or severe compression injury.
- Axonal ("Wallerian") degeneration occurs distal to the injury and is followed by nerve regeneration (by sprouting from the severed nerve end) after 10 days.
- Nerve growth occurs at a rate of 1 mm/day.
- Prognosis is generally good as the cylinder is intact, but the more proximal the lesion the less the distal recovery.
- Sensation recovery is generally better than motor recovery, especially if the lesion is proximal and muscle wasting occurs while it is "denervated."

Neurotemesis

- The nerve is completely divided or irreparably damaged with loss of apposition of the severed nerve bundles and their respective distal parts.
- Neurotemesis is usually caused by high-energy injury, penetrating trauma, severe traction, ischemia, or high-pressure injection injury.
- Minimal recovery is possible without operative intervention to repair or graft a new nerve to the injury.
- Surgical repair may allow axon regeneration to the correct end organ, but recovery will not be complete, as often "mis-wiring" occurs.

Diagnosis

- What is the injury? Is there an open wound, fracture, recent surgery, or prolonged immobility?[1]
- Conduct a complete neurological examination.[2] You must know the motor and sensory supplies of peripheral nerves! Use a pin or your finger for sensory testing. Compare the area of normal and injured side sequentially. Assess two-point discrimination as well.
- *Tips.* Anesthetic skin looks shiny and does not sweat. Denervated skin will not wrinkle in water.

---

1 Soloman L, Warwick D, Nayagam S (2001). *Apley's System of Orthopaedics and Fractures*, 8th ed. London: Hodder Arnold, pp. 229–254.

2 Flores AJ, Lavernia CJ, Owens PW (2000). Anatomy and physiology of peripheral nerve injury and repair. *Am J Orthop* **29**(3):167–173.

- There are specific features of different levels of injury in peripheral nerves of the upper limb.
- ⚠ Examination very soon after injury can be misleading, as sensory loss may take time to appear.

Treatment

Closed injuries

- Injuries in continuity (the vast majority) can be expected to recover spontaneously, so exploration is not indicated.
- Compression injuries should have compressive forces removed, e.g., external ones such as plaster, or internal ones such as carpal tunnel syndrome.
- Wait 6 weeks to 3 months after injury before obtaining an EMG.

Open injuries

- *Primary repair* (suture) within 24 hr is ideal, but an uncontaminated operative field, adequate skin coverage, and proper equipment (e.g., microscopes) must be present.
- Delayed *secondary repair* can be done at any time after injury once the soft tissues have healed (3–6 weeks acceptable). The nerve can be mobilized to allow a no-tension repair after resection of the cut nerve stumps. Usually, however, a nerve graft has to be used to bridge the defect (the sural nerve as a donor is the most common).

Brachial plexus injuries

Knowledge of brachial plexus anatomy is vital to diagnosis and treatment of these injuries.[1]

Causes

- **Child**. Obstetric—i.e., traction on the plexus associated with difficult delivery, large babies, shoulder dystocia, forceps delivery, breech presentation, prolonged labor. Such injuries occur at a rate of 2/1000.
- **Adult**. Almost all brachial plexus injuries are traumatic.[2]
  - Usually closed, e.g., motorcycle accidents, falls, and traction injuries with forced abduction of the arm
  - May be open, e.g., stab or gunshot wounds
- Always look for associated injuries, e.g., head, neck, chest, abdominal, and vascular injuries.

Types

- *Erb–Duchenne (upper)* involves C5 and C6 ± C7. The arm classically hangs at the side with the arm flaccid, internally rotated, adducted, and the wrist flexed (waiter's tip position).
- *Klumpke's (lower)* involves C8 and T1 ± C7. The hand is clawed from intrinsic muscle paralysis and, if the sympathetic trunk is involved, there is a Horner's syndrome.
- The lesion can be at the spinal cord, roots, trunks, or trunk divisions.
- Try to localize the lesion to preganglionic (intraspinal) or postganglionic (extraspinal). If histamine is injected into the skin of the supplied area, vasodilatation, weal, and flare indicate a positive result and a preganglionic injury is present. If there is no flare, the lesion is postganglionic.

Prognosis

- The majority resolve without surgical intervention.
- If there are no EMG abnormalities at 3–4 weeks, prognosis is good with conservative treatment.
- No biceps function at 6 months of age, causalgic pain, Horner's syndrome, and the presence of root avulsion on myelogram (hence intraspinal lesion) indicate a poor prognosis.
- Recovery is generally very slow and often unsatisfactory.

Treatment

Child

Use physiotherapy to prevent joint contracture and stiffness. If there is no return of function at 2 months, consider myelography or histamine tests to localize the injury level.

- Open injuries should be explored acutely but not if there are more life-threatening injuries (which is usually the case). Primary repair may be possible in this group.
- Delayed surgery (if required at all) is normal for most patients.
- Preganglionic injuries are irreparable and should not be explored.

1 Birch R (1996). Brachial plexus injuries [review]. *J Bone Joint Surg Br* **78-B**:986–992.
2 Shin AY, Spinner RJ, Steinmann SP, Bishop AT (2005). Adult traumatic brachial plexus injuries. *J Am Acad Orthop Surg* **13**(6):382–389.

- Postganglionic injuries may be explored for up to 6 months post-injury. Secondary repair with nerve grafting can then be attempted if a clear lesion is isolated.
- Salvage surgery with tendon transfers or shoulder arthrodesis may improve function and give better results than amputation.

Adult

- EMG at 3–6 weeks
- If there is no recovery, surgery should be done within 6 months of injury.
- A variety of treatment options exists, including primary nerve repair, nerve grafting, or tendon transfers depending on the location of the injury.

Osteoarthritis

This is degenerative joint disease: it is a disease of cartilage, not the joint.
- It is limited to the joint itself and there is no systemic effect.
- It may involve any synovial joint but is most common in weight-bearing joints such as the hip and knee.[1]
- It is the most common form of arthritis.
- Approximately 2 million people visit their primary care physician for osteoarthritis per year, and it is predicted that there will be a 66% increase in the number of people with osteoarthritis-related disability by 2020.

Types

Primary osteoarthritis
This type mainly affects the following joints: distal interphalangeal, first carpometacarpal, hips, knees, and apophyseal joints of the spine. Women are more affected than men and there may be a hereditary component, but the etiology is unknown.

Secondary osteoarthritis
This type affects previously damaged joints and is more common in weight-bearing joints. Both sexes are equally affected. Local causes are fractures, acquired or congenital deformities, joint injury (chondral lesions), diabetic neuropathy (Charcot joints), and avascular necrosis.

Clinical features
- Characteristic pain, swelling, and deformity
- Dull, aching pain with morning stiffness of the affected joint
- Pain becomes steadily worse throughout the day and may disturb sleep.
- Acute onset is marked by a swollen, hot, and painful joint with raised inflammatory markers.
- Look for Heberden's nodes at the distal and Bouchard's nodes at the proximal interphalangeal joints.
- Physical symptoms may not correlate with the severity of radiographic changes, so judge each patient on an individual basis.

X-ray changes
- Joint space narrowing
- Subchondral bone sclerosis
- Cyst formation (especially at the hip)
- Osteophyte formation

Treatment
Relieve pain, improve mobility, and correct deformity, in that order.

---

1 Felson DT (2006). Clinical practice. Osteoarthritis of the knee. *N Engl J Med* **354**(8):841–848. Erratum in: *N Engl J Med* (2006) **354**(23):2520.

Medical

- Pain relief with simple analgesics in combination with NSAIDs helps control symptoms and increase mobility. Beware of GI bleeding, especially in the elderly, and of worsening asthma.
- Weight loss, physical therapy, and aids to daily living such as walking sticks, heel raises, raised chair, and household aids should all be in place before contemplating surgery.
- Intra-articular injection with a combination of steroid (Kenalog or methylpredisone) and 1% lidocaine without epinephrine aids in symptomatic relief. Patients should be made aware that this is not a cure!
- In general, it is safe for patients to receive up to three steroid injections in a 12-month period.
- Oral medications such as glucosamine and chondroitin sulfate and supplemental injections such as Synvisc have yet to show a proven benefit in randomized controlled trials.

Surgical treatment

This is indicated for pain relief, improved mobility, and correcting deformity only after conservative measures have failed.

Surgical options include the following:

- *Osteotomy*: realignment of a joint to unload an arthritic area
- *Arthrodesis*: permanent stiffening of a joint by excision and fusion to stop pain
- *Excision*: removal of the joint without fusion, i.e., hip girdlestone procedure
- *Arthroplasty*: replacement of all or part of the joint surface by an artificial material

Carpal tunnel syndrome

- Carpal tunnel syndrome (CTS)[1] is caused by compression of the median nerve as it enters the palmer surface of the hand under the flexor retinaculum.
- Incidence is 1–3.5/100,00 people
- It is most common in middle age, with a female:male ratio of 5:1.
- CTS is often bilateral but when unilateral it most commonly affects the dominant hand.
- Over 500,000 surgeries are performed each year for CTS.

Etiology

- CTS is caused by an increase in pressure in the carpal canal.
- The most common cause is idiopathic.

Compression of the tunnel wall

- Trauma, e.g., distal radius fracture
- Inflammatory conditions—i.e., rheumatoid arthritis (thickening of the surrounding synovium and tissues)
- Subluxation or dislocation of the wrist
- Anomalous structures such as muscles, vessels
- Acromegaly (soft-tissue thickening and enlargement)

Compression within the tunnel

- Fluid retention, e.g., during pregnancy
- Myxoedema
- Space-occupying lesion, e.g., benign tumor
- Chronic proliferative synovitis

Changes in the median nerve

- Diabetes mellitus
- Peripheral neuropathies

Clinical features

Symptoms

- Aching pain and paraesthesia (pins and needles) over radial three and a half fingers
- Pain typically occurs at night and can disturb sleep.
- Relieved by shaking the hand
- Patient may notice dropping items (weak pinch grip)
- It can be made worse by activity.
- Atypical symptoms can be common.

Signs[2]

- The hand looks normal.
- There is thenar muscle wasting if CTS is chronic and severe.
- Weakness of thumb abduction

1 Cranford CS, Ho JY, Kalainov DM, Hartigan BJ (2007). Carpal tunnel syndrome. *J Am Acad Orthop Surg* **15**:537–548.
2 Tetro AM, Evanoff BA, Hollstien SB, Gelberman RH (1998). A new provocative test for carpal tunnel syndrome: assessment of wrist flexion and nerve compression. *J Bone Joint Surg Br* **80-B**:493–498.

- *Tinnel's test*: Tapping over the nerve at the wrist in neutral position produces symptoms.
- *Phalen's test*: Rest elbows on the table and passively flex the wrist. If symptoms appear within 60 sec, the test is positive.
- *Median nerve compression test*: Extend elbow, supinate forearm, flex wrist to 60°, press on carpal tunnel. The test is positive if symptoms occur within 30 sec.

Investigations

Nerve conduction studies are the gold standard but still show only 90% accuracy.

Treatment

Conservative

- Splinting
- Injection of corticosteroids
- Avoidance of precipitating factors

Surgical

- Surgical decompression
- Use a tourniquet.
- Perform skin incision in line with the ulna border of the tunnel in line with the web space in between the third and fourth ray. This is to avoid the motor branch of the median nerve.
- Protect the nerve and visualize the nerve directly throughout.
- Do not extend the skin incision beyond the wrist crease, so as to protect the palmar cutaneous branch of the median nerve.

Complications

- Complex regional pain syndrome
- Tender, hypertrophic scar giving pillar pain (pain in the heel of the scar on pressure)
- Neuroma of the palmar cutaneous branch
- Recurrence
- Bowstringing of flexor tendons

Ganglion cyst

A ganglion cyst[1] is a degenerative mucinous cyst swelling that can arise from a tendon sheath or joint. It contains clear, colorless, gelatinous fluid.

Common sites

- Dorsum of the wrist, arising from the scapholunate ligament or midcarpal joint (70% of all cases)
- Radial aspect of the volar wrist, normally from the scaphotrapezial joint (20% of all cases)
- Base or distal interphalangeal joint of finger
- Dorsum of the foot
- Around the knee

Clinical features

- A slow-growing, cystic lump commonly presents as dorsal wrist pain.
- The cyst is firm, smooth, and rubbery and will usually transilluminate.
- It may be more obvious with the wrist in palmar flexion.

Diagnosis

- Needle aspiration produces gelatinous fluid. If no fluid can be aspirated then investigate further, since a soft tissue tumor (including sarcoma) is possible.
- MRI scanning should be used if there is serious concern about a soft tissue tumor.
- Occult ganglia (no palpable lump) can yield symptoms in the wrist or foot. An ultrasound scan will confirm the diagnosis.

Treatment

- 50% will disappear spontaneously. Therefore, treat conservatively unless pressed by the patient.
- Aspiration may be curative in 50% of cases.
- Deliberately induced traumatic rupture often leads to recurrence.

Surgery

- Excision is not a guaranteed success (recurrence is approximately 10%; painful scar, approximately 10%).
- Use a tourniquet.
- If the cyst is not occult or excessively large, a day-case procedure with local anesthesia is appropriate.
- Excise thoroughly and transfix the base to prevent recurrence.

---

1 Nahra ME, Bucchieri JS (2004). Ganglion cysts and other tumor-related conditions of the hand and wrist. *Hand Clin* **20**(3):249–260.

Bone tumors

The most common bone tumor is metastatic (breast, prostate, lung, thyroid, and kidney). The second most common bone tumor is multiple myeloma. Primary tumors (most common is osteosarcoma) are rare but more common in young adults. They have a poor prognosis and may involve extensive surgery as well as radiation or chemotherapy. Most bone tumors require a multidisciplinary team (orthopedic surgeon, oncologist, musculoskeletal radiologist, soft tissue pathologist).

Excellent summaries of bone tumors can be found at: http://www.bonetumor.org.

Metastatic tumors

- *History*: age, prior medical problems, exposure to radiation, complaints of "bone pain" being worse with rest or at night
- Look for other areas of disease, particularly the spine. Get a full medical workup for metastases including chest X-ray and CT of the chest, abdomen and pelvis. A bone scan and/or MRI may also be indicated.

Treatment

- Internal fixation for weight-bearing areas (ideally prophylactic before fracture occurs) allows early weight-bearing and perhaps early discharge from the hospital.
- Use radiation ± chemotherapy for non-weight-bearing lesions or metastases in difficult locations.

Benign tumors

- *Osteochondroma* (exostosis) is a cartilaginous capped outgrowth of bone from the cortex, normally near an epiphysis. It is usually solitary. Multiple lesions require close follow-up. Any sudden increase in size may indicate malignant transformation to chondrosarcoma.
- *Chondroma* is a non-calcified cartilaginous growth in the medulla (enchondroma) of tubular bones such as phalanges and metacarpals or metatarsals.
- *Osteoid osteoma* is an exquisitely painful area in the long bone of a young adult, usually male, that is classically relieved by NSAIDs. Radiology shows a "nidus," which is a small osteolytic area surrounded by a rim of dense sclerosis.
- *Non-ossifying fibroma* is a fibrous tissue tumor, which usually appears radiologically as an oval cortical defect with a sclerotic rim. It is a common incidental finding on X-rays, and usually needs no treatment.

Treatment

Surgical treatment of bone tumors should be conducted at a tertiary-care orthopedic oncology center.

- Obtain a biopsy for histological diagnosis prior to surgery.
- Principles of treatment are simple local excision or removal by curettage if the patient is symptomatic or surgery is likely to cause pathological fracture (likely if >50% diameter of bone involved).
- Cavities should be packed with bone graft or bone cement.
- Internal fixation may be necessary to stabilize the bony defect.

Primary malignant tumors (rare)

Diagnosis

- Painful swelling of part of a limb (especially at night)
- Blood tests are rarely diagnostic and often nonspecific (e.g., ↑ alkaline phosphatase, ↑ ESR, ↑ Ca^{2+}).

Radiological investigations

- *Plain X-ray* may help to make diagnosis through typical features.
- *CT/MRI* is used to stage and assess local or systemic spread (CT is better for bones; MRI is better for soft tissue).
- *Angiography* helps in planning radical surgery and possible limb salvage.

Pathological diagnosis

- Open biopsy is required to achieve diagnosis.
- This must be performed by the surgeon who will do the definitive surgery. The biopsy track must be excised as part of the definitive excision and placed to maximize the chance of limb-salvage surgery.

Osteosarcoma

This is the most common primary bone tumor.

- Tumor occurs in long bones of young adults (peak incidence 10–20 years) or as a consequence of Paget's disease in the elderly (see 📕 p. 640).
- X-ray features include bone destruction, soft tissue invasion, radiating spicules of bone ("sunray" appearance), subperiosteal elevation with new bone formation (Codman's triangle).
- Metastasis is via blood to the lungs.

Treatment

- Wide local resection with limb salvage is the goal.
- Preoperative systemic chemotherapy is commonly used.

Chondrosarcoma

- Usually seen in older patients (30–60 years)
- Is metaphyseal as well as seen in flat bones, e.g., ilium of pelvis, ribs
- May present de novo, or arise from a preexisting osteochondroma.
- Metastasis is uncommon. Local invasion occurs, but is slow growing.

Treatment

- Wide local resection without chemotherapy or radiation
- Limb salvage is rare for pelvic tumors.
- Occasionally radiotherapy may be used in the elderly.

Five-year survival >75% (low grade) or >25% (high grade) with surgery.

Giant cell tumor

- This tumor is rare before the age of 20 years.
- It is usually benign but may undergo malignant transformation (~10%).
- It rarely metastasizes; usually it is to the lungs, but it may be locally invasive.
- Treatment is with local excision and the defect is filled with bone graft or cement.
- Recurrence is common (~20%), especially with malignancy.

Ewing's sarcoma
- Affects children and young adults; tends to present as a large mass
- Radiological feature ("onionskin" appearance). The MRI scan shows soft tissue involvement.
- Metastasis to the lung is very fast and common.
- Treatment is with preoperative chemotherapy (12 weeks) and then reevaluation and restaging. Wide excision or amputation is necessary.
- Prognosis is generally poor.

Low back pain

Low back pain is extremely common, with 60%–80% of adults suffering from this during their lifetime. The vast majority of patients have a self-limiting condition of a degenerative or traumatic nature and require no surgical or orthopedic intervention. This can easily be ascertained in a 10-min focused consultation in general practice.[1]

Types of pain

Discogenic pain
- Typically midline and made worse by lordotic postures, e.g., bending and lifting
- Pain is from the annulus fibrosis layer of the disc when it is being stretched.

Neurogenic pain (sciatica)
- Pain radiates down the leg from the buttock to the calf or foot.
- It is commonly caused by a lumbar disc herniation or "bulge" compressing and irritating the nerve root as it exits the spinal foramina.
- Radiation should match the sensory dermatome of the nerve root involved.
- Numbness or paraesthesia in the dermatome of the affected root may also be present.
- Other features are pain on sneezing, coughing, and straining.

Referred pain
- May arise from retroperitoneal pathology (aortic aneurysm, pancreatic pathology, rectal pathology, lymphadenopathy, or hip/sacroiliac joint osteoarthritis)

Psychogenic pain (nonorganic)
- This is a diagnosis of exclusion, i.e., exclude all other pathology.
- Typical features of nonorganic pain are pain on axial compression or pelvic rotation, nondermatomal sensory loss, nonanatomical tenderness, cogwheel (give way) weakness, and overreaction (Waddell's signs).[2]

Common pathological (organic) causes
- Lumbar disc herniation
- Spinal stenosis (reduction in diameter of the spinal canal)
- *Spondylolisthesis.* A forward slip of one vertebra on another below it, leading to pain and neurologic symptoms. Slip greater than 50% is deemed unstable.
- *Spondylosis.* Degenerative disc disease
- *Spondylolysis.* Defect in the neural arch. This usually causes a stress fracture.
- *Coccydynia.* Pain in the coccyx may be due to lumbosacral disc disease.
- *Metabolic bone disease.* Osteomalacia, osteoporosis ± fracture.
- *Inflammation.* Joint disease especially ankylosing spondylitis.
- *Infection.* TB (rare now), staphylococcus-induced discitis.
- Cauda equina syndrome

Tests

- *History*. Be wary of the "red flags" of serious spinal pathology, e.g., thoracic pain, fever or unexplained weight loss, history of cancer, progressive neurologic compromise.
- *Physical examination*: motor strength, sensation, reflexes, rectal tone
- *Spine X-rays*: AP, lateral, oblique views, lumbar-sacral spine
- *CT scan*: Assesses bony architecture.
- *MRI scan* is used to evaluate for nerve, disc, and soft tissue pathology.

Treatment

Nonoperative

- Most patients require nonoperative treatment.
- Initial rest (1–2 days only), analgesia, early mobilization with encouragement and physical therapy
- This may also involve evidence-based patient education[3] and counseling. 90% of cases resolve in 6 weeks and 75% of patients may experience symptoms and disability 1 year after initial consultation, but require no further management.

Surgery

- Few patients require surgery—focus should be on proven pathology demonstrated by imaging where possible.
- Procedures used include the following:
  - Discectomy
  - Nerve root decompression
  - Spinal decompression
  - Spinal decompression and fusion

1 Shen F, Samartzis D, Andersson G (2006). Nonsurgical management of acute and chronic low back pain *J Am Acad Orthop Surg* **14**: 477–487.
2 Waddell G, McCulloch JA, Kummel E, Venner RM (1980). Nonorganic physical signs in low-back pain. *Spine* **5**:117–125.
3 Royal College of General Practitioners (2002). *The Back Book*. London: The Stationary Office Books.

Paget's disease

First described by Sir James Paget (1876), the incidence of Paget's disease increases with age. It is most commonly seen in the spine, skull, pelvis, and femur.

For more information go to: http://www.paget.org.

Pathological features

- Increased osteoclastic bone resorption id followed by compensatory bone formation, i.e., there is an overall increase in bone turnover.
- The bone is softer but thickened and is liable to pathological fracture.

Clinical features

- Most patients are completely asymptomatic and diagnosis is via an incidental finding on X-ray or raised alkaline phosphatase found on investigation of other pathologies.
- The patients may note an increase in size of their forehead, or difficulty in wearing hats.
- Increased thickness of bone may be the only symptom or sign that the patient complains of.
- Subcutaneous bones may be deformed, classically the tibia when it becomes saber shaped.
- Pain may be present but is unusual. It may represent high turnover at the time or more likely a pathological fracture. In patients known to have Paget's disease, an increase in pain must be taken seriously as it may be a marker of sarcomatous change in the bone.

Investigations

- Serum calcium and phosphorus are normal.
- Alkaline phosphatase is high (due to ↑ osteoblast activity).
- Urinary excretion of hydroxyproline is high (↑ bone turnover).
- Bone scan shows "hot spots" in affected areas.
- X-ray shows both sclerosis and osteoporosis. The cortex is thickened and the bones are deformed. Pathological fracture is a feature and the normal bone architecture is lost with coarse trabecular pattern.

Complications

- Pathological fractures
- Malignant deformation into sarcoma (<5%; prognosis is *very poor*)
- High-output cardiac failure may develop from the increased vascularity of Paget's bone. Functionally the bone is acting as an arteriovenous fistula.
- Deafness—bony deformation in the ear causes damage to the cranial nerve.
- Osteoarthritis
- Leontiasis ossea—thickening of facial bones (rare).
- Paraplegia due to vertebral involvement (rare)

Treatment
- Most patients require no treatment.
- Fractures will heal normally but bony deformity with a fracture can be a difficult challenge!
- Drugs that reduce bone turnover (fight osteoclasts), such as calcitonin or the bisphosphonates,[1] are effective in relieving pain and may also relieve neurological complications such as deafness.

1 Rendina D, De Filippo G, Mossetti G (2005). Paget's disease and bisphosphonates. *N Engl J Med* **353**(24):2616–2618.

The great toe

Hallux valgus (bunions)

- Hallux valgus is lateral deviation of the big toe.[1]
- There is prominence of the head of the first metatarsal medially, with lateral angulation of the great toe (hence valgus) from the pull of the extensors.
- As time passes, a protective bursa develops over the metatarsal head (the bunion) and the great toe begins to crowd or even overlap its neighbors.

Causes

- *Congenital.* Often familial, related to metatarsus primus varus where the first metatarsal is angled more medially, i.e., splayed, than usual and is rotated
- *Acquired.* The most common form. It is probably due to weak intrinsic muscles, with age. Inappropriate footwear is also a cause, as there is a higher incidence in shoe-wearing cultures.

Symptoms

- Often asymptomatic, even in cases of severe deformity
- Pain typically will appear at the site of the bunion, due to pressure.
- Later, symptoms of joint pain may present from osteoarthritis and subluxation of the joint.

Treatment

Conservative

- Correct footwear with a wider toe box and padding to protect the bunion. This measure should always be tried and have failed before surgery is considered.

Surgical

- *Exostectomy.* Removal of the bunion alone. This is a simple procedure but does not remove the underlying deformity and the problem may recur.
- *Distal metatarsal osteotomy.* The bunion is removed and the metatarsal head or neck is cut. The distal fragment is then realigned anatomically and the fracture held with a K wire. There are many types or shapes of osteotomy described, but the most common eponyms are Mitchell's, Wilson's, and Chevron. This procedure is only suitable for smaller deformities.
- *Proximal metatarsal osteotomy.* This is an osteotomy just proximal to the base of the metatarsal and the metatarsocuneiform joint. Larger bony deformities can be corrected this way. It may be combined with a distal soft-tissue release where the lateral constraints by the metatarsophalangeal joints (MTPJs) are also released through a small, separate dorsal excision.
- *Excision arthroplasty.* Removal of the metatarsal head (Mayo) or base of the proximal phalanx (Keller) can be attempted but is fraught with a lot of long-term complications and is only an operation for the elderly.

- *Arthrodesis*. This is suitable for severe deformity and degenerative change and is tolerated well by males. Females may have a problem with footwear (they must wear flat shoes afterward). This procedure is normally reserved for salvage surgery.

Hallux rigidus

The great toe is straight (not valgus) and there may be a callosity over the dorsum of the first MTPJ. The main symptom is a stiff, painful first MTPJ.[2]

Causes
- *Congenital*: due to a shortened metatarsal
- *Acquired*: normally traumatic or idiopathic degeneration

Symptoms
There is pain on walking over the first MTPJ along with profound stiffness. There may also be weakness with pushing off.

Treatment
Adolescents and the young
- Provide a rocker sole to relieve pain.

Adults
- Arthrodesis almost always occurs after failed conservative treatment.
- MTPJ replacement (rare)
- Excision arthroplasty (elderly only)

1 Coughlin MJ (1996). Hallux valgus [instructional course lecture]. *J Bone Joint Surg Am* **78-A**:32–66.
2 Coughlin MJ, Shurnas PS (2003). Hallux rigidus: demographics, etiology, and radiographic assessment [review]. *Foot Ankle Int* **24**(10):731–743.

Arthroplasty

Arthroplasty is the surgical reconstruction or replacement of a malformed or degenerate joint. The primary goal is to relieve pain. Increases in mobility and function are secondary aims.

Classification

- *Excision/resection*—e.g., Keller's at the first MTPJ
- *Interposition*. A joint is excised and then a piece of tissue is implanted in the gap to cause a thick scar.
- *Partial (hemi-) or total replacement*. All or one-half of the articular surface is removed and replaced with other material. This procedure has been made possible by the massive advances in both biomaterials and bioengineering that have produced inert, sterilizable materials of acceptable strength to perform the joint functions.

Example: total hip replacement[1]

Indications

- Osteo- and rheumatoid arthritis when pain affects sleep, quality of life, and normal daily activities
- Avascular necrosis of the head of the femur with secondary joint degeneration
- Failed conservative management

Prevention of infection

Deep infection is a potentially devastating complication of hip or any arthroplasty and its incidence should be ≤1% in all units. Prevention of infection is achieved by the following:

- *Ultraclean air systems and exhaust body suits*. A unidirectional laminar flow system and body suits provide the best physical barrier between the patient and the surgical team.
- *Prophylactic antibiotics*. These are given IV within an hour of the induction of anesthesia. Broad-spectrum antibiotics are usually used, i.e., cefazolin (1 g IV given q8hr x 23 hr).

Procedure

The surgical approach exposes both the femoral head and acetabulum. The head of the femur is exposed, dislocated, and either reshaped (resurfacing) or, more commonly, removed at the neck. The acetabulum is then deepened and reshaped to allow a cup to be placed (the new "socket"). A cavity is then created within the cut surface of the femur going downward to allow a stem to be placed (the new "ball"). The stem and cup are usually grouted in place with polymethylmethacrylate bone cement or "press fit" without cement, and the two components are reduced and stability is tested.

The wound is then closed. Patients are mobilized on day 1 postoperatively, fully weight bearing, and usually discharged within 2–5 days.

Complications

Operative
- Dislocation of the prosthesis if incorrectly aligned, or if the patient does not follow hip precautions
- Nerve injury (sciatic nerve most common)
- Profound hypotension can be seen with absorption of the monomer in the cement, causing cardiotoxicity.

Postoperative
- Mortality (1%)
- Thromboembolic disease (DVT or PE)
- Deep infection (1%)
- Dislocation (4%) is usually due to patient noncompliance with physiotherapy guidelines.
- Aseptic loosening ("wearing out"). Most total hip replacements would be expected to have ≥90% survival rates 10 years after surgery.

1 Huo MH, Muller MS (2004). What's new in hip arthroplasty. *J Bone Joint Surg Am* **86-A**:2341–2353.

Useful reading

Online orthopedic hyperbooks (free)
http//:www.wheelessonline.com

Reference textbooks
Review
Miller M (2004). *Review of Orthopaedics*, 4th ed. Philadelphia: Saunders.

Soloman L, Warwick D, Nayagam S (Eds.) (2001). *Apley's System of Orthopaedics and Fractures*. London: Hodder Arnold.

Elective
Canale T (Ed.) (2002). *Campbell's Operative Orthopaedics,* 9th ed. (4 vols). London: Mosby.

Trauma
Rockwood CA (Ed.) (2001). *Rockwood and Green's Fractures in Adults*, 5th ed. Philadelphia: Lippincott, Williams, and Wilkins.

Rockwood CA (Ed.) (2001). *Rockwood and Wilkin's Fractures in Children*, 5th ed. Philadelphia: Lippincott, Williams, and Wilkins.

Surgical exposures
Hoppenfeld S, Deboer P (2004). *Surgical Exposures in Orthopaedics: The Anatomic Approach*, 2nd ed. Philadelphia: Lippincott, Williams, and Wilkins.

Urology

Francis J. McGovern, MD

Symptoms and signs in urology

Symptoms

Pain

- May be located over the site of pathology, e.g., testes
- May radiate in accordance with enervation of the structure involved.
  - Kidney pain is in the renal angle (between the lower border of the 12th rib and the spine).
  - Ureteric pain is between the renal angle and the groin.
  - Bladder pain is in the suprapubic region.
  - Prostatic pain is in the perineum, but may radiate along the urethra to the tip of the penis.
- Pain may be related to function, e.g., suprapubic pain exacerbated by bladder filling.

Hematuria (macroscopic)

- Frequently this is a sinister symptom of malignant disease, especially the bladder, when it is normally painless.
- When associated with painful voiding it is usually due to bladder infection or stones.

Lower urinary tract symptoms

- This is a group of symptoms that typically affect the older male.
- They are often caused by bladder outflow obstruction related to prostatic enlargement.
- Symptoms are related to both voiding and storage.
- *Voiding symptoms*: poor urine flow, hesitancy, post-micturition dribbling
- *Storage symptoms*: frequency, nocturia, urgency, urge incontinence
- The International Prostate Symptom Score (IPSS) is a validated questionnaire to estimate the patient's perception of severity of symptoms.

Urinary incontinence

- Affects women more commonly than men
- *Stress incontinence* is urine leakage that occurs at times of increased intravesical pressure, e.g., during coughing, sneezing, lifting
  - It results from incompetence of the urethral sphincter and bladder neck mechanism. It is usually related to pregnancy and childbirth.
- *Urge incontinence* is urine leakage that occurs in association with a strong desire to void.
  - Urine leaks from the bladder before the patient is able to reach a toilet.
  - The usual cause is overactivity of the detrusor muscle.
  - It may be idiopathic or secondary to other bladder disease.
  - It may be secondary to neurogenic disease.
  - Stress and urge incontinence frequently coexist.
- *Insensible urine leakage* occurs without any associated symptoms.
  - Urine leaks from the bladder continuously and the patient is sometimes unaware.

- *Causes*: overflow incontinence from chronic retention, fistulation (commonly between the bladder and vagina), gross sphincter disturbance resulting from surgery or neurological disease

Male sexual dysfunction
- Erectile dysfunction (ED), commonly known as impotence
  - ED is the inability to attain and maintain an erection adequate for satisfactory sexual intercourse.
  - There are degrees of ED.
  - Men with incomplete ED respond more satisfactorily to treatment.
  - Most cases have an organic basis.
  - 20% of cases are primarily psychogenic.
- Premature ejaculation
  - More common in younger men
  - Often associated with performance anxiety
- Loss of libido
  - Loss of normal sex drive
  - Either psychogenic or related to hypogonadal states

Hemospermia
- Presence of blood in ejaculate
- Rarely associated with significant pathology

Signs
Inspection
- Examination of the penis must include retraction of the foreskin (if possible) and inspection of the glans and external meatus for signs of infection, inflammation, or tumor.

Palpation
- Tenderness in the renal angle or a palpable flank mass may indicate renal pathology.
- Suprapubic dullness to percussion is an indication of a bladder mass or the bladder being full of urine.
- Check for testicular asymmetry, masses, or tenderness (underdevelopment, tumors, and infection).
- An intrascrotal mass may include the testis (e.g., cancer) or be separate from it (e.g., epididymal cyst).
- Do a digital rectal examination to determine the size, consistency, regularity, and symmetry of the prostate.

Standard testing in urinary tract disease

Laboratory tests

Urinalysis

- Dipstick analysis for blood, leukocytes, protein, nitrites, and glucose
  - Nitrites, blood, and leukocytes are tested for infection.
  - Blood can indicate microscopic hematuria.
  - Protein and leukocytes area analyzed for intrinsic renal disease. Or signs of infection
- Microbiology for presence of urinary infection or cytology to look for malignant cells. Midstream urine (MSU) specimens are required for bacteriological culture: take care to avoid contamination, particularly in women.
- Matched urine and serum biochemistry to assess glomerular function, e.g., matched osmolarities, sodiums, and potassiums.

Blood

- Serum creatinine levels provide a crude assessment of overall renal function.
- Creatinine (Cr) clearance (requires 24-hr urine collection and measurement of serum creatinine):

$$\text{Cr clearance (mL/min)} = u \times v/p$$

  - where u is urine Cr concentration, v is 24 hr urine volume, and p is plasma Cr concentration.
- Serum prostate-specific antigen (PSA) is an indicator of prostate disease.
  - It is interpreted according to an age-specific reference range.
  - High levels are found in benign prostatic hyperplasia (BPH), prostate cancer, acute retention, and urinary infection. False elevations can occur in men with recent ejaculation, instrumentation, or bicycling.
- Sex hormone measurements are occasionally useful in the assessment of male sexual dysfunction and infertility.

Radiology

Ultrasound

- Renal and bladder scans are for hydronephrosis and urinary tract infections.
- A transrectal ultrasound scan measures the prostate accurately and allows systematic biopsy for detection of cancer.
- Scrotal ultrasound with color-flow Doppler is used to evaluate acute scrotum for testicular torsion or testicular cancer.

Intravenous urogram (IVU)

- Provides greater functional information than ultrasound
- Provides superior imaging of the ureter

Computerized tomography (CT)

- Pre- and post-contrast scans provide some functional information with regard to arterial and venous blood flow and excretory function of the kidneys.
- CT is vital for the staging of renal cell carcinoma, transitional cell carcinoma of the renal pelvis, ureter, or bladder, and testicular cancer.

Magnetic resonance imaging (MRI)

- Provides greater accuracy than CT in assessment of the prostate capsule and seminal vesicles
- MRI is a sensitive test for the presence of bone metastases.

Bone scan

- Demonstrates abnormal area of bone turnover
- A useful screening test for the presence of bone metastases
- Plain films are taken to aid interpretation if the site or pattern of hot spots is indeterminate.

Nuclear renography

- Provides anatomical and functional information about the kidneys
- A DMSA scan provides an image of functioning renal parenchymal tissue.
- An MAG3 renogram provides dynamic information regarding excretion from the kidneys and determines whether or not obstruction is present.

Endoscopy

Flexible cystoscopy

- Examines urethra and bladder
- Performed using local anesthetic gel
- There is limited potential for intervention.

Rigid cystoscopy

Under GA this technique permits biopsy or placement of ureteral stents and the resectoscope allows resection of tissue.

Ureteroscopy

- Rigid and flexible ureteroscopes provide access to the ureter and pelvicalyceal system.
- This technique enables the passage of instruments and laser fibers for treatment of stones and upper-tract tumors.

Urinary tract stones

Key facts
- The prevalence of stones in the population is around 3%.
- They are the most common reason for emergency urological visits.
- Peak presentation is in the summer months.
- The most common age of presentation is 20–50 years.
- 90% of urinary calculi are radio-opaque.

Etiology
- *Metabolic*: hyperparathyroidism, idiopathic hypercalciuria, disseminated malignancy, sarcoidosis, hypervitaminosis D
- *Familial metabolic causes*: cystinuria, errors of purine metabolism, hyperoxaluria, hyperuricuria, xanthinuria
- Infection
- Impaired urinary drainage, e.g., medullary sponge kidney, pelviureteric junction obstruction, ureteric stricture, extrinsic obstruction

Pathological features
Calcium stones
- Calcium stones comprise 75% of all urinary calculi.
- They are usually combined with oxalate or phosphate, are sharp, and may cause symptoms even when small.

Triple-phosphate stones (struvite stones)
- Compounds of magnesium, ammonium, and calcium phosphate
- They comprise 15% of all calculi.
- They commonly occur against a background of chronic urinary infection and may grow rapidly.
- "Staghorn" calculi (fill the calyceal system) are a form of struvite.

Uric acid stones
- These stones occur as a result of high levels of uric acid in the urine.
- They comprise 5% of all urinary stones and are radiolucent.

Cystine stones
- These are relatively rare: 1%–2% of all cases.
- They are difficult to treat because of their extremely hard consistency.

Other stones
- Xanthine, pyruvate, and other stones; 1% of all calculi

Clinical features
- "Ureteric/renal colic." Severe, intermittent, stabbing pain radiates from loin to groin.
- Microscopic or, rarely, frank hematuria
- Systemic symptoms such as nausea, vomiting, tachycardia, and pyrexia
- Loin or renal angle tenderness is due to infection or inflammation.
- Iliac fossa tenderness occurs if calculus has passed into distal ureter.

Basic tests
- Raised WBC suggests infection (this should be confirmed by urinalysis [UA] and culture); raised Cr suggests renal impairment.

- Stones are often visible on plain abdominal X-ray (KUB).
- Serum calcium, phosphate, and uric acid
- 24 hr urine for Ca, phosphate, oxalate, urate, cystine, and xanthine

Advanced tests
- Non-contrast spiral CT is the gold standard for locating stones and assessing evidence of complications.
- IVU will show stones' location and any proximal obstruction.
- Renal ultrasound scan is used for assessing hydronephrosis.

Treatment

Acute presentations (renal colic, ureteric obstruction)
- Analgesia, e.g., diclofenac 100 mg PR; antiemetic, e.g., metoclopramide 10 mg IV; IV fluids
- Small stones (<0.5 cm) may be managed expectantly as most will pass spontaneously.
- Emergency treatment with percutaneous nephrostomy and/or ureteric stent insertion is necessary if pain, fever, or obstruction is persistent.

Elective presentations
- Extracorporeal shock-wave lithotripsy (ESWL)
  - Focused, externally generated electrohydraulic or ultrasonic shock waves
  - Targeted onto the calculus with ultrasound, X-ray, or a combination
  - ESWL causes stone disintegration and the fragments are then voided.
- Percutaneous nephrolithotomy (PCNL)
  - Used for large stones in the renal pelvis and occasionally for large stones impacted in the upper ureter
  - Provides percutaneous track into the renal pelvis with fluoroscopic guidance
  - The nephroscope is inserted and the calculus visualized.
  - Stone is removed either in total or, if large, following fragmentation.
- Endoscopic treatment
  - The ureteroscope is inserted and the stone visualized.
  - The stone is fragmented using ultrasound, electrohydraulic intracorporeal lithotripsy, or laser.
- Open nephrolithotomy/ureterolithotomy.
  - Used for for large staghorn calculi or complex stones, e.g., above the ureteric stricture

Prevention of recurrence
- Increase oral fluid intake and reduce calcium intake.
- Correct metabolic abnormalities.
- Treat infection promptly.
- Urinary alkalization, e.g., with sodium bicarbonate 5–10 g/24 hr po in water (mainly for cystine and urate stones)
- Give thiazide diuretics (for idiopathic hypercalciuria).

Obstruction of the ureter

Key facts
Ureteric obstruction leads to hydronephrosis (ureteric and pelvicalyceal dilatation).

Pathological features
Hydronephrosis can be unilateral or bilateral (see Fig. 19.1).

Unilateral
- Extramural
  - Aberrant vessels at the pelviureteric junction (PUJ)
  - Extrinsic tumor: carcinoma of the cervix, prostate, large bowel, or retroperitoneal endometriosis
  - Idiopathic retroperitoneal fibrosis
  - Post-radiation fibrosis
  - Retrocaval ureter
  - Abdominal aortic aneurysm
- Intramural
  - Transitional cell carcinoma of the renal pelvis or ureter
  - Sloughed papillae secondary to papillary necrosis
  - Urinary calculi
  - Ureteric stricture
  - Aperistaltic segment is almost always congenital.

Bilateral
- All causes of unilateral obstruction may cause bilateral hydronephrosis.
- Congenital posterior urethral valve
- Congenital or acquired urethral stricture
- Benign enlargement of the prostate
- Locally advanced prostate cancer
- Large bladder tumors
- Gravid uterus

Clinical features
- Flank pain
- Fever and/or rigors (if complicated by infection)
- Symptoms and signs of renal failure (if obstruction is long-standing)

Investigation and diagnosis
- Serum biochemistry and hematology
- UA and culture
- KUB X-ray/IVU
- Ultrasound scan and/or CT scan
- Isotope renogram.
- Retrograde pyelogram

Complications
- Infection, pyonephrosis
- Hypertension
- Renal failure

Treatment

Emergency presentation
- Emergency treatment is indicated if there are signs of infection, established renal failure, or uncontrollable symptoms.
- Treatment is drainage of the kidney via a percutaneous nephrostomy or retrograde ureteral stent.

Elective presentation
Definitive treatment is directed at the underlying cause. Possible interventions include the following:
- Treatments of calculi (📖 p. 653)
- Ureteric stenting (unilateral or bilateral)
- Ureterolysis and ureteric transfer (for retroperitoneal fibrosis)
- Prostatic resection
- Bladder drainage using a urethral or suprapubic catheter

In cases where renal function cannot be restored, a nephrectomy is considered.

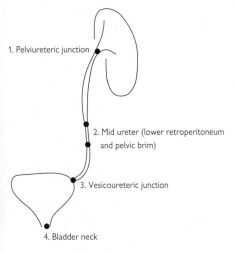

1. Pelviureteric junction

2. Mid ureter (lower retroperitoneum and pelvic brim)

3. Vesicoureteric junction

4. Bladder neck

Fig. 19.1 The most common sites of renal stone impaction. 1, pelvoureteric junction; 2, pelvic brim; 3, vesicoureteric junction.

Benign prostatic hyperplasia

Key facts

- Benign prostatic hyperplasia (BPH) is a nonmalignant enlargement of the prostate gland. There is an increase in both stromal and glandular components.
- The incidence of BPH is ~25% in 40- to 60-year-olds, and 40% in those over 60.
- BPH is the most common cause of lower urinary tract symptoms (LUTS) in middle-aged and elderly men.

Pathological features

The etiology is largely unknown. Possible factors include the following:

- Androgens—there is no BPH in those who have had early castration.
- Estrogens—The estrogen–testosterone ratio increases with age.
- Growth factors, e.g., a high concentration of TGF-α occurs in BPH.

Clinical features

Symptoms

- Storage symptoms such as frequency, urgency, nocturia, and incontinence
- Voiding symptoms include hesitancy, poor stream, intermittency, terminal dribble, and abdominal straining.
- Superimposed infection may cause dysuria and hematuria.
- Incomplete emptying and chronic or acute retention of urine

Signs

- Smooth enlargement of the prostate is detected by digital rectal examination.
- Possible palpable bladder if there is chronic retention
- Always examine for neurological signs in those with LUTS.

Complications of BPH

- Intractable LUTS
- Hematuria
- Urinary tract infection
- Stone formation
- Acute retention of urine
- Chronic retention of urine
- Overflow incontinence
- Obstructive renal failure

Diagnosis and tests

- Use prostate symptom score to assess severity.
- Use digital rectal examination and serum PSA measurement to assess for features of malignancy.

Basic tests

- Serum creatinine, urinalysis: all patients
- Urine flowmetry and residual volume estimation: those considered for intervention

Advanced tests

- Cystoscopy: to exclude bladder disease
- Transrectal ultrasound-guided biopsy: if there is concern of underlying malignancy
- Renal ultrasound, invasive urodynamic studies

Treatment

Treatment is recommended for patients with LUTS that are affecting quality of life or for those patients with complications.

Medical treatment

- Patients with mild symptoms and no complications may be observed (watchful waiting).
- α-Adrenergic antagonists relax smooth muscle of the prostatic urethra to decrease outlet resistance. Side effects include dizziness and hypotension (especially postural).
- 5α-Reductase inhibitors block conversion of testosterone to dihydrotestosterone (DHT) and are shown to cause involution of BPH. Side effects include loss of libido and erectile dysfunction.
- Combination drug therapy with both of the above agents may reduce the clinical progression and decrease the need for surgery.

Surgical treatment

- Reserved for those with any complications or symptoms not responding to medical therapy.
- Surgical options include the following:
    - Transurethral resection of the prostate (TURP) is the most commonly performed procedure for BPH.
    - Open retropubic prostatectomy for large glands
    - Transurethral incision in the prostate (TUIP)
    - Bladder neck incision
    - Laser "prostatectomy"
    - Microwave thermotherapy ablation of the prostate

Stricture of the urethra

Key facts

- These are classified according to site and etiology, e.g., post-inflammatory bulbar stricture or traumatic membranous stricture.
- They are graded according to length and (in the anterior urethra) degree of fibrosis of corpus spongiosum (spongiofibrosis).
- Any part of the urethra may be involved.
- The propensity for stricture recurrence parallels the severity (grade).

Etiology

- Trauma
  - Pelvic fracture
  - Falls astride, e.g., on bicycle crossbar
  - Urinary tract instrumentation/surgery
- Infection
  - *Neisseria gonorrhoea* and *Chlamydia trachomatis*
  - Catheter-associated UTI
- Lichen sclerosis et atrophicus

Pathological features

- Annular narrowing by scar tissue composed of dense collagen and fibroblasts, which may extend into corpus spongiosum
- Lichen sclerosus (balanitis xerotica obliterans) consists of dermal sclerosis with epidermal atrophy. Urethral lesions are usually confined to the meatus and fossa navicularis.

Clinical features

- History of urethritis, trauma, or urinary tract instrumentation
- LUTS, divergent or diminished stream, straining to void, urgency, frequency
- Hematuria ("initial" or "terminal," i.e., at the beginning or end of the stream)
- UTI (often recurrent)
- Urinary retention, acute or chronic
- Overflow incontinence

Complications

- Urinary-tract calculi formation
- Infection including UTI, prostatitis, epididymitis, and (rarely) Fournier's necrotizing fasciitis
- Renal failure secondary to chronic obstruction

Diagnosis and tests

- Urinalysis (microbiology, biochemistry, and cytology)
- Urea and electrolytes
- Urodynamics and measurement of post-void residual bladder volume
- Voiding cystourethrogram with or without retrograde urethrogram
- Endoscopy

- Ultrasound scan (transperineal or endoluminal) to assess extent of spongiofibrosis
- Magnetic resonance tomography

Treatment

Initial

- Treat infection before going to surgical treatment.
- For acute urinary retention, severe symptoms, or renal failure use temporary suprapubic catheterization.

Definitive

- All urethral reconstructive surgery has an attrition rate.
- Initial internal urethrotomy may cure up to 30% of cases, but repeat procedures are rarely successful and may cause progression.
- Urethroplasty may be used for some cases.
  - Short strictures are excised and the urethra primarily reanastomosed.
  - For longer or complex strictures pedicled flap reconstruction or graft reconstruction is used. The graft or flap may be applied as an onlay (to augment the native urethra) or as a tube.
  - For free grafts, buccal mucosa is currently favored.
  - More complicated repairs are best managed with staged repairs.
- Perineal urethrostomy may be required.

Scrotal swellings

Major causes

Intratesticular lesions
- Malignant testicular tumors
- Benign intratesticular lesions: simple intratesticular cyst or epidermoid cysts and benign teratoma (especially in the prepubertal testis)

Inflammatory lesions
- Acute epididymo-orchitis or viral orchitis
- Chronic tuberculous epididymo-orchitis, schistosomal epididymitis, sperm granuloma

Traumatic lesions
- Scrotal hematoma
- Hematocele (hematoma within tunica vaginalis)
- Testicular hematoma (within tunica albuginea testis)

Derangement of testicular, adnexal, or cord anatomy
- Epididymal cysts or spermatocele of the epididymis
- Varicocele (varicosities of the pampiniform plexus)
- Inguinal hernia (patent processus vaginalis in children)
- Hydrocele (vagina = within tunica vaginalis, or cordal)
- Late (missed) or prenatal torsion of the spermatic cord
- Persistence of embryological vestigial structures
  - Müllerian duct remnant (appendix testis)
  - Wolffian duct remnants (appendix epididymis, vas aberrans of Haller, paradidymis)

Miscellaneous
- Acute idiopathic scrotal edema
- Cutaneous lesions, e.g., sebaceous cysts
- Henoch–Schönlein purpura

Clinical features and diagnosis
- Testicular tumors
  - Firm intratesticular or progressively enlarging lesions are tumors until proven otherwise.
  - Do not be misled by painful testicular swelling following relatively trivial trauma—tumors may present this way.
- Tuberculous epididymitis may occur with or without evidence of pulmonary, systemic, or other genitourinary involvement.
- Hydroceles, patent processus vaginalis, and large spermatoceles are transilluminable, may be fluctuant, and are usually confined to the scrotum.
- Varicocele is often associated with reduced fertility or dragging discomfort that worsens on standing and settles when recumbent. It is more obvious as a fluctuant swelling with the patient standing. A cough impulse may be felt. Ipsilateral testis may be atrophied. Examine the abdomen to exclude an associated renal tumor.

- Inguinal hernias tend to be intermittent and associated with groin discomfort, and, when "out," the examining hand cannot get above the swelling in the cord/inguinal canal. A history of long-standing enlargement is typical.

Tests

- Urinalysis
- Blood tests. Consider tumor markers (AFP, β-HCG) and inflammatory markers (CRP, WCC).
- Ultrasound scanning of the scrotal contents has several important uses:
  - It distinguishes intratesticular from paratesticular swellings, solid from cystic lesions, and cellulites from abscess.
  - For examining impalpable testes, e.g., within large hydroceles
  - It can indicate rupture of the tunica albuginea testis.
  - Examination of the abdomen can identify a renal mass associated with varicocele or ascites with hydrocele or scrotal edema, etc.
  - Color-flow Doppler ultrasound can show hyperemia, torsion (underperfusion), and varicocele.

Treatment

For testicular tumors and acute epididymo-orchitis, 🕮 p. 677.

- Testicular tumors are removed surgically via an inguinal incision.
- Suspected paratesticular tumors are approached surgically in the same way as testis tumors. Surgery may be conservative with benign testicular and paratesticular tumors.
- Sperm granuloma may be excised, or epididymectomy may be performed. Reassurance may be all that is required in many cases. Recurrence rates after surgery are high.
- Epididymal cysts and spermatocele may be aspirated but recurrence is common. Excision risks loss of epididymal patency, is associated with risk of recurrence, and should probably be discouraged in men who have not completed their family.
- Hydroceles: Treat if symptomatic.
  - Procedures usually reconfigure the serosal remnant of tunica vaginalis so as to allow lymphatic drainage via scrotal lymphatics. Reduction, inversion (Jaboulay), or imbrication (Lord's) of the tunica vaginalis is used.
- Embryological remnants require no treatment if asymptomatic.
- Varicocele: Treat if symptomatic or if associated with infertility or failure of testicular growth.
  - Venous embolization and retroperitoneal ligation (laparoscopic or open) of the testicular vein have similar results. Minimally invasive treatments are preferable. Gubernacular veins and other collaterals may account for failures. Use open surgical ligations via an inguinal incision.
  - Acute idiopathic penoscrotal edema of childhood usually settles with conservative treatment. Antihistamines and antibiotics are frequently prescribed, but there is little evidence to support this treatment.

Disorders of the foreskin

Phimosis

Key facts

- Narrowness of the preputial opening prevents retraction and exposure of the glans.
- Phimosis may be physiological in infants and young children and will resolve.
- Pathological phimosis is secondary to scarring such as balanitis xerotica obliterans (BXO) or following monilial balanoposthitis.
- Pathological phimosis may be associated with discomfort, UTI, balanoposthitis, and (perhaps) carcinogenesis.

Clinical features

- In childhood, physiological phimosis may be identified by absence of scarring of the preputial tip, and by pouting of the inner layer of the prepuce when a gentle attempt is made to retract it.
- A whitish sclerotic preputial tip and no pouting characterize BXO.
- Parents may complain of ballooning of their child's foreskin or of recurrent balanoposthitis. In adults, the diagnosis is obvious.

Treatment

- Physiological phimosis needs no treatment.
- Early BXO may be treated by application of topical steroid cream.
- Surgical treatment of phimosis includes circumcision and dorsal slit.

Paraphimosis

Key facts and diagnosis

- The retracted foreskin acts as a constricting ring, reducing lymphatic and venous drainage of tissues distal to the ring (glans, inner layer of foreskin). Subsequent edema makes reduction more difficult.
- Involved tissues typically appear edematous and inflamed with progression to infection, ulceration, and necrosis if left untreated. This condition can occur in normal penises.

Treatment

- *Early cases:* Gentle manual compression of the edematous tissues within a saline-soaked swab will allow reduction of the foreskin after a few minutes, without anesthesia.
- *Established cases:* LA penile block or anesthesia may be necessary. Hyaluronidase can be injected under the constriction.
- *Neglected or severe cases:* A relaxing dorsal incision may be made through the constriction and the tissues immediately proximal and distal to it. Subsequent circumcision is often offered.

Common conditions of the penis

Peyronie's disease
Key facts
- Damage to tunica albuginea penis, forming inelastic penile plaques mostly in the dorsal midline, causing local pain and deformity
- This disease is associated with Dupuytren's contractures, plantar fascial contractures, and tympanosclerosis.
- One-third of patients have erectile dysfunction.

Clinical features
History and examination
- Gradual or sudden development of palpable penile plaques with painful distortion of the erect penis occurs in two-thirds of patients.
- Occasional history of penile trauma, urethral instrumentation
- Erectile dysfunction may involve the whole or part of the penis.
- Pain usually resolves but deformity does not.
- Penetrative sexual intercourse may be more difficult or impossible because of pain, angulation, or buckling.
- The plaque is palpable with the flaccid penis stretched.
- Erection is induced pharmacologically and a photo record kept.

Tests
Plain-film soft-tissue radiography or grayscale ultrasound may demonstrate calcification, an indicator of plaque maturity.

Treatment
Medical
Medical treatment is indicated for those able to engage in intercourse and whose disease is still evolving.
- *Oral treatment options*: colchicine, vitamin E, or Potaba®
- *Intralesional injections*: verapamil or collagenase (investigational)
- Treatment of associated erectile dysfunction

Surgical
Surgery is indicated for those with stable lesions or severe deformity.
- Plication techniques involve plication of the tunica opposite the deforming plaque.
- Grafting techniques: The plaque is excised, and the defect grafted.
- Prosthesis insertion within corpora cavernosa is generally reserved for patients with severe erectile dysfunction refractory to medical therapy.

Priapism
Key facts
Priapism is an abnormally sustained erection unrelated to sexual stimulation. It is classified as high flow (arterial) or low flow (veno-occlusive).

Low-flow priapism
Congestion secondarily reduces arterial blood flow, leading to local hypoxia, acidosis, and hypercapnea. Causes include the following:
- Drugs (intracavernosal prostaglandin and papaverine, psychotropics, e.g., trazodone, chlorpromazine)

- Abnormal blood viscosity (sickle cell, myeloma, leukemia, thalassaemia, total parenteral nutrition)
- Neurological disease, e.g., spinal or cerebrovascular disease
- Miscellaneous causes, e.g., infiltration by solid tumor

This condition is characterized by painful, persistent erection, not involving the glans and corpus spongiosum.

High-flow priapism

- This most commonly follows blunt trauma to the penis or perineum, but has been caused by intracavernosal injection or revascularization
- The mechanism is arteriocavernosal fistula with unregulated arterial inflow, and increased venous outflow.
- It is characterized by partial, painless swelling of the glans and corpus spongiosum.

Tests

- Color Doppler ultrasonography or cavernosal blood gases
- pH <7.25, pO_2 <30mmHg, and pCO_2 >60 mmHg suggest low-flow priapism.
- FBC and differential; hemoglobin electrophoresis

Treatment

Low flow

- Correct underlying abnormalities, e.g., sickle cell (rehydration, oxygen, transfusion), myeloma (plasmapheresis)
- Oral beta-agonists, e.g., terbutaline 5 mg + further 5 mg 15 min later
- Intracavernosal phenylephrine
- Corpora cavernosa aspiration (up to 50 mL) + manual pressure
- Surgical techniques augment venous drainage of the corpora cavernosa.

High flow

- Selective pudendal arteriography and embolization

Erectile dysfunction

Key facts

Erectile dysfunction (ED) is the inability to achieve or maintain an erection satisfactory for sexual intercourse. It is distinct from premature, retrograde, or delayed ejaculation. Causes include the following:

- *Psychogenic*: anxiety, depression
- *Drugs*: antihypertensives, recreational drugs, tobacco, alcohol
- *Vascular*: hypercholesterolemia, atheroma, diabetes mellitus (DM)
- *Metabolic/endrocrine*: azotemia, hypercholesterolemia, hypogonadism, hyperthyroidism, hyperprolactinemia, DM
- *Neurological*: Parkinson's disease, CVA, spinal injury, neurological damage following pelvic surgery, pelvic fracture, autonomic neuropathies
- *Penile*: cavernositis, Peyronie's disease, previous priapism

Clinical features

- Specific validated questionnaires have been developed as investigational tools and can be used in practice.
- The presence of morning erections strongly suggests psychogenic cause.
- Small testicles and lack of secondary sexual characteristics suggest an endocrine cause.
- Lack of lower limb pulses suggests a possible vascular cause.
- Neurological deficits in S2, 3, and 4 distribution suggest a neurological cause.

Investigations and diagnosis

- Check blood glucose, lipids and serum electrolytes, hormone profiles (testosterone, FSH/LH, prolactin), and thyroid function for an underlying cause.
- Dynamic cavernosometry confirms if there is a true vasculogenic cause (venous or arterial).
- Angiography demonstrates arterial anatomy if revascularization is contemplated.

Treatment

- Psychotherapy or specialist sexual counseling for psychogenic causes
- Oral phosphodiesterase-5 inhibitors: sildenafil (Viagra), vardenafil, tadalafil
- Apomorphine sublingual
- Intracavernosal: prostaglandins, α-blockers, papaverine
- Intraurethral: prostaglandin
- Vacuum-device-induced pseudoerection
- Prosthesis

Adenocarcinoma of the kidney

Key facts
- Accounts for 2% of all cancers
- Incidence is 2–5/100,000

Clinical features
- This condition may be asymptomatic at presentation, the tumor being detected during imaging of the abdomen for an unrelated condition (e.g., CT scan or ultrasound scan).
- Symptoms include painless hematuria, groin pain, and awareness of a mass arising from the flank.
- Chest symptoms and bone pain may be present with metastases to these sites.
- A positive family history or clinical evidence of neurological or ocular disease should raise the possibility of von Hippel–Lindau disease (VHL).
- Renal carcinomas are often small and may be multiple.
- Local spread often includes spread via intravascular invasion into the renal vein and the IVC in ~5% of cases.

Diagnosis and investigations
- Blood tests. Obtain Hb and ferritin to check for anemia (iron deficiency), and electrolytes and creatinine to check for overall renal function. Raised corrected calcium and alkaline phosphatase suggest possible bony metastases.
- The diagnostic and staging investigation of choice is a pre- and post-IV contrast-enhanced CT scan of the abdomen and chest (CT delineates the size, local extent, local invasion, and likely sites of possible metastases).
- Obtain a bone scan if there is clinical or biochemical evidence of bony metastases. Obtain a chest film to rule out lung metastasis.

Treatment
Surgery
- Recommended as the only curative treatment except in the very elderly or those with extensive (inoperable) local invasion
- May be via open or laparoscopic approach
- Radical nephrectomy is recommended for large tumors.
- Partial nephrectomy may be suitable for peripheral tumors <4 cm in size.
- Resection of the primary cancer is occasionally appropriate with the presence of metastasis (the deposit must be solitary and itself amenable to complete local resection, e.g., in the liver or lungs).
- Minimally invasive ablative techniques such as radiofrequency ablation or cryosurgery can be used in selective cases with small cancers.

Medical therapy
- Used for metastatic disease
- Biological therapy can be with immune modulators such as interferons (IFNs) and interleukins (ILs). Partial response rates of 15%–20% can be achieved, but the treatment carries significant morbidity. This is reserved for patients with a good performance status.
- Angiogenesis inhibitors are currently being studied
- Chemotherapy is rarely used, as the tumors are not chemosensitive.
- Hormonal therapy (androgens and tamoxifen) may have some benefit.
- Radiotherapy is useful to palliate painful bony metastases.

Prognosis
- The outcome following nephrectomy is unpredictable.
- Tumors pathologically confined to the kidney confer a good prognosis. Adverse risk factors include extracapsular spread, invasion of the renal vein, and lymph node involvement.
- Cure is likely if the tumor is less than 4 cm in diameter and if there are no adverse pathological features.
- Periodic radiological follow-up is recommended in most cases so that locally recurrent or metastatic disease can be detected at an early stage.

Transitional cell tumors

Key facts

- Transitional cell tumors (TCT) may affect any part of the urinary epithelium (renal pelvis, ureter, bladder, or, very rarely, urethra).
- TCT have a spectrum of disease from benign superficial "papilliferous" growths to frankly invasive transitional cell carcinoma (TCC). Progression may occur from benign to more malignant forms with time.
- TCC of the bladder is the fifth most common cause of cancer deaths.
- TCC of the upper urinary tract is similar in spectrum of disease and management to bladder tumors but is much less common.
- TCC is associated with the following:
  - Exposure to aromatic hydrocarbons, e.g., workers in petrochemical, industrial-dye, and rubber industries, chimney sweeps
  - Smoking (especially in women)
- Risk is probably due to carcinogenic products excreted and concentrated in the urine, and tumors are more likely in locations exposed to urine for the longest periods, i.e., bladder.

Pathological features

- The majority (70%) of cases are superficial in nature at diagnosis, being confined to the mucosa.
- Invasion into the lamina propria, muscle, and perivesical fat can occur, with lymphatic and distant spread occurring in advanced cases.
- TCC in situ is preinvasive and associated with a high risk of muscle-invasive disease if not adequately treated.
- TCC must be differentiated from other forms of bladder cancer:
  - Squamous cell carcinoma, usually caused by chronic irritation due to schistosomiasis infestation (bilharzia), indwelling catheter, and repeated previous surgical interventions
  - Adenocarcinoma, which is rare, presenting in middle age, and is usually located in the dome of the bladder in association with the urachus

Clinical features

- Most cases present with painless hematuria.
- Other features are painful micturition, renal colic due to blood clot, disturbance of urinary stream, and retention of urine.

Diagnosis

Urine cytology

Urine cytology may reveal malignant cells. If there are malignant cells, TCC or carcinoma in situ will probably be present.

Cystoscopy

- This is usually carried out using a fiber-optic flexible cystoscope and local anesthetic gel.
- It images the bladder and urethra. Suspected lesions usually require transurethral resection under GA for diagnosis.

Transurethral resection
- This is usually carried out using a rigid endoresectoscope under GA.
- It permits resection of all or part of the tumor using a diathermy loop, with the tumor resected piecemeal. Resection may be carried out into deep tissue (the muscle wall of the bladder beneath the tumor).
- Subsequent pathological examination will determine the histological grade and the pathological stage, e.g., depth of invasion.
- Following resection, bimanual examination determines whether or not a residual mass is present.

Upper-tract imaging
- This technique is used to identify and assess pelviureteric tumors.
- It consists of intravenous urogram (IVU) or ultrasound scan.
- Ultrasound scan permits examination of the renal cortex and will detect tumors 1 cm in diameter in the pelvicalyceal system, ureter, and bladder.
- Bladder tumor may show as a filling defect in the cystogram phase.

Local staging
MRI and CT scanning are used to detect local or systemic spread.

Treatment
Superficial TCC
- Removal is completed by endoscopic resection.
- Recurrence is common and regular endoscopic surveillance with check cystoscopy is performed.
- Intravesical chemotherapy reduces the risk of tumor recurrence (a single dose of mitomycin C is instilled after resection of the tumor).
- For multiple or recurrent TCC, six intravesical treatments are given.

Carcinoma in situ
- Requires thorough therapy to prevent invasive TCC
- Immunotherapy with intravesical BCG is effective in 60% of cases.
- Needs close endoscopic surveillance with regular bladder biopsy

Invasive TCC
- Muscle-invasive tumors are high grade and the prognosis is poor.
- Curative therapy can be offered with radical cystectomy (combined with a urinary diversion via an ileal conduit) or radical radiotherapy.

Squamous cell and adenocarcinoma
- Radical cystectomy can be done, provided general condition allows.
- This condition is usually resistant to radiotherapy and chemotherapy.

Prognosis
- Approximately 30% of patients develop muscle-invasive disease.
- The 5-year survival rate for muscle-invasive bladder cancer is 40%–50%.
- Metastatic TCC has a poor prognosis with a median survival of 13 months.
- Systemic chemotherapy with cis-platinum-containing regimes provides a long-term response in 15% of cases.

Adenocarcinoma of the prostate

Key facts

- This is the most commonly diagnosed cancer affecting men in the Western world.
- Peak incidence is in eighth decade.
- Approximately 75% of cases present with early disease; 20% of cases have metastases at presentation.

Clinical features

- The majority of men present with lower urinary tract symptoms.
- Bone pain, pathological factures, and features of hypercalcemia are occasional presenting features due to metastases.
- May be diagnosed by digital rectal examination. Areas of firmness or palpable nodules are suggestive of malignant change.

Diagnosis and investigations

- *Serum prostate-specific antigen* (PSA) can be used as a screening test. It has high sensitivity but low specificity. Elevated age-specific levels are an indication to consider prostate biopsy.
- *Transrectal ultrasound* (TRUS) permits detailed imaging of the prostate. Systematic needle biopsy is performed, guided by ultrasound images with antibiotic prophylaxis. Images are graded using the Gleason grading system, which assigns a numerical score to adverse features from a minimum of 2 to a maximum of 10.
- *Pelvic MRI* is used to detect the presence of extracapsular extension or the presence of pelvic lymphadenopathy (suggests spread).
- *Laparoscopic node biopsy* may be performed to sample enlarged nodes prior to considering radical treatment.
- *Bone scanning* will detect the presence of bone metastases.

Treatment

Localized disease (confined to prostate)

Patients with a life expectancy of <10 years

- Active monitoring with treatment deferred until there is evidence of disease progression (rising serum PSA)
- Hormonal therapy or α-blocker treatment offered for troublesome lower urinary tract symptoms
- TURP is considered for severe symptoms with features of obstruction.

Life expectancy of >10 years

- Counseled in detail about radical treatment aimed at cure
- The options are as follows:
  - *Radical prostatectomy* is an operation to remove the prostate and seminal vesicles. Complications include incontinence and erectile dysfunction.

- *External beam radiotherapy.* Radiation is delivered at a radical dose of 55–70 Gy in 20–25 fractions over a 6- to 8-week period. Complications include cystitis, proctitis, and erectile dysfunction.
- *Brachytherapy.* Radioactive seeds are placed into the prostate using transrectal ultrasound guidance. A relatively new technique and long-term follow-up data are lacking.

Locally advanced disease (spread beyond the prostate)

- This is incurable and treatment is therefore palliative.
- 80% of cases are androgen-dependent. Hormone therapy reduces androgenic drive to the prostate cancer cell via two methods:
  - Luteinizing hormone-releasing hormone (LHRH) agonists, given by 3-monthly depot injections. LHRH suppresses testosterone production by the testes. Side effects include hot flushes, lethargy, and loss of sexual function.
  - Anti-androgens, given orally. These act as competitive inhibitors at the level of the androgen receptor. They reduce androgenic stimulus to the prostate cancer cell without reducing serum testosterone levels. Side effects include gynecomastia and nipple tenderness (60%). Potency is sometimes preserved.

Metastatic disease

This is treated with hormonal therapy with LHRH analogues. Addition of an anti-androgen provides a secondary response in some cases of PSA relapse. Pain from bone metastases usually responds to radiotherapy.

Hormone-resistant disease

- All prostate cancers will eventually become hormone resistant.
- Chemotherapy is appropriate for patients who have a good performance status.
- Palliative radiotherapy and bisphosphonates are used for bony metastases.

Prognosis

- *Localized prostate cancer:* excellent prognosis with 70%–90% 10-year disease-specific survival figures
- *Locally advanced, nonmetastatic disease:* median survival of 7 years
- *Metastatic disease:* median survival of 2–3 years
- Once the state of hormone-resistant disease has been reached, the median survival is 6–12 months.

Carcinoma of the penis

Key facts
- This is the rarest of the urological cancers.
- It occurs primarily in older men.

Clinicopathological features
- More than 95% of cases are squamous cell carcinoma.
- Carcinoma usually affects the glans but may involve the shaft.
- It is associated with chronic infection of the penis, particularly in the presence of phimosis.
- Early cases present with a painless ulcer, nodule, or "warty" outgrowth on the penis that may also involve the foreskin.
- Advanced disease presents with a fungating mass, usually ulcerated. Inguinal lymphadenopathy may be present on examination. Nodes are often reactive rather than being metastatic, and antibiotics should be given prior to further assessment.

Diagnosis and investigations
- Biopsy lesion to confirm the diagnosis.
- Pelvic and abdominal CT or pelvic MRI scanning provides further evidence of nodular involvement in cases with positive inguinal nodes.

Treatment
- If primary tumor is confined to the glans, treatment involves either partial amputation or radiotherapy.
- Superficial lesions can be treated by excision of the glans, followed by glans reconstruction.
- More advanced carcinomas require total penectomy. Inguinal and iliac lymph node dissections are considered.

Prognosis
- Early-stage penile cancer has a high cure rate with either surgery or radiotherapy.
- Long-term survival is sometimes seen even in cases of lymph node involvement.

Testicular tumors

Key facts

- This is the most common malignancy in men between the ages of 18 and 40.
- Annual incidence is 6/100,000 males per year.
- Testicular cancer is associated with undescended testicles.
- Increased risk is associated with higher levels of exogenous estrogens either prenatally or in childhood.
- An increased level of awareness has led to more tumors being detected on self-examination, particularly among younger men.

Pathological features

- Common types are seminoma and non-seminomatous germ cell tumors (NSGCTs). Lymphoma is a rare testicular tumor unless patients are over the age of 50, when it is the most common type.
- Seminoma
  - Peak incidence is at age 30–40 years.
  - Lymphatic spread is more common than hematogenous spread.
  - Lymphatic type spreads to para-aortic, paracaval, and iliac nodes.
- NSGCTs
  - Peak incidence is at 20–30 years of age.
  - Spread to retroperitoneal lymph nodes or lung
- Lymphomas: Peak incidence is at over 60 years of age.
- Marsden staging (after investigations and treatment):
  - Stage 1: confined to testis
  - Stage 2: abdominal nodal spread
  - Stage 3: nodal disease outside the abdomen
  - Stage 4: extralymphatic spread

Clinical features

- The usual presentation is with a painless testicular mass.
- Typical features are irregular, firm, and fixed, and the mass does not transilluminate.
- Palpate the abdomen for intra-abdominal masses (either para-aortic node masses or hepatomegaly).
- Check for supraclavicular lymphadenopathy and signs of lung or neurological disease.

Diagnosis

- Any clinically suspicious mass requires an urgent testicular ultrasound scan. Typical features are a nonhomogeneous mass with increased vascularity.
- Serum tumor markers are β-HCG and AFP. Increased levels suggest metastatic disease in NSGCTs but may be normal in localized or metastatic disease. In some cases of seminoma there will be a mild elevation in β-HCG; however, the AFP level should be normal.
- CT scan of abdomen and chest to assess presence of metastases
- CT scan of brain, bone scan only if clinically indicated

Treatment

- Orchidectomy is carried out at the earliest opportunity. This is performed via an inguinal approach so that the spermatic cord can be clamped prior to mobilization of the testis.
- Seminoma is radiosensitive; even widespread local disease responds well to radiotherapy.
  - Stage 1 may be treated by orchidectomy only, orchidectomy + prophylactic iliac, paracaval, and para-arotic radiotherapy, or orchidectomy + prophylactic chemotherapy.
  - Stage 2, 3, or 4 is treated with orchidectomy + radiotherapy to involved node groups, and chemotherapy.
  - Visceral metastases are treated with a combination of chemotherapy and radiotherapy.
- NSGCT is chemosensitive; even widespread metastatic disease responds well to chemotherapy.
  - Stage 1 is treated with orchidectomy.
  - Stage 2, 3, or 4 is treated with orchidectomy + chemotherapy. If lymphadenopathy is still present following chemotherapy, a retroperitoneal lymph node dissection is performed.

Prognosis

- Cure rates are over 95% for stage 1 tumors.
- Metastatic disease also has excellent long-time survival rates with combination therapy.

Hematuria

Causes and features

Hematuria may be microscopic or macroscopic.
- Urinary tract infection is the most common cause. It is usually associated with lower urinary tract symptoms, particularly cystitis.
- Renal stones are often associated with pain (renal colic).
- Malignancy (transitional cell tumor, renal adenocarcinoma, prostate adenocarcinoma) is most likely to be macroscopic, often with few other acute symptoms.
- Post-interventional, e.g., post-TURP, post-cystoscopy, post-catheterization
- Enlarged prostates can cause hematuria in the elderly.
- Renal disease, e.g., glomerulonephritis, vasculitis, usually causes microscopic hematuria, is often asymptomatic, and rarely presents as an emergency.

Complications
- Suprapubic colicky pain or acute retention of urine suggests clots in the bladder or urethra.
- Cardiovascular collapse is rare.

Emergency management

Resuscitation
- Establish large-caliber IV access if the bleed is large. Give crystalloid fluid up to 1000 mL if patient is tachycardic or hypotensive.
- *Do not* catheterize without seeking advice if there is any suggestion of lower urinary tract pathology or post-interventional bleeding.
- Whistle tip catheters can be used to irrigate clots from the bladder.
- Irrigation (three-way) catheters may be used to relieve acute symptoms of clot colic or clot retention but should be placed by experienced staff.
- Send blood for CBC (Hb, WBC), electrolytes, blood bank sample, coagulation studies, and platelet count.

Establish diagnosis
- Conduct a full clinical examination. Particularly check the prostate on PR exam.
- Use cystoscopy (usually rigid, may be flexible) to identify bladder tumors.
- Obtain CT scan with IV contrast if there is normal renal function.

Early treatment
- Ensure that all clotting abnormalities are corrected.
- Ensure that fluid balance is correct. Promote an active diuresis to prevent clot formation and retention.
- Transfuse blood only if Hb <8 g/dL or if the patient is symptomatic or high risk.
- Send a urine culture and then start antibiotics according to local protocol if infection is suspected.

Definitive management

Transitional cell tumors (📖 p. 671)
Transurethral resection will help to control symptoms, establish a diagnosis, and start treatment.

Renal stones (📖 p. 653)
- These may pass spontaneously.
- They may need endoscopic removal, lithotripsy, or percutaneous treatment.

Post-interventional
Flexible cystoscopy may be required.

Acute urinary retention

Causes and features

Acute urinary retention is defined as a painful inability to pass urine.

Local causes

- Prostatic enlargement (BPH or carcinoma) (📖 p. 657) is often acute on chronic retention.
- Posturological surgery, e.g., post-TURP, clot impaction
- Bladder or urethral stone impaction
- Pressure on the bladder, e.g., late pregnancy, fecal impaction
- Urinary tract infection

General causes

- Pharmacological, e.g., the following:
  - Anticholinergic side effects of many drugs
  - Anesthetic drugs
  - Alcohol intoxication
  - α-sympatheticomimetics
- Post-nonurological surgery
  - Precipitated by recent catheterization
  - Abdominal surgery with lower abdominal pain
  - Epidural or spinal anesthesia
- Loss of normal neurological control
  - Spinal injury (trauma, slipped disc, neurological disease)
  - Epidural or spinal anesthesia

Symptoms

- Suprapubic pain, inability to pass urine despite desire
- Patient may dribble urine in small volumes, especially if there is underlying chronic retention.
- Palpable or percussible bladder strongly suggests preexisting chronic retention or lower urinary tract disease.

Signs

- Prostatic enlargement on PR examination
- Check for signs of neurological disease.

Emergency management

Resuscitation

- A warm bath may aid micturition in drug-induced retention.
- Catheterize patient if retention persists. Seek advice prior to catheterization if there are concerns about local pathology as a cause or if there is a history of previous surgical instrumentation of the urethra.
- Suprapubic catheterization may be required for known or suspected urethral disease or failed urethral catheterization (📖 p. 210).
- Document initial urine volume passed after the catheter is inserted. Large volumes suggest underlying chronic retention.
- Send urine for Gram stain, culture and sensitivity (C & S).
- Send blood for CBC and electrolytes.

Establish a diagnosis
- Check medications, especially recent changes.
- Cystoscopy may be required.
- Review the full clinical examination, including neurological findings and rectal examination.

Early treatment
- Monitor renal function, especially if there is underlying chronic retention. Renal function may deteriorate even after relief of the obstruction.
- Monitor fluid balance in the first 48 hr if there is associated chronic retention. A secondary diuresis may occur.
- Start antibiotics if there is evidence of a UTI.

Definitive management
Prostatic disease (📖 p. 657)
- TURP may be required.
- 5-α-reductase inhibitors may help to slowly induce atrophy.
- α-blocker may enable successful trial of voiding.

Acute testicular pain

Causes and features

This is an acute emergency in men of childbearing age. Torsion of the testicle must be dealt with immediately to preserve testicular function. It is the most common cause of referral for acute testicular pain.

Torsion of the testicle

Key facts

- Torsion is the result of anatomical variants in testicular anatomy, e.g., "bell clapper" testicle with pronounced meso-orchium, allowing rotation within the tunica vaginalis.
- Peak age of incidence is at 12–18 years.
- Torsion initially causes venous obstruction, but with prolonged increased venous pressure, arterial compression occurs and the testicle rapidly develops irreversible ischemia and necrosis.
- Testicular salvage depends on the degree of torsion and time spent torsed. Speed of presentation, diagnosis, and treatment are all important. Torsion greater than 360° and lasting longer than 24 hr results in near-universal complete or severe atrophy.
- Spermatogenic cells are more susceptible to ischemia than Leydig cells. Decreased fertility may occur even if the testicle is macroscopically normal after treatment.

Features

- Sudden onset of moderate to severe, constant, unilateral scrotal pain often with nausea, vomiting, and abdominal pain.
- There may have been preceding episodes of intermittent pain that suddenly resolved.
- The testis is globally tender, high in the scrotum, may have a transverse axis, and be slightly enlarged. If it is infarcted, scrotal wall edema and tenderness may be present. Absence of ipsilateral cremasteric reflex is the most reliable sign.

Torsion of the testicular appendages

- This occurs in testicular appendix "hydatid of Morgagni" or epididymal appendages (e.g., cysts, ductal remnants).
- Features and symptoms are similar to those of testicular torsion.
- The "blue dot sign" is said to be diagnostic when present.
- The testis and epididymis may be non-tender, and the cremasteric reflex should be preserved.

Acute epididymo-orchitis

- Peak incidences vary according to cause, at ages 35 and >55 years.
- Common organisms include *Chlamydia trachomatis,* and *Neisseria gonorrhoea* in the young (sexually transmitted infections [STI]).
- *Escherichia coli* and proteus occur in chronic bladder outflow obstruction, or urinary tract instrumentation.
- One-third of male adolescents with mumps develop orchitis, which is unilateral in 80%. A third of these testes will atrophy.

Features
- Gradual onset of pain (hours or days)
- Dysuria, urethral discharge, and pyrexia are common.
- Tenderness and induration are localized to the epididymis and spermatic cord in epididymitis.
- Cremasteric reflex is preserved.
- Prehn's sign (relief of pain with scrotal elevation)

Idiopathic scrotal edema
- Often less painful and tender than it appears
- Swelling is mostly cutaneous and a normal-sized and textured testicle may be palpable with care.

Acute inguinal lymphadenopathy
- May occur secondary to lower-limb, buttock, or perineal infections.
- Rarely part of systemic infection of lymphatic disorder

Emergency management
Resuscitation
- Give analgesia (e.g., morphine 5–10 mg IV).

Establish a diagnosis
- Order testicular color duplex ultrasound immediately.
- Immediate surgical exploration is indicated for all cases where the diagnosis of torsion is considered possible and the history is short (i.e., testicular viability is still at issue).
- Send UA and culture, urethral swab, and chlamydia serology if infection is suspected.

Definitive management
If a torsed testicle is found at surgery
- A viable testicle is detorsed and fixed.
- A clearly nonviable testicle is excised.
- The opposite testicle is fixed (orchidopexy) to prevent the opposite side torsing in the future.

Torsion of testicular or epididymal appendage
- Excise appendage.

Epididymo-orchitis
- Suspected STD, e.g., ceftriaxone 250 mg IM single dose, doxycycline 100 mg po bid 7 days
- Suspected UTI-related: ciprofloxacin 500 mg po bid 10–14 days
- Scrotal elevation, local ice therapy, and oral NSAIDs may help.
- Abscess formation may require drainage or orchidectomy.
- Treatment of acute viral orchitis is symptomatic.

Eponymous terms

David L. Berger, MD

Acanthosis nigricans Pigmentation of the axillary skin associated with breast or gastric cancer.

Achondroplasia Familial dwarfism in which growth of the long bones and skull is defective.

Adenomyomatosis, gallbladder Thickening of the gallbladder wall with occasional intramural sinuses that may partially occlude the gallbladder lumen.

Adiposa dolorosa Multiple lipomas, usually on the arms and trunks, that are occasionally painful.

Adrenogenital syndrome A condition, usually with autosomal recessive inheritance, affecting 1:5000 to 1:15,000 births, characterized by cortisol and/or aldosterone deficiency due to an enzymatic defect in cortisol synthesis. This results in secondary adrenal hyperplasia through loss of feedback on the pituitary gland. Diversion of precursors into the synthesis of other steroids, particularly androgens, results in virilization and ambiguous genitalia (through clitoral hypertrophy) of the female fetus and pseudo-precocious puberty in the male. Early closure of the epiphyseal plates leads to short stature. Impaired aldosterone secretion can cause a salt-losing state that requires replacement therapy.

Aerocele The collection of air in one or more tissue layers of the cranium due to injured or inflamed cranial air sinuses.

Albers–Schönberg disease See Osteopetrosis.

Albright's hereditary osteodystrophy An X-linked form of pseudo-hypoparathyroidism characterized by mental retardation, low serum calcium, cataracts, and tetany. Patients tend to be of short stature and have short first, fourth, and fifth metacarpals. Metastatic calcification of the basal ganglia is a feature.

Albright's syndrome, or polyostotic fibrous dysplasia A condition thought to be due to disordered bony development, featuring fibrodysplastic bony changes, patchy skin pigmentation, and precocious puberty in girls. Affected bones become soft and deformed from childhood onward.

Allen's test Assesses the adequacy of the collateral circulation to the hand. Digital pressure is applied to both the radial and ulnar arteries at the wrist and the patient repeatedly clenches a fist. Adequate collateral supply exists if there is complete palmar flushing with 15 sec of release of each vessel in turn.

Amastia Absence of both breast and nipple. Some 90% of patients with unilateral amastia have absent or hypoplastic pectoral muscles.

Amaurosis fugax Episodes of transient blindness due to central retinal artery embolization from carotid vessel disease or proximal vessel atherosclerosis.

Amazia Congenital absence of breast tissue but not the nipple. It is now known as hypoplasia of the breast, to differentiate it from amastia.

Angiodysplasia Vascular lesions of unknown etiology, most frequently found in the right colon, occasionally associated with cutaneous and oral lesions. They occur with increasing age and present with bleeding that may be torrential, but more often as a series of small bleeds.

Angiomyoneuroma (glomus tumor) A small, painful, benign tumor of blood vessels, rarely larger than a few mm in size, found mainly in the extremities. Half arise in the digits, predominantly subungually. They are exquisitely painful and tender and appear blue–purple in color. Treat by excision with a wide margin.

Angiosarcoma A soft-tissue tumor of young men and women that produces a bulky tumor with a tendency to bleed and metastasize to the lungs.

Ankyloglossia Also known as tongue-tie, it is due to a short lingual frenulum. It rarely affects speech, but frenectomy is recommended when food control and oral hygiene are a problem.

Antibioma A hard, edematous swelling containing sterile pus following treatment of an abscess with long-term antibiotics rather than with incision and drainage.

Aortoenteric fistula A connection between the aorta and small intestine, resulting in hemorrhage heralded by a sentinel bleed, and may culminate with exsanguination. It is most commonly due to infection of a prosthetic graft rather than a primary spontaneous fistula.

Apert's syndrome Occurs in 1:160,000 births; 30% of cases are autosomal dominant. The skull is tower shaped (oxycephaly) with premature fusion of all the sutures. Mild face aplasia and syndactyly of the middle three fingers occur. Other associations include esophageal atresia, and renal and congenital heart anomalies.

Aphthous ulcers The most common disorder affecting the oral mucosal membranes, of unknown etiology. They are painful, recurrent, and occur most commonly in childhood, rarely in the edentulous. Large ulcers, present for 3 months or more, may mimic carcinomas and should be biopsied if doubt exists about their status.

Arnold–Chiari malformation A hindbrain abnormality in which the cerebellum and medulla are found to lie below the level of the foramen magnum. Compression of the foramen of Magendie results in obstructive hydrocephalus in 80%–90% of cases. Syringomyelia and spina bifida are commonly associated.

Askanazy cell tumor, or Hurtle cell adenoma, thyroid A tumor consisting of featureless granular cells of varying size distributed in the fibrous stroma of the thyroid. They are difficult to differentiate from malignant tumors but are regarded as benign.

Asplenia Absence of the spleen, associated with cardiac anomalies, including situs inversus.

Athelia Absence of the nipple. It is exceedingly rare.

Baker's cyst A central swelling of the popliteal fossa, most evident when the patient stands. It represents a synovial membrane diverticulum, almost always associated with knee joint pathology such as arthritis or torn meniscus.

Balanitis xerotica obliterans A disease of unknown etiology characterized by keratotic lesions with inflammatory changes leading to phimosis and occasional meatal stenosis. It has the appearance of a white stenotic band at the end of the foreskin and minor trauma often results in hemorrhage.

Ballance's sign Fixed dullness in the left flank with shifting dullness best appreciated in the right flank, resulting from intraperitoneal and extraperitoneal bleeding following splenic rupture.

Barrett's esophagus The presence of columnar lined mucosa in the anatomical esophagus. BE may be due to acid or biliary reflux. It is found in 10% of patients undergoing endoscopy for reflux symptoms. Strictures, ulceration, bleeding, dysplasia, and malignant transformation may occur.

Battle's sign Bruising over the mastoid process following a base-of-skull fracture that involves the petrous temporal bone.

Bazin's disease See Erythrocyanosis frigida.

Bezoars Masses of ingested human hairs (trichlobezoars) or indigestible vegetable matter and fiber (phytobezoars) that form in the stomach and interfere with digestion, or may migrate into the small bowel and cause intestinal obstruction.

Bier spots The presence of white patches among the mottled blue–purple appearance of an acutely ischemic limb that has been in a warm environment for several hours.

Blind loop syndrome Malabsorption due to colonization of a blind-ending segment of bowel by abnormal bacteria that prevent the digestion and absorption of food. Causes include congenital abnormalities (e.g., small bowel diverticula), strictures, or, more commonly, surgical construction of small bowel anastomoses and loops.

Blue nevus Results when embryonic melanocyte migration from the neural crest is arrested in the dermis.

Bochdalek hernia A posterior diaphragmatic hernia in which the septum transversum fails to unite with the intercostal part of the diaphragm. It occurs in infants and is characterized by gross herniation of abdominal contents and associated lung hypoplasia.

Boerhaave's syndrome Spontaneous esophageal rupture following an episode of intense vomiting or retching, characterized by severe upper abdominal and chest pain, tachycardia, tachypnea, and subcutaneous emphysema.

Bowen's disease An irregular reddish-brown, cutaneous plaque, occasionally ulcerated and commonly found on the trunk. It is an intraepidermal carcinoma in situ and may develop into squamous cell carcinoma.

Branham's test When a pneumatic tourniquet is inflated around the root of a limb with a suspected arteriovenous malformation, a significant fall in the pulse rate suggests a significant arteriovenous shunt.

Budd–Chiari syndrome Posthepatic venous obstruction that may result from spontaneous thrombosis, extrinsic compression by tumor, or a web in the vena cava.

Calot's triangle An essential landmark in laparoscopic cholecystectomy surgery. Its boundaries are the common hepatic duct, cystic duct, and inferior border of the liver.

Campbell de Morgan spots Small, red spots that commonly occur on the trunk in middle age and do not blanch. They are of no significance.

Cancer en cuirasse Multiple malignant nodules on the chest wall in breast cancer that mimic the breast plate on a suit of armor.

Caput medusa Engorged veins radiating from the periumbilical region, resulting from extrahepatic portosystemic shunting from portal hypertension.

Carbuncle Multiple, adjacent follicular infections with *Staphylococcus aureus*, commonly seen in diabetics. Treat with antibiotics and surgical drainage as required.

Cardiac myxoma A rare primary cardiac tumor, commonly arising in the left atrium, that can present either with obstruction mimicking mitral stenosis or tumor emboli.

Carnett's test Determines whether an abdominal lump lies intraperitoneally or within the abdominal wall. The patient lies flat and raises the extended legs off the couch. An intraperitoneal lump disappears, whereas one in the abdominal wall persists.

Caroli's disease An anatomical abnormality characterized by intrahepatic cystic changes with an increased risk of bile duct cancer.

Carr's concretions Microscopic calculi within the papilla of the kidney thought to be involved in the pathogenesis and propagation of renal calculi.

Charcot's triad Fever, rigors, and jaundice characteristic of acute cholangitis. Right hypochondrial pain is often an additional feature. This is a serious and potentially fatal condition, caused by ascending infection of the biliary tree associated with partial biliary obstruction.

Chemodectoma A carotid body tumor extending from the carotid bifurcation that presents with solitary or bilateral lumps anterior and deep to sternocleidomastoid. Characteristically they can be displaced laterally but not vertically, and are associated with bruits and thrills in 20% of cases. The risk of malignancy increases with size.

Chopart's amputation An amputation made through the tarsal bones.

Churg–Strauss syndrome Affects young and middle-aged adults, often with a history of atopy, asthma, and allergic rhinitis, in which there is a marked eosinophilia. Clinical manifestations include peripheral neuropathy, cardiac involvement (heart failure and myocardial infarction), and vascular involvement affecting the stomach, small bowel, kidneys, and CNS due to aneurysm formation, thrombosis, and infarction.

Chvostek's sign Hyperexcitability of the facial nerve to local percussion over the parotid gland in patients with a reduced serum calcium concentration. It can also occur in 10% of people with normal calcium levels.

Chylothorax The accumulation of lymphatic fluid (which can have the appearance of pus) within the pleural cavity, following thoracic duct trauma (blunt and penetrating injuries or surgical procedures), obstruction by malignant disease (particularly lymphomas and carcinomas of the lung and breast), and congenital defects (usually also associated with ascites).

Cloquet's (Callisen's) hernia A deep femoral hernia that cannot protrude from the saphenous opening as it lies deep to the femoral vessels.

Contre-coup injury Injury to the brain on the opposite side of the initial injury, due to transmitted movements of the cerebral tissue within the skull.

Cooper's hernia A rare multilocular, deep-femoral hernia that enters the thigh via deep investing fascia.

Corrigan's pulse A collapsing pulse found in the presence of an arteriovenous fistula.

Courvoisier's sign Painless, palpable jaundice due to a distended gallbladder, which is more likely from malignant disease obstructing the bile ducts than from gallstones (where the gallbladder tends to be fibrotic and contracted).

Craniofacial dysostosis or Crouzon's syndrome A condition characterized by stenotic cranial sutures, maxillary hypoplasia and prognathism, beaked nose, exophthalmos, and mental retardation.

Crigler–Najjar syndrome Prehepatic jaundice due to an inability to conjugate bilirubin within the liver. There are two types, autosomal recessive (type I) and autosomal dominant (type II).

Cronkhite–Canada syndrome A triad of GI polyps, alopecia, and fingernail atrophy. The changes are not neoplastic, but due to an unidentified deficiency state.

Crueveilhier's sign (saphena varix) Is positive if an impulse is felt at the saphenofemoral junction when the patient stands and coughs.

Cullen's sign Periumbilical bruising seen in acute, severe necrotizing pancreatitis or other form of severe intraperitoneal bleed, i.e., ectopic pregnancy, abdominal trauma.

Curling's ulcer Acute gastroduodenal ulceration associated with severe burns.

Cushing's ulcer Acute gastroduodenal ulceration associated with stress, such as severe hemorrhage, myocardial infarct, and multiple trauma, and in critically ill patients.

DeQuervain's disease Inflammation around the extensor pollicis brevis and abductor pollicis longus tendons, often associated with thickening of the extensor retinaculum. This results in pain on movement of the thumb and tenderness where the tendons cross the radial styloid.

DeQuervain's thyroiditis Self-limiting viral inflammation of the thyroid gland, which usually follows a recent upper respiratory tract infarction, characterized by giant cell infiltration.

Dermatomyositis A condition of insidious onset characterized by proximal muscular weakness, pain, and tenderness. There is a characteristic purple skin rash that affects the cheeks and light-exposed areas. There is association with occult malignancies of the colon, lung, breast, and genitourinary tract.

Desmoid tumor A locally expanding tumor of mesenchymal tissue often found in the infraumbilical abdominal wall muscles or intrabdominal mesenchymal tissue. It commonly affects middle-aged females and requires wide excision. It is associated with familial adenomatous polyposis.

Dysplastic nevus Dysplastic nevi are considered precursors of malignant melanoma, when there is a family history; solitary lesions in the absence of a family history are not. All patients should avoid excessive sunlight.

Ectopia vesicae (bladder extrophy) Occurs in 1:30,000 live births, more commonly in males. There is an open bladder and defective anterior abdominal wall associated with separated pubic bones and penile epispadias or bifid clitoris. It is associated with glandular metaplasia and the risk of squamous carcinoma of the bladder remnant.

Ehlers–Danlos syndrome A rare collagen disorder characterized by the development of saccular or dissecting aneurysms.

Emphysematous cholecystitis A rapidly progressive infection of the gallbladder due to anaerobic organisms, characterized by air in the wall of the gallbladder and a high risk of perforation.

Empyema—gallbladder A pus-filled gallbladder resulting from impaction of a gallstone in the neck of the gallbladder.

Encephalocele The protrusion of cranial meninges, cerebrospinal fluid, and brain tissue through an opening in the skull.

Epidermal nevus syndrome The presence of extensive light-brown, warty lesions in association with skeletal and CNS developmental abnormalities.

Epidural hematoma The formation of a hematoma in the epidural space, most commonly following a fracture of the parietal or temporal bones with rupture of the middle meningeal artery or its branches that traverse them.

Epispadias A rare condition characterized by failure of development of the anterior wall of the lower urogenital tract, affecting the glans and penis alone (1:120,000) or the whole urinary tract, when it is commonly associated with bladder extrophy (1:30,000). It most commonly affects males and is characterized by the urethra exiting from the dorsal penile surface at varying sites.

Erythrocyanosis frigida Also known as Bazin's disease. It affects healthy females with fat and often hairless legs. Capillary dilatation alongside arteriolar constriction results in dusky red–purple blotches that blanch on pressure and rapidly refill. They can be painful. Ulceration and persistent edema may occur in severe cases.

Erythromelalgia A condition characterized by erythema and pain in the dependent extremities, relieved by elevation. The inappropriate release of local vasodilators has been implicated.

Exophthalmos Proptosis (sticking out of the globe of the eye), lid retraction, conjunctival edema, and, in severe cases, ophthalmoplegia or optic nerve damage. It affects 2%–3% of patients with Graves disease.

Fallot's tetralogy Congenital cyanotic heart disease with four features: (1) ventriculoseptal defect, (2) pulmonary stenosis, (3) overriding aorta, and (4) right ventricular hypertrophy. The infant becomes cyanotic on exertion and adopts a classical squatting position, which raises their systemic vascular resistance, thereby increasing pulmonary blood flow.

FAP (familial adenomatous polyposis) An autosomal dominant syndrome characterized by multiple colorectal and intestinal polyps as well as other intestinal and mesenchymal lesions.

Felty's syndrome An association between rheumatoid arthritis, splenomegaly, and granulocytopenia, which may be complicated by leg ulcers and recurrent infections.

Finkelstein's test Used to identify cases of stenosing tenosynovitis. The patient places their thumb in the palm and clenches a fist. The examiner pushes the hand into ulnar deviation and, if the test is positive, pain is felt at the radial styloid, radiating down the forearm.

FitzHugh–Curtis syndrome Severe right hypochondrial pain due to perihepatitis from *Chlamydia trachomatis* or gynococcus infection.

Fournier's gangrene A form of necrotizing fasciitis involving the perineal or scrotal skin, leading to subcutaneous necrosis. Synergy appears to occur between normal nonpathogenic organisms, leading to local vascular thrombosis and necrosis. It is associated with uncontrolled diabetes mellitus.

Frey syndrome Gustatory sweating of the cheek following accidental or surgical trauma of the parotid region. It results from cross-regeneration of the transected sympathetic and parasympathetic fibers and develops over about 12 months.

Galactocele A cystic lesion containing breast milk, occurring in women who suddenly stop breast-feeding.

Gamekeeper's thumb A sprain of the metacarpophalangeal joint of the thumb, leading to rupture of the ulnar collateral ligament. Non-healing leads to chronic instability and weakened pinch grip.

Gardner's syndrome A variant of FAP involving an association between multiple epidermal cysts, intestinal polyposis, desmoid tumors, and osteomas.

Gaucher's disease A genetic abnormality leading to active storage of abnormal glucocerebrosides in the spleen, resulting in massive childhood splenomegaly.

Gilbert's syndrome Congenitally acquired mild jaundice, due to a failure of transport of bilirubin to the liver, which can be precipitated by episodes of starvation. There is an absence of urinary bilirubin, although fecal and urinary urobilinogen levels are increased. It is of little clinical significance.

Glomus tumor See Angiomyoneuroma.

Glucagonoma A tumor of the pancreatic islet cells that is characterized by mid-maturity-onset diabetes, an erythematous rash that tends to blister and crust, glossitis, and raised glucagon levels.

Grawitz tumor Adenocarcinoma of the kidney.

Grey Turner sign Bruising in the flanks resulting from retroperitoneal hemorrhage (e.g., hemorrhagic pancreatitis).

Gynecomastia The benign growth of breast tissue in males. The breast is uniformly enlarged and soft. The condition may be physiological (e.g., maternal estrogens, estrogen–androgen imbalance of puberty), due to hypogonadism (pituitary disorders, androgen blockade), neoplasms (adrenal or gonadotrophic tumors, bronchogenic, renal cell), or systemic disease (hepatic failure, renal dialysis, hypothyroidism), or drug induced (androgen blockers, estrogens, cimetidine, spironolactone, ketoconazole, methyldopa, metoclopramide).

Hamartoma Overgrowths of one (or more) cell type normally found within the organ from which they arise, e.g., neurofibromas.

Hammer toe Hyperextension of the metatarsophalangeal joint and distal interphalangeal joint with flexion of the proximal interphalangeal joint.

Hand–Schüller–Christian disease Multiple visceral and lytic skeletal lesions, characteristically also involving the skull, that are associated with diabetes insipidus and exophthalmos.

Hangman's fracture Traumatic disruption of the pars interarticularis of the atlas (C2) following a hyperextension injury.

Hashimoto's disease A diffusely enlarged, painless thyroid gland due to lymphocyte infiltration. It is rubbery in nature and often mimicking a multi-nodular goiter. If enlargement is asymmetrical, other causes must be excluded. Clinically the patient is euthyroid or mildly hyperthyroid.

Henle–Coenen sign If an arteriovenous fistula is occluded and the distal vessels still pulsate, this indicates that the fistula can be safely treated by ligation.

Hereditary osteodystrophy An X-linked form of pseudo-hypoparathyroidism characterized by hypoparathyroidism, low serum calcium, mental retardation, cataracts, and tetany. Metastatic calcification of the basal ganglion is also a feature.

Hesselbach's hernia A rare form of external femoral hernia that enters the thigh lateral to the deep epigastric and main femoral vessels.

Hibernoma A lipoma consisting of brown fat cells.

Hidradenitis suppurativa A chronic, recurrent, deep-seated skin infection of the axilla or perineum.

Howship–Romberg sign Pain referred to the inner aspect of the knee via the genicular branch of the obturator nerve, which may arise from an obturator hernia that strangulates.

Hydatid of Morgagni Also known as the appendix testis. It is a remnant of the Müllerian duct found at the upper pole of the testis, situated in the groove between the testis and epididymis. It may undergo torsion.

Hyperhidrosis Excessive sweating of the axilla, palms, and feet, which can be socially embarrassing and distressing.

Hypersplenism A combination of splenomegaly, anemia, leukopenia, and/or thrombocytopenia with bone marrow hyperplasia. Splenectomy may be required.

Inspissated bile syndrome Inspissation of bile in the common bile duct during early infancy (usually from hemolysis), resulting in proximal bile duct and gallbladder dilatation.

Insulinoma A rare tumor of pancreatic-islet beta cells that is characterized by hypoglycemic attacks. These are both unpredictable and worsen in severity with time. Diagnosis is based on Whipple's triad.

Intraperitoneal rupture of bladder Is usually traumatic in origin, from surgical instrumentation or abdominal trauma in the presence of a full bladder.

Jefferson's (burst) fracture Disruption of the ring of atlas (C2) following traumatic injury to the neck. Spinal column damage is uncommon, as the fragments tend to open outward.

Kantor's string sign Is indicative of Crohn's disease. Involvement of the terminal ileum leads to structuring of the lumen. This gives the radiological appearance of a thread-like structure on barium follow-through.

Kaposi's sarcoma Painless red–brown macules on the limbs and anal and oral mucosa. Occasionally they may ulcerate. They can be found in the elderly, endemically (e.g., in Africa), and in immunosuppressed patients (e.g., transplant patients, HIV patients).

Kartagener's syndrome Bronchiectasis and sterility resulting from abnormal ciliary action.

Kehr's sign Left shoulder pain referred from splenic injury and rupture.

Keratoacanthoma See Molluscum sebaceum.

Killian's dehiscence The weak point between the cricopharyngeal and thyropharyngeal muscles through which pharyngeal mucosa can herniate, leading to formation of a pharyngeal pouch.

Klein's sign Right iliac fossa pain that moves to the left when the patient turns on to his or her left side. It can be associated with mesenteric lymphadenitis and Meckel's diverticulum.

Klippel–Trenaunay syndrome A condition of the lower limb, characterized by congenital varicose veins, deep-vein abnormalities, bony and soft-tissue deformity, limb elongation, and capillary nevi.

Köhler's disease Osteochondritis of the navicular bone. This can be one of the causes of a painful limp in a child under 5 years of age.

Krukenberg tumor An ovarian tumor arising from spread of a primary gastric carcinoma.

Ladd's bands Persistent fibrous bands between the small bowel mesentery and liver that can lead to obstruction of the second part of the duodenum. They are commonly associated with incomplete rotation of the bowel.

Laugier's hernia A rare form of femoral hernia that enters the thigh through a defect in the pectineal part of the inguinal ligament.

Li–Fraumeni syndrome An inherited predisposition to cancer thought to be due to mutation of the p53 tumor suppressor genes.

Linitis plastica Also known as leather bottle stomach. Submucosal proliferation of fibrous tissue secondary to carcinoma of the stomach leads to gastric-wall thickening and a reduction in stomach volume and plasticity. Because it spreads readily along the mucosa plane and presents late, its prognosis is poor.

Lipodystrophy Excessive fat deposition in the legs. It may be mistaken for edema.

Livedo reticularis Cyanotic skin mottling due to vasospasm of the arterioles with concomitant capillary dilatation.

Malgaigne bulges Bulges seen above the inguinal ligament in thin individuals on coughing or straining. They are variants of normal and do not represent inguinal hernias.

Mallory–Weiss syndrome or tear Hematemesis resulting from prolonged, violent vomiting leading to mucosal tears at the gastroesophageal junction.

Marfan syndrome A rare inherited collagen disorder characterized by tall stature, arachnodactyly (webbed fingers), lens subluxation, and the development of saccular and dissecting aneurysms—particularly of the thoracic aorta. Aortic regurgitation may occur due to aortic root dilatation.

Marjolin's ulcer A long-standing venous ulcer that fails to heal, in which squamous cell carcinoma develops.

McBurney's point Lies one-third of the way along a line drawn from the right anterior superior iliac spine to the umbilicus. It is the classical point of maximal tenderness in acute appendicitis and the center point for the (McBurney's) incision used in open appendectomy.

McMurray's test Is used to identify medial meniscal tears. With the patient supine, the knee is flexed and foot rotated medially and laterally, while bringing the knee to 90° of flexion. Discomfort or a click is noted in the presence of a tear.

Medullary sponge kidney Is due to dilatation of the terminal collecting ducts of the kidney, which predisposes to the formation of renal calculi.

Meigs syndrome Ascites and pleural effusions associated with benign ovarian tumors.

Ménétrier disease Hypertrophy of the gastric mucosa, most typically proximally, resulting in hypochlorhydria and hypersecretion of gastric juices, leading to protein loss. Patients may present with epigastric discomfort and peripheral edema. There is no associated increased risk of gastric cancer.

Meralgia paraesthetica Numbness and hyperalgesia around the lateral thigh following entrapment of the lateral cutaneous nerve of the thigh as it passes beneath the inguinal ligament.

Milia Small, white, superficial facial spots derived from hair follicles. They appear in newborn babies and following skin grafting and dermabrasion and are treated by expression.

Mirrizi syndrome Obstructive jaundice resulting from impaction of a gallstone in the cystic duct, which presses against the common hepatic duct, causing extrinsic compression.

Molluscum contagiosum Small, pale, firm nodules with a characteristic central depression that follow infection with the pox virus. They tend to regress with time, although they can be treated by curettage.

Molluscum sebaceum A solitary skin tumor that grows rapidly over 6–8 weeks and involutes over about 6 months to leave a residual scar. It has the appearance of a dome-shaped lesion with a central keratin-filled crater, and can be mistaken both clinically and histologically for a well-differentiated squamous cell carcinoma.

Mondor disease of the breast Superficial thrombophlebitis affecting the veins of the breast. Initially, there may be tenderness, which is followed by fibrosis and contraction, resulting in skin dimpling.

Morgagni hernia A congenital diaphragmatic hernia that presents in early adult life with dyspnea or as an incidental mediastinal mass. Abdominal contents expand into the anterior mediastinal compartment through a persistent defect in the anterior diaphragm.

Murphy's sign Cessation of inspiration while holding pressure in the right upper quadrant. It is due to an inflamed gallbladder and the patient may be unable to fully inspire because of the pain.

Myositis ossificans Ectopic bone formation arising within hematoma in muscle following soft-tissue injury.

Nelson syndrome The presence of skin hyperpigmentation and accelerated growth of a pituitary tumor following bilateral adrenalectomy for pituitary-dependent Cushing's syndrome. It results from loss of pituitary feedback.

Nutcracker esophagus Alternative name for diffuse esophageal spasm—the presence of long-duration, high-intensity peristaltic contractions in the esophagus, which may be associated with chest pains and dysphagia.

Obturator sign The aggravation of right iliac fossa pain upon passive internal rotation of the right hip in patients with appendicitis in whom the appendix lies adjacent to obturator internus.

Osteogenesis imperfecta An inherited collagen disorder resulting in fragile bones that fracture easily, blue sclera, deafness, and soft teeth.

Osteopetrosis (Albers–Schönberg disease, marble bone disease) An inherited disorder of bone resulting in increased bone density, fractures, and anemia. The recessive form is less severe than the autosomal dominant form.

Pancreas divisum Arises when the ventral and dorsal pancreatic buds fail to fuse during embryological development. Consequently, the main pancreatic duct drains via an accessory ampulla. The vast majority of patients are asymptomatic, although this may be one of the causes of chronic pancreatitis.

Peau d'orange Localized edema found in breast cancer, in which the skin of the breast has the pitted appearance of an orange skin.

Phalen's test The reproduction of discomfort and paraesthesia of the fingers in the distribution of the median nerve (lateral 3 1/2 fingers) when the wrist is held in flexion. These results are due to compression of the median nerve as it passes beneath the flexor retinaculum through the carpal tunnel.

Phlegmasia alba dolens A swollen, white, edematous limb, occasionally seen in patients with severe iliofemoral venous thrombosis. Progression to phlegmasia cerulea dolens may occur.

Phlegmasia cerulea dolens A blue, swollen, edematous limb following severe proximal venous thrombosis. This may progress to venous gangrene as circulatory congestion and stasis occur.

Pneumatosis cystoides intestinalis Gas-filled cysts within the intestinal and mesenteric walls, most commonly affecting the small intestine. These can be seen on plain abdominal X-rays.

Pneumaturia The passage of flatus in urine, which can arise from a colovesical fistula (e.g., diverticular disease, carcinoma, inflammatory bowel disease) or urinary tract infection in diabetics, where the glucose is fermented by the infecting organism.

Poland's syndrome An association between pectoral muscle abnormality, absence or hypoplasia of the breast, and characteristic hand deformity of hypoplasia of the middle phalanges and skin webbing (synbrachydactyly).

Pott's carcinoma of scrotum Squamous cell carcinoma of the scrotum, associated with chronic exposure of the scrotal skin to aromatic carcinogens in coal-derived chimney soot. It is now more commonly associated with exposure to heavy metals and mineral oils, particularly those used in the cotton industry.

Pott's disease of the spine Tuberculosis of the spine leading to bony destruction and vertebral collapse. This in turn results in kyphosis and spinal compression.

Proctalgia fugax Severe, recurrent rectal pain in the absence of any organic disease. Attacks may occur at night, after bowel actions, or following ejaculation. Anxiety is said to be an associated feature.

Pseudomyxoma peritonei Disseminated mucinous tumor within the peritoneal cavity, commonly due to ruptured ovarian or appendiceal mucinous neoplasms. This condition is locally recurrent and potentially fatal even with heroic surgery and chemotherapy.

Red currant jelly stool A description attributed to the blood-stained stool found in intussusception.

Reidel's thyroiditis Thyroiditis characterized by a marked fibrotic reaction leading to a hard, non-tender thyroid gland. Thyroid function tends to be normal, and differentiation from malignant disease can be difficult as fine-needle aspirates tend to be acellular.

Reinke's edema The presence of generalized edema of the upper vocal cords in response to noxious stimuli.

Reiter's syndrome The triad of polyarthritis, conjunctivitis, and urethritis as a result of venereal infection, usually chlamydia. The initial attack lasts for 4–6 weeks, although some patients develop chronic symptoms.

Rendu–Osler–Weber syndrome Hereditary hemorrhagic telangectasia. This is a rare autosomal dominant condition characterized by the presence of hemangiomas affecting the lips, buccal cavity, nasopharynx, and whole GI tract. These may bleed, resulting in episodes of hematemesis, hematuria, melena, epistaxis, or anemia that are self-limiting.

Richter's hernia A form of strangulated hernia in which only part of the bowel lumen becomes strangulated, leading to incomplete intestinal obstruction with ischemia and gangrene of the strangulated part.

Rovsing's sign Pain and tenderness in the right iliac fossa produced by palpation of the left iliac fossa. It may be found in acute appendicitis.

Sister Mary Joseph's node The appearance of umbilical nodules in the presence of advanced intra-abdominal carcinoma, typically stomach but also large bowel, ovarian, or, occasionally, breast.

Sjögren's syndrome The presence of keratoconjunctivitis sicca, salivary gland involvement (leading to xerostomia, i.e., dry mouth), and rheumatoid arthritis or other mixed connective-tissue disorder. Primary Sjögren's syndrome is characterized by the first two features, whereas secondary Sjögren's has all three.

Spigelian hernia A rare type of hernia due to defects within the internal oblique aponeurosis as it interdigitates with the anterior and posterior rectus sheath. Peritoneum and visceral contents may herniate through these defects.

Stevens–Johnson syndrome Also known as erythema multiforme, characterized by ulceration that has a characteristic target appearance and results from drug allergies (particularly to sulphonamides and barbiturates) or mycoplasmal infections or occurs idiopathically. The lesions may be associated with conjunctivitis, tracheitis, and dysphagia.

Sump syndrome Is due to the collection of stones and debris in the distal common bile duct following choledochoduodenostomy, resulting in epigastric pain, cholangitis, and pancreatitis.

Thrombophlebitis migrans Increased coagulability of blood associated with visceral cancers, particularly adenocarcinomas.

Tinel's sign Transient finger paraesthesia that follows percussion of the median nerve proximal to the wrist in patients with median nerve compression due to carpal tunnel syndrome.

Trichobezoars See Bezoars.

Troisier's sign Enlargement of the left supraclavicular lymph node due to advanced metastatic gastric carcinoma.

Trousseau's sign Phlebothrombosis of the superficial leg veins that is associated with cancer.

Ureterocele A cystic dilatation of the intravesical submucosal ureter. It is often associated with other congenital anomalies, including duplicated ureters.

VACTERL syndrome The association of vertebral (V), anorectal (A), cardiovascular (C), tracheo-esophageal (TE), renal (R), and limb (L) anomalies. Progesterone and estrogen intake during early pregnancy has been implicated.

Vermooten's sign Digital rectal examination reveals a doughy, displaced, or absent prostate in the presence of an intrapelvic rupture of the prostatic urethra.

Von Hippel–Lindau disease An inherited disorder characterized by cerebellar and spinal cord hemangioblastomas, retinal angiomas, and an increased risk of visceral cancers, particularly renal cell carcinoma.

Von Recklinghausen's disease (neurofibromatosis type I) Autosomal dominantly inherited nodular thickening of nerve trunks, associated with patchy skin pigmentation (café-au-lait spots). Malignant transformation of these neurofibromas tends to occur only in this particular subgroup of patients, and their prognosis is poor.

Waterhouse–Friedrichsen syndrome Bilateral adrenal cortical necrosis due to septicemia (meningococcal, pneumococcal, streptococcal), hemorrhage, or burns.

Whipple's triad Fasting hypoglycemic attacks with a blood glucose level of less than 2.5 mmol/L, relieved by glucose and associated raised insulin levels. These are characteristic of an insulinoma.

Zenker's diverticulum A pharyngeal pouch that occurs through the dehiscence of Killian, between cricopharyngeus and inferior constrictors of the pharynx. There is usually a history of food sticking and regurgitation. Progressive weight loss, dysphagia, and aspiration pneumonia can also occur.

Zollinger–Ellison syndrome Intractable duodenal ulceration due to elevated levels of circulating gastrin levels. There is an association with multiple endocrine neoplasia (MEN) type I. Diagnosis is confirmed by acid secretion tests, which show elevated resting levels. Secretin challenge elevates gastrin levels in G-cell hyperplasia but not G-cell tumors.

Index